Pediatric
Orthopaedics
and Sports Injuries

A QUICK REFERENCE GUIDE

John F. Sarwark, MD, FAAP
Cynthia R. LaBella, MD, FAAP

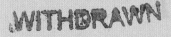

American Academy of Pediatrics
141 Northwest Point Blvd
Elk Grove Village, IL 60007-1098
www.aap.org

American Academy of Pediatrics
Department of Marketing and Publications Staff

Maureen DeRosa, MPA, Director, Department of Marketing and Publications

Mark Grimes, Director, Division of Product Development

Diane E. Lundquist, Senior Product Development Editor

Sandi King, MS, Director, Division of Publishing and Production Services

Theresa Wiener, Manager, Editorial Production

Jason Crase, Editorial Specialist

Peg Mulcahy, Manager, Graphic Design and Production

Library of Congress Control Number: 2010904536

ISBN: 978-1-58110-284-0

MA0428

9-205/0410   1 2 3 4 5 6 7 8 9 10

*To the pediatricians and primary care providers who devote their careers
to the well-being of our children.*

Table of Contents

Editors

John F. Sarwak, MD, FAAP
Professor of Orthopaedic Surgery
Northwestern University Feinberg School
of Medicine
Martha Washington Professor of
Orthopaedic Surgery and
Head, Pediatric Orthopaedic Surgery
Children's Memorial Hospital
Chicago, IL

Cynthia R. LaBella, MD, FAAP
Assistant Professor of Pediatrics
Northwestern University Feinberg School
of Medicine
Medical Director, Institute for Sports
Medicine
Children's Memorial Hospital
Chicago, IL

Contributors

Michael C. Ain, MD
Associate Professor, Orthopaedics
and Neurosurgery
Johns Hopkins University
Baltimore, MD

John Batson, MD, FAAP
Clinical Associate Professor of Pediatrics
Moore Orthopaedics, University of
South Carolina School of Medicine
Columbia, SC

Holly J. Benjamin, MD, FAAP, FACSM
Associate Professor of Pediatrics
and Surgery
Section of Academic Pediatrics
Section of Orthopedic Surgery and
Rehabilitation Medicine
Director of Primary Care Sports Medicine
University of Chicago
Chicago, IL

David T. Bernhardt, MD, FAAP
Professor
Department of Pediatrics/Orthopedics
and Rehabilitation
Division of Sports Medicine
University of Wisconsin School of
Medicine and Public Health
Madison, WI

Jennette L. Boakes, MD, FAAP
Pediatric Orthopaedic Surgeon
Shriner's Hospital for Children,
Northern California
Clinical Professor of Orthopaedic Surgery
University of California Davis Schook
of Medicine
Sacramento, CA

Susannah M. Briskin, MD, FAAP
Assistant Professor of Pediatrics
Primary Care Sports Medicine Rainbow
Babies and Children's Hospital/
University Hospitals Case
Medical Center
Cleveland, OH

Alison Brooks, MD, MPH, FAAP
Sports Medicine Fellow
University of Wisconsin
Madison, WI

Roy Cardoso, MD
Department of Orthopaedic Surgery
University of California Davis School
of Medicine
Sacramento, CA

Rebecca L. Carl, MD, FAAP
Assistant Professor of Pediatrics
Northwestern University
Attending Physician, Institute for
    Sports Medicine
Children's Memorial Hospital
Chicago, IL

Joseph Congeni, MD, FAAP
Associate Professor of Pediatrics
Northeastern Ohio Universities College of
    Medicine and Pharmacy
Clinical Associate Professor of Pediatrics
    and Sports Medicine
Ohio University College of Osteopathic
    Medicine

Steven C. Cuff, MD
Clinical Assistant Professor
Department of Pediatrics
Division of Sports Medicine
Nationwide Children's Hospital
The Ohio State University College
    of Medicine
Columbus, OH

Jon R. Davids, MD, FAAP
Chief of Staff
Medical Director Motion Analysis
    Laboratory
Shriners Hospital for Children
Greenville, SC

**Lindsay Davidson, MD, MSc, MEd,
FRCSC**
Associate Professor
Department of Surgery
Division of Orthopaedics
Queen's University
Kingston, ON

Rebecca A. Demorest, MD, FAAP
Pediatric and Young Adult Sports
    Medicine
Associate Director, Sports Medicine
Children's Hospital & Research Center
    Oakland
Oakland, CA

Martin S. Decintio
Department of Pediatric Orthopaedic
    Surgery
Children's Hospital Medical Center
    of Akron
Akron, OH

Emalee Flaherty, MD, FAAP
Director, Child Abuse Pediatrics
Associate Professor of Pediatrics
Northwestern University Feinberg School
    of Medicine
Chicago, IL

Gaia Georgopoulos, MD
Associate Professor Orthopaedic Surgery
University of Colorado Health
    Sciences Center
Medical Director Orthopaedic Surgery
The Children's Hospital
Denver, CO

Matthew Grady, MD, FAAP
Pediatric and Adolescent Sports Medicine
Department of Orthopedics
Children's Hospital of Philadelphia
Philadelphia, PA

Andrew John Maxwell Gregory, MD, FAAP
Assistant Professor of Orthopaedics
    and Rehabilitation
Vanderbilt Team Physician
Vanderbilt University
Nashville, TN

Bettina Gyr, MD
Assistant Professor of Orthopaedic Surgery
Baylor College of Medicine
Houston, TX

Mark Halstead, MD
Assistant Professor, Departments of
    Pediatrics and Orthopedics
Team Physician, St Louis Rams
Washington University School of Medicine
St Louis, MO

Henry J. Iwinski, Jr, MD
Associate Professor of Orthopaedic Surgery
University of Kentucky
Assistant Chief of Staff
Shriners Hospital for Children
Lexington, KY

Neel Jain, MD
Senior Resident
Department of Orthopaedic Surgery
Northwestern University Feinberg School
    of Medicine
Chicago, IL

Michelle A. James, MD
Chief
Department of Orthopaedic Surgery
Shriners Hospital for Children Northern
    California
Chief
Division of Pediatric Orthopaedics and
    Professor of Clinical Orthopaedic
    Surgery
University of California Davis School
    of Medicine
Sacramento, CA

James N. Jarvis, MD, FAAP
Professor of Pediatrics
CMRI/Arthritis Foundation Research
    Chair
Section Chief, Pediatric Rheumatology
University of Oklahoma College of
    Medicine
Oklahoma City, OK

Kerwyn Jones, MD
Assistant Director Orthopedic Surgery
Akron Children's Hospital
Akron, OH

Najeeb Khan, MD
Senior Resident
Department of Orthopaedics
Northwestern University Feinberg School
    of Medicine
Chicago, IL

Amanda Weiss Kelly, MD, FAAP
Director of Pediatric Sports Medicine
Rainbow Babies and Children's Hospital
Assistant Professor of Pediatrics
Case Western Reserve University
Cleveland, OH

Young-Jo Kim, MD, PhD, FAAP
Assistant Professor of Orthopaedic
    Surgery
Children's Hospital—Boston
Harvard Medical School
Boston, MA

Mininder S. Kocher, MD, MPH
Associate Director
Division of Sports Medicine
Children's Hospital Boston
Associate Professor of Orthopaedic Surgery
Harvard Medical School
Boston, MA

Chris G. Koutures, MD, FAAP
Pediatrics and Sports Medicine
Gladstien & Koutures
Anaheim Hills, CA

Michelle Labotz, MD, FAAP
Sports Medicine Clinic
Intermed PA
Portland, ME

Gregory L. Landry, MD, FAAP
Professor of Pediatrics and Orthopedics
University of Wisconsin School of
    Medicine and Public Health
Head Team Physician
University of Wisconsin-Madison
    Athletic Teams
Madison, WI

**Claire M. A. LeBlanc, MD, FRCPC,
    FAAP, Dip. Sports Med**
Associate Professor of Pediatrics
University of Alberta
Edmonton, Alberta
Canada

Joel A. Lerman, MD
Department of Orthopaedics
Shriners Hospital for Children,
    Northern California
Clinical Associate Professor
Department of Orthopaedic Surgery
University of California-Davis
Davis, CA

Robert H. Listernick, MD
Director, Diagnostic and Consultation
    Services
Professor of Pediatrics
Northwestern University Feinberg School
    of Medicine
Chicago, IL

Megan M. May, MD, FAAP
Senior Resident
Department of Orthopaedic Surgery
Northwestern University Feinberg School
    of Medicine
Children's Memorial Hospital
Chicago, IL

Teri M. McCaimbridge, MD, FAAP
Primary Care Sports Medicine
Towson Orthopedics Associates
Assistant Professor of Pediatrics
The Johns Hopkins School of Medicine
Baltimore, MD

Jordan Metzl, MD, FAAP
Sports Medicine Service, Hospital for
    Special Surgery
Associate Professor of Pediatrics
Cornell Medical College
Cofounder
The Sports Medicine Institute for
    Young Athletes
New York, NY

Todd A. Milbrandt, MD, MS
Assistant Professor of Pediatric
    Orthopaedics
University of Ketucky
Shriners Hospital for Children
Lexington, KY

Jeffrey Mjaanes, MD, FAAP
Assistant Professor
Department of Pediatrics and
    Orthopedic Surgery
Rush University Medical Center
Midwest Orthopaedics at Rush
Chicago, IL

Kathleen Y. Moen, MD
Assistant Professor
Dartmouth Hitchcock Medical Center
Lebanon, NH

Jose A. Morcuende, MD, PhD
Associate Professor
Department of Orthopaedic Surgery
　and Rehabilitation
University of Iowa
Iowa City, IA

Teresa Mosqueda, MD
Department of Orthopaedic Surgery
University of Iowa Hospitals and Clinics
Iowa City, IA

Blaise A. Nemeth, MD, MS, FAAP
Assistant Professor
Departments of Pediatrics and
　Orthopedics and Rehabilitation
University of Wisconsin
Madison, WI

Kurt J. Nilsson, MD, MS
Intermountain Orthopaedics
Boise, ID

Andrew R. Peterson, MD, FAAP
Assistant Professor of Pediatrics and
　Orthopedics/Rehabilitation
University of Wisconsin
Madison, WI

Stephen G. Rice, MD, PhD, MPH,
　FAAP, FACSM
Director
Jersey Shore Sports Medicine Center
Program Director
Pediatric Sports Medicine Fellowship
Jersey Shore University Medical Center
Neptune, NJ
Clinical Associate Professor of Pediatrics
UMDNJ-Robert Wood Johnson
　Medical School
Piscataway, NJ

Kevin Shea, MD
Intermountain Orthopaedics
Boise, ID

Eric D. Shirley, MD
LCDR, MC USN
Pediatric Orthopaedic Surgeon
Naval Medical Center Portsmouth
Portsmouth, VA

Peter A. Smith, MD, FAAP
Associate Professor Orthopaedic Surgery
Rush University Medical Center
Staff Orthopedist
Shriners Hospital for Children
Chicago, IL

Anthony A. Stans, MD
Chair
Division of Pediatric Orthopedic Surgery
Mayo Clinic
Rochester, MN

Daniel J. Sucato, MD, MS
Staff Orthopaedic Surgeon
Texas Scottish Rite Hospital for Children
Dallas, TX

Vishwas R. Talwalker, MD
Assistant Professor of Orthopaedic Surgery
Shriner's Hospital for Children and
　University of Kentucky
Lexington, KY

Jeffrey D. Thomson, MD
Director
Department of Orthopaedic Surgery
Connecticut Children's Medical Center
Hartford, CT
Associate Professor, Orthopaedic Surgery
University of Connecticut School
　of Medicine
Farmington, CT

John Tis, MD
Director, Pediatric Orthopaedics
Walter Reed Medical Center

Michael Vitale, MD, MPH, FAAP
Associate Chief
Division of Pediatric Orthopaedics
Chief
Pediatric Spine and Scoliosis Service
Morgan Stanley Childrens Hospital of
    New York–Presbyterian
Ana Lucia Associate Professor of Pediatric
    Orthopaedic Surgery
Columbia University Medical Center
New York, NY

Kelly M. Waicus, MD
Team Physician
UNC Sports MedicineAssistant
    Clinical Professor
Departments of Orthopedics and
    Pediatrics
University of North Carolina–Chapel Hill
Chapel Hill, NC

Jeffrey L. Young
Senior Resident
Department of Orthopaedic Surgery
Northwestern University Feinberg School
    of Medicine
Chicago, IL

Preface

The purpose of this book is to provide primary care physicians, pediatricians, residents, medical students, and health care professionals with a brief but complete discussion of orthopaedic problems in children. The book can serve as a desk reference and a quick reference guide for physicians who care for children to help them diagnose and treat pediatric musculoskeletal problems.

The book offers an overview approach, and includes differential diagnosis and work-up of patients with orthopaedic injuries and bone and joint conditions. A limited number of specific references and a few key ones are included for further in-depth reading. Cross-referencing is extensively provided to avoid repetition and redundancy. We have presented the material in a simple and practical manner.

We thank the contributors for their authoritative contributions to this guide. We are thankful for the outstanding editorial assistance of Diane Lundquist, senior product development editor, and to the publishing staff of the American Academy of Pediatrics for their help and support. We hope that our readers—everywhere—will find this book highly useful.

John F. Sarwark, MD, FAAP
Cynthia Rose LaBella, MD, FAAP

Part 1: Growth and Motor Development

TOPICS COVERED

1. **Normal Growth and Motor Development**
   Somatic Growth
   Normal Motor Development
   Gender Differences in Motor Development
   Sports Readiness
2. **Abnormal Musculoskeletal Growth and Motor Development**

CHAPTER 1

Normal Growth and Motor Development

- Normal growth and maturation of the child's musculoskeletal system and development of motor skills are determined by numerous factors, including genetic (familial inheritance), nutritional, hormonal, illness, physical activity, social conditions, race, culture, climate, and geographic location.
- This chapter describes normal growth and maturation of the pediatric musculoskeletal system; normal patterns of motor skill development; and methods of evaluating growth, maturation, and development and identifying abnormalities.

Somatic Growth

- Somatic growth refers to the increase in weight, height, and organ size.
  — Assess somatic growth by comparing a child's height and weight to a population of other children at the same chronologic age using Centers for Disease Control and Prevention growth charts.
  — These charts include the range of height, weight, head circumference, and body mass index (BMI) measured in a sample of American children aged birth to 20 years.
  — While frequently used as a marker of health and nutritional status, somatic growth is not a reliable indicator of biological maturity. There is significant individual variation in the timing (when the growth spurt occurs) and tempo (rate or speed at which growth spurt occurs) of growth.
- Growth rate varies with age, is greatest from birth to 2 years, declines during childhood, and briefly increases again during the adolescent growth spurt (Table 1-1, Figure 1-1).
- During the prepubertal stage between 6 and 12 years of age, growth averages 3 to 3.5 kg and 6 cm per year, with minimal difference between boys and girls (Figure 1-1).

Table 1-1. Rates of Growth in Weight and Height by Age

Age	Daily Weight Gain (g)	Monthly Weight Gain	Growth in Length (cm/mo)
0–3 mo	30	2 lb	3.5
3–6 mo	20	1.25 lb	2.0
6–9 mo	15	1 lb	1.5
9–12 mo	12	13 oz	1.2
1–3 y	8	8 oz (0.5 lb)	1.0
4–6 y	6	6 oz	3 cm/y

Adapted from Behrman RE, Kliegman RM, Jenson HB, eds. *Nelson Textbook of Pediatrics.* 17th ed. Philadelphia, PA: W.B. Saunders Co; 2004: 35, with permission from Elsevier.

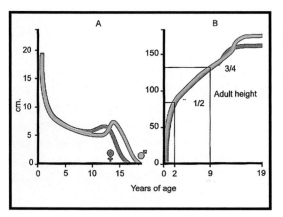

Figure 1-1. Growth rates for girls and boys: A; by age; B, as fraction of adult height. From Staheli LT. *Fundamentals of Pediatric Orthopedics.* Philadelphia, PA: Lippincott Williams & Wilkins; 2008:8. Reprinted by permission.

ADOLESCENT GROWTH SPURT

- The adolescent growth spurt begins at about 9 to 10 years of age for girls and 11 to 12 years of age for boys.
  - — Males experience a growth spurt about 2 years after the onset of puberty, heralded by the onset of gonadal enlargement.
  - — Girls experience a growth spurt 6 months after the appearance of breast buds. The growth spurt starts peripherally with enlargement of the hands and feet, then progresses centrally to the arms and legs, and lastly the trunk.
  - — The peak growth rate occurs earlier for trunk length and later for leg length compared with stature; thus the late childhood growth spurt is characterized by rapid trunk growth and the early adolescent growth spurt is characterized by rapid growth of the legs.

HEIGHT

- The rate of height growth accelerates until it reaches a maximum, termed the peak height velocity (PHV), which occurs about 2 years after the start of the adolescent growth spurt.
- The growth spurt lasts anywhere from 24 to 36 months (Figure 1-2).

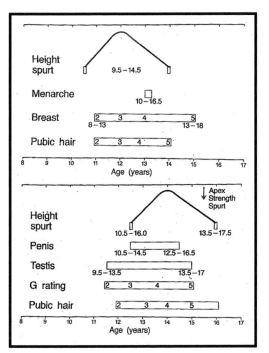

Figure 1-2. Sequence of events at puberty for the average adolescent male and female aged 8 to 17 years. The onset of menses generally follows peak height velocity by 1 year. Adapted from Tanner JM. *Growth at Adolescence.* Oxford, England: Blackwell Scientific Publications; 1962. Reprinted by permission from John Wiley & Sons, Inc.

- Standard deviations of age at PHV range from 0.7 to 1.2 years, indicating significant individual variation in the timing of the growth spurt.
- Age at PHV is a reliable indicator of somatic maturity in boys and girls.
- In boys PHV occurs at an average age of 14 years at a rate of 10.3 cm (4.3") per year and then decelerates to a stop by age 18 years.
- Girls start their growth spurt at an average age of 12 years at a rate of 9 cm (3.8") per year, reach PHV, and stop growing approximately 2 years earlier than boys (usually by age 16 years).
- The onset of menses generally follows maximum growth in height (PHV) by 1 year and therefore indicates a rapid deceleration in growth and limited additional gains in stature (Figure 1-2).
- Peak height velocity and magnitude of height gained is 3 to 5 cm greater in boys than in girls.
- Girls achieve a final mean adult height of 163.8 cm compared with 176.8 cm for boys, for an average adult height difference of 13 cm between men and women. This difference in final adult stature is because of the smaller PHV and the earlier termination of growth in girls compared with boys.
- Pubertal growth accounts for almost 25% of final adult height.
- The genetic contribution to final adult height is approximately 60%.
- There is a trend for youth who attain PHV at an earlier age to be slightly taller at that age, but ultimately there seems to be no relationship between age at PHV and final adult stature.

- Early maturers generally have a higher PHV than late maturers, and late maturers on average are taller when the growth spurt begins; consequently the mean adult height of early and late maturers is usually the same.
- Height differences among boys with differences in age of pubertal onset will generally disappear by late adolescence.
- Similarly, children with constitutional growth delay will "catch up" with their peers by late adolescence.

ESTIMATING ADULT HEIGHT

- *Mid-parental height* is a frequently used method to estimate a child's genetic height potential based on the child's gender and the biological parents' height, with a standard deviation of approximately 2".
  — Mid-parental height for boys = paternal height + maternal height + 5 (inches)/2
  — Mid-parental height for girls = paternal height + maternal height − 5 (inches)/2
- *Multiplier method*
  — Height at given chronological age (cm) X multiplier = adult height (Figure 1-3)

HEIGHT MULTIPLIER FOR BOYS				HEIGHT MULTIPLIER FOR GIRLS			
AGE (Y + MO)	M	AGE (Y + MO)	M	AGE (Y + MO)	M	AGE (Y + MO)	M
Birth	3.535	8 + 6	1.351	Birth	3.290	8 + 6	1.254
0 + 3	2.908	9 + 0	1.322	0 + 3	2.759	9 + 0	1.229
0 + 6	2.639	9 + 6	1.298	0 + 6	2.505	9 + 6	1.207
0 + 9	2.462	10 + 0	1.278	0 + 9	2.341	10 + 0	1.183
1 + 0	2.337	10 + 6	1.260	1 + 0	2.216	10 + 6	1.160
1 + 3	2.239	11 + 0	1.235	1 + 3	2.120	11 + 0	1.135
1 + 6	2.160	11 + 6	1.210	1 + 6	2.038	11 + 6	1.108
1 + 9	2.088	12 + 0	1.186	1 + 9	1.965	12 + 0	1.082
2 + 0	2.045	12 + 6	1.161	2 + 0	1.917	12 + 6	1.059
2 + 6	1.942	13 + 0	1.135	2 + 6	1.815	13 + 0	1.040
3 + 0	1.859	13 + 6	1.106	3 + 0	1.735	13 + 6	1.027
3 + 6	1.783	14 + 0	1.081	3 + 6	1.677	14 + 0	1.019
4 + 0	1.731	14 + 6	1.056	4 + 0	1.622	14 + 6	1.013
4 + 6	1.675	15 + 0	1.044	4 + 6	1.570	15 + 0	1.008
5 + 0	1.627	15 + 6	1.030	5 + 0	1.514	15 + 6	1.009
5 + 6	1.579	16 + 0	1.021	5 + 6	1.467	16 + 0	1.004
6 + 0	1.535	16 + 6	1.014	6 + 0	1.421	16 + 6	1.004
6 + 6	1.492	17 + 0	1.010	6 + 6	1.381	17 + 0	1.002
7 + 0	1.455	17 + 6	1.006	7 + 0	1.341	17 + 6	—
7 + 6	1.416	18 + 0	1.005	7 + 6	1.309	18 + 0	—
8 + 0	1.383	Mature Heights = Ht x M		8 + 0	1.279	Mature Heights = Ht x M	

Figure 1-3. Height multiplier tables. Paley J, Talor J, Levin A, Bhave A, Paley D, Herzenberg JE. The multiplier method for prediction of adult height. *J Pediatr Orthop.* 2004;24:732–737.

WEIGHT

- On average, peak weight velocity (PWV) is greater in boys than girls. Peak weight velocity coincides with PHV in boys, but occurs about 6 to 9 months after PHV in girls.
- During puberty, girls reach PWV at age 13 years at a rate of 8.5 kg per year followed by a decrease to less than 1 kg per year by 15 years.
  — Pubertal weight gain in girls is caused primarily by continuous increase in fat mass rather than an increase in skeletal and muscle mass.
- Boys reach PWV at age 14 years at a rate of 9.5 kg a year followed by a decrease to less than 1 kg per year by 17 years.
  — Pubertal weight gain in boys primarily is caused by increases in height (skeletal mass) and muscle mass with a stable fat mass.
- Weight gains during puberty account for approximately 40% to 50% of ideal adult weight in both sexes.

BONE GROWTH

- Primary ossification centers develop before birth in the long bones.
- Primary ossification centers develop during infancy in small bones such as the patella and tarsal bones.
- Secondary ossification centers, within the epiphysis of long bones, develop during infancy and early childhood and fuse with primary ossification centers during late childhood, adolescence, and early adult life.
- The cartilage between the primary and secondary ossification centers of long bones becomes the epiphyseal growth plate.
  — The epiphyseal plate is responsible for longitudinal growth and is subject to pressure or axial forces.
  — Long bones of the upper and lower extremities (femur, tibia, fibula, humerus, radius, ulna) grow in length through the process of *endochondral ossification*, the proliferation of cartilage cells in the epiphyseal growth plate which then ossify to bone.
- The growth in diameter of bones around the diaphysis occurs by *appositional ossification*, the deposition of bone beneath the periosteum.
  — The pelvis, carpals, and tarsals grow by appositional ossification.
  — The phalanges, metacarpals, and spine grow by appositional and endochondral ossification.
- The clavicle is formed through *intramembranous ossification*, which unlike endochondral ossification, does not require a preexisting cartilage model.
- At the ends of each long bone the epiphysis is covered by articular cartilage and forms the joint surface.
  — The development of normal joints requires a functioning neuromuscular system to allow normal motion.
- Ring epiphyses surround the periphery of round bones, such as the tarsal bones and vertebrae, which grow circumferentially.

- Apophyses are growth plates at the surface of bones such as the iliac crest.
  — Traction apophyses are growth plates at the sites of muscle-tendon attachments, such as the tibial tubercle or ischial tuberosity, and thus are subject to traction forces.
  — Apophyses contribute to adult bone shape and may look like a bony outgrowth or bump.
- Ossification begins first in the scapula, humerus, radius, and ulna, and then additional ossification centers develop in a predictable order (Table 1-2).
- On average, ossification centers develop earlier in girls than boys.
- Long and short tubular bones are mature when the diaphyses and the epiphyses fuse.
- Round or irregularly shaped bones are mature when they achieve final adult shape.
- During the fetal period, the metaphyses are composed of *woven bone* that has a high collagen content, giving it the flexibility needed for birth. By 4 years of age, the majority of woven bone has been converted to lamellar bone.
- Cortical bone thickness increases throughout childhood, resulting in increased diaphyseal thickness with age. Conversion to lamellar bone gives mature bone greater tensile strength but much less flexibility.
- The peak velocity of bone mineral accumulation lags behind PHV by an average of 1 year.
- Greater than 90% of peak skeletal bone mass is present by age 18 years.
- The rate of bone growth is precisely regulated, and each growth center contributes a specific percentage of final bone length.
- The trunk grows most rapidly during childhood.
- Growth of the upper limbs occurs earlier than the lower limbs, which grow the fastest during adolescence.
- The foot grows earlier than the rest of the lower limb and achieves its adult length earlier than the rest of the body; half of the adult foot length is achieved between 12 and 18 months of age.
- From infancy through early childhood, a child's lower extremities progress from a varus to valgus position.
- Lateral bowing of the tibia is common during the first year, and bowlegs are common during the toddler years.

Table 1-2. Appearance of Important Ossification Centers in Girls and Boys

	Girls	Boys
Humeral head	0–2 mo	0–3 mo
Capitellum	1–6 mo	0–8 mo
Radial head	3–5 y	4–5 y
Femoral head	1–6 mo	2–8 mo
Patella	1.5–3.5 y	2.5–6 y
Navicular	1.5–3 y	1.5–5.5 y

From Staheli LT. *Fundamentals of Pediatric Orthopedics.* Philadelphia, PA: Lippincott Williams & Wilkins; 2008. Reprinted by permission.

- Knock-knees are most prominent between 3 and 4 years of age.
- The normal bowlegged position evolves into a maximum average valgus angle of 12 degrees between ages 2 and 3 years and then eventually self-corrects to the average adult valgus angle of 5 degrees.
- A child's level of habitual physical activity does not affect the rate of skeletal maturation and has no effect on final adult body stature.

GROWING PAINS

- Growing pains are defined as limb pains that cannot be traced to trauma or disorders of bone, muscle, or joints, and are common in the pediatric age group, with an incidence of 4% to 36%.
- They most commonly occur from 3 to 5 years of age and from 8 to 12 years of age and more often in females than males.
- Pain is usually in the lower extremities and occurs at rest or during the night and not with physical activity.
- The children have a normal physical examination and no evidence of other systemic disease.
- The etiology is unknown; growing pains are benign and self-limited, with no effect on growth velocity.

ASSESSING SKELETAL MATURITY

- Level of ossification, or skeletal maturation, is the best indicator of biological maturity.
- Progression from a cartilaginous skeleton to a fully ossified adult skeleton is radiographically visible.
- Assessment of skeletal age (SA), or bone age, is based on bone development.
- A single radiograph of the left hand is most commonly used to assess skeletal maturity.
  — The bones are compared with those in a standard radiographic atlas, either Greulich-Pyle or Tanner-Whitehouse, using a defined set of criteria.
  — The skeletal ages derived from the different atlases are not equivalent and cannot be used interchangeably.
- Skeletal age may be compared to chronological age (CA), expressed as a difference between SA and CA or as a ratio of SA to CA.
  — For example, a child with an SA of 11.8 years and a CA of 10.1 years is said to have advanced skeletal maturity for CA. Skeletal age minus CA yields a difference of +1.7 years, and SA divided by CA yields 1.2. A ratio above 1.0 indicates advanced skeletal maturity; conversely, a ratio below 1.0 indicates delayed skeletal maturity.
- Children may be classified as having an SA that is advanced, average, or delayed.
  — Children whose SA is within 1 year of CA are classified as average maturers.
  — Children whose SA is 1 year or more behind CA are classified as delayed or late maturers.
  — Children whose SA is 1 year or more ahead of CA are classified as advanced or early maturers. Early maturers tend to be heavier and taller compared with late maturers at all ages, but final adult height typically is similar.

- Skeletal age is better correlated with stage of pubertal development than with CA and can be useful in predicting adult height in early or late maturers.
- Height, weight, and stages of pubertal development have become the main clinical tools for monitoring adolescent development because of the cost, inconvenience, and radiation exposure associated with using radiographs to assess skeletal age.

CHANGES IN BODY COMPOSITION

- Body composition is most often described as a two-compartment model, a combination of lean or fat-free mass (FFM) and fat mass (FM).
- The primary components of FFM are bone, skeletal muscle, and nonskeletal muscle soft tissue; the primary component of FM is adipose or fat tissue.
- Subcutaneous "baby fat" develops during the first year of life and gradually is burned up by increased mobility in early childhood.
- Fat mass and FFM gradually increase as body size increases between 2 and 6 years of age, but on average FM decreases more in boys than in girls due to increased energy expenditure and decreased caloric intake.
- Body physique remains relatively stable from 6 to 12 years of age, and FFM on average is 80% in a prepubertal child.
- Body mass index is **weight divided by height squared (kg/m²)** and is related to FFM in children and adolescents.
  — Body mass index increases in infancy, decreases through early childhood to a low point around 5 or 6 years of age, then rises again through rest of childhood and adolescence.
  — Children with the same BMI can have significantly different percentages of fat and FFM, and therefore elevated BMI is not uniformly a good indicator of fatness in childhood and adolescence.
- Fat-free mass undergoes a well-defined spurt during adolescence (Figure 1-4).

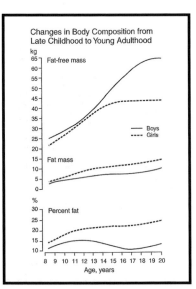

Figure 1-4. Growth curves for fat-free mass, fat mass, and relative fatness. From Malina RM, Bouchard C, Beunen G. Human growth: selected aspects of current research on well-nourished children. *Ann Rev Anthropol.* 1988;17:187–219. Reprinted by permission of Annual Reviews, Inc.

- Throughout adolescence lean or fat-free body mass increases from 80% to 90% in boys but decreases from 80% to 75% in girls as they accumulate more subcutaneous fat.
- During the interval of PHV, boys gain approximately twice as much FFM as girls (14 kg vs 7 kg), while girls gain twice as much fat mass as boys (3 kg vs 1.5 kg).
- Women have almost twice the percentage of body fat as men.
- Girls continue to gain FM but not FFM into late adolescence (16–20 years of age).
  — Girls enter puberty with 15.7% average body fat, and as adults average 26.7%.
  — Boys enter puberty with 4.3% average body fat, and as adults average 11.2%.
- Adult males have 150% of the FFM of an average adult female.
- Young women have more subcutaneous fat deposits in the pelvis, breast, upper back, and arms, compared with young men.
- The effect of heredity on body mass and composition is about 40%.
- Children who have more fat after 6 years of age have a higher risk of retaining fat through childhood and into adulthood.

CHANGES IN MUSCLE MASS AND STRENGTH

- The percentage of muscle, or muscle mass, increases with age.
- During middle childhood, muscle strength, coordination, and endurance increase through maturation and training.
- Small differences in muscle strength begin to appear between boys and girls in middle to late childhood.
- The greatest gains in muscular mass and strength occur during adolescence in girls and boys, with boys showing greater gains in both.
- The muscular strength gains in early adulthood occur at a much slower rate than in puberty.
- In boys, muscle strength increases linearly with age from early childhood through age 13 or 14 years and then experiences a marked acceleration through late adolescence into early or mid-20s.
- In girls, muscle strength also increases linearly through age 15 years but without an adolescent spurt.
- For boys this increase in muscle is a dominant change during puberty. The increase in strength is more than predicted from growth in stature.
- On average, the peak gains in muscular strength and power occur after PHV but around PWV. The peak increase in muscle strength lags behind the increase in mass, occurring in the final stage of pubertal development.
- Muscle mass peaks around 3 months after height spurt in boys and girls, and the increase in mass is double that in boys compared with girls.
- The sex difference in strength is more marked in the upper extremity and trunk than in the lower extremity.
- Boys who are early maturers tend to be taller and have greater muscle mass and greater strength than boys who are late maturers.
- Girls who mature early tend to only have a minimal increase in strength.

FLEXIBILITY AND JOINT MOBILITY

- Joint hypermobility, or ligamentous laxity, is defined as the ability to extend a joint beyond its normal range of motion.
  - The most commonly used method to screen for generalized joint hypermobility is the Beighton score (see Figure 4-2a).
- During ages 6 to 12 years, muscle flexibility and joint mobility may be increased. The prevalence of joint hypermobility is highest in school-aged children, approximately 5% to 7%.
- During puberty there is increased tightness of the hamstrings and calf muscles, which is greatest during the height spurt for boys and girls.
- In general, girls show greater muscle flexibility and joint mobility at all ages compared with boys.

EXERCISE CAPACITY

- In middle childhood, aerobic and anaerobic exercise capacity increase slowly and are limited compared with adolescence.
- When maximum aerobic capacity is expressed relative to body weight, mean values remain constant for boys but decrease with age for girls from 6 to 16 years of age because of greater accumulation of fat.
- Increases in maximum aerobic capacity are strongly related to physical maturity, specifically heart, lung, and muscular growth.
- For boys, there is evidence of an adolescent growth spurt in maximum aerobic capacity, with maximum gain around PHV. There is no evidence for this in girls.
- Anaerobic capacity increases more gradually than aerobic capacity, and aerobic capacity continues to increase into early adulthood but at a slower rate than in puberty.

Normal Motor Development

- Average age for acquisition of motor skills in first years of life is shown in Table 1-3.
- Many variables regulate fundamental and complex motor skill development, including somatic growth and maturation, heredity or inherent skill, and environmental experiences such as socioeconomic status, quality of instruction, child and parent interest, and opportunities to engage in physical activity.
- Children achieve or improve their motor skills with age in a similar sequence but at different rates, resulting in wide variability in motor skills at specific ages.
- Fundamental motor skills are common motor activities with specific, observable patterns that are prerequisites for acquiring more complicated skills necessary for sports, games, and other physical activities. These fundamental motor skills can be divided into 3 basic categories:
  1) locomotive skills (walking, running, jumping, hopping)
  2) non-manipulative skills (turning, balancing, leaping, sliding)
  3) manipulative skills (kicking, throwing, catching, striking, bouncing, pulling, pushing).

Table 1-3. Acquisition of Motor Skills in First 5 Years of Life

Milestone	Age of Attainment (mo)
Gross Motor	
Head steady in sitting	2
Pull to sit, no head lag	4
Hands together in midline	4
Rolls back to stomach	7
Sits without support	10
Crawls	10
Walks alone	15
Crawls up stairs	15
Sits on small chair	18
Runs well	24
Goes up stairs alternating feet	30
Rides tricycle	36
Climbs well	48
Skips	60
Fine Motor	
Reaches for and grasps objects	4
Transfers object hand to hand	7
Grasps object with thumb and forefinger	10
Turns pages of book	12
Builds tower of 3 cubes	15
Imitates vertical stroke	18
Circular scribbling	24
Makes vertical and horizontal strokes	30
Copies a circle	36
Copies a square	48
Copies a triangle	60

- Beyond the basic skills of walking and running, children exhibit a wide range of ability with more advanced activities such as throwing, catching, and kicking.
- Adeptness in motor skills is incremental and related to body size, maturity, agility, and balance.
- The prepubertal period from infancy through 9 years of age is critically important for the acquisition and development of motor skills in a growing child.
- Handedness is usually established firmly by age 3 or 4 years.
- By 5 to 7 years of age, most children demonstrate mature fundamental movement patterns, which are coordinated and mechanically efficient.

- Children younger than 7 to 8 years cannot perform complex tasks requiring much coordination, but by 11 to 12 years of age, children can perform high-level motor skills, including faster and more precise performance of complicated tasks and foot skills.
- Puberty is the final critical period for motor skill development.

GAIT

- Early gait is characterized by a fast cadence with short steps and a wide-based gait, with the knees and arms flexed and the trunk rotating with each stride.
- After several months of walking, toddlers walk more slowly with a longer stride, a more stable torso, extended knees, and arms swinging at the side for balance.
- By 3 or 4 years of age most children walk with adult gait patterns, although continued changes in gait velocity, stride length, and cadence occur into adulthood.

Gender Differences in Motor Development

- Girls generally perform better than boys in fine motor tasks, while boys perform better than girls in gross motor tasks. These differences in motor ability increase with age and are primarily explained by specific gender-oriented types of sports and activities, encouragement, opportunity, and expectations.
- Certain fundamental motor skills (skip, catch, hop) initially appear in girls ahead of boys, but the most mature developmental stages of other skills (run, throw, kick, strike, jump) are attained sooner in boys than in girls (Table 1-4).
- Motor performance levels in girls are relatively stable across time, but boys may experience a temporary disruption of motor coordination during their growth spurt, termed *adolescent awkwardness* or *overgrown, clumsy age*.
- Gender differences in motor performance are relatively low or moderate before puberty but quite large after puberty.

Table 1-4. Age at Which Highest Developmental Level of Fundamental Motor Skills Is Achieved in Boys and Girls

Motor Skill	Boys (y)	Motor skill	Girls (y)
Running	4	Running	5
Throwing	5	Skipping	6
Skipping	6.5	Catching	6.5
Catching	7	Hopping	7
Kicking	7	Kicking	8
Striking	7	Striking	8.5
Hopping	7.5	Throwing	8.5
Jumping	9.5	Jumping	10

Data are derived from Seefeldt V HJ. Patterns, phases, and stages: an analytical model for the study of developmental movement. In: Kelso JA Scott, Clark JE, eds. *The Development of Movement Control and Coordination*. New York, NY: John Wiley & Sons; 1982.

- While environmental influences primarily account for the gender differences in prepubertal motor performance prior to puberty, environmental and biological factors account for the rapid and large increases after puberty.

Sports Readiness

- Children acquire motor skills in similar sequence but at different rates, so sport readiness must be assessed individually.
- Many children younger than 7 years cannot perform the complex motor tasks necessary for competitive sports.

CHAPTER 2

Abnormal Musculoskeletal Growth and Motor Development

- Most children usually remain within 1 or 2 growth lines (eg, between the 50th and 90th percentile).
- Appropriate nutrition is the critical environmental factor affecting normal biological maturation; adequate food intake parallels normal increase in body size.
- *Failure to thrive:* Weight is less than the 5th percentile or declines more than 2 major percentile lines (eg, declines from the 80th percentile to the 40th percentile).
- *Undernutrition:* Weight for age typically declines (wasting) before height for age (stunting) and weight for height.
- *Undernutrition* is associated with more delay in skeletal age relative to chronologic age and later ages at peak height velocity and menarche, while obesity is associated with advanced maturation.
- *Other non-nutritional causes of abnormal growth:* Length often declines first or at the same time as weight.
- *Constitutional growth delay:* Weight and height decrease toward the end of infancy, remain stable during middle childhood, and then increase toward the end of adolescence, resulting in normal adult stature.
- *Familial short stature:* The child and parents are small, and the child's growth remains below but parallels the normal curves.
- There is a risk of overdiagnosing or underdiagnosing growth abnormalities in children with extremely tall or short parents if parental height is not taken into account.
- Musculoskeletal problems account for about one third of congenital defects, with hip dysplasia and clubfeet accounting for half of the primary musculoskeletal defects.
- Three percent of newborns have major defects and infants with multiple minor defects should be thoroughly evaluated to exclude a major malformation.

- *Abnormal morphogenesis* can be classified into 4 categories of defects: malformations, disruptions, deformations, dysplasias.
  — *Malformations*, such as limb hypoplasia, arise during organogenesis and are of teratogenic or genetic origin.
  — *Disruptions*, such as ring constriction bands, occur later in gestation when teratogenic, traumatic, or other factors interfere with normal fetal growth.
  — *Deformations*, such as calcaneovalgus foot deformity caused by molding in the breech position, occur at the end of gestation and are due to intrauterine crowding or position.
  — *Dysplasias* result from altered growth that occurs before and after birth.
- Most musculoskeletal problems are caused by *environmental factors* such as malnutrition, infection, or trauma that can alter bone growth in children.
  — Growth plate compression or injury, metabolic disorders such as rickets, and nutritional deficiencies can retard growth.
  — Inflammatory disorders or trauma may damage the growth plate or articular cartilage and result in malunion, shortening, or angular deformity.
  — Pituitary tumors, Marfan syndrome, chronic osteomyelitis, and foreign body reaction may accelerate growth.
- Developmental variations, which resolve with time and seldom require any treatment, should be differentiated from deformities. Examples include flatfeet, in-toeing, out-toeing, bowlegs, and knee-knees.
- Adolescents with delayed puberty or secondary amenorrhea may not have normal bone mineral accrual and thus may have reduced bone mineral density as adults.

Abnormal Motor Development

- Abnormalities with visual-spatial information that guides gross motor actions can lead to ineptitude at skills such as catching or throwing.
- Some children have difficulty planning complex motor procedures needed for tasks such as dancing, and others lack adequate proprioception and are impaired with activities requiring balance and control of body movement.
- Abnormalities with fine motor skills, caused by impaired hand-eye coordination, can lead to problems with rapid and precise hand movements and impair tasks such as drawing, writing, or playing an instrument.
- Limited competence in fundamental motor skills at an early age can negatively affect future performance in physical and motor activities.
- *Developmental deviation* is when children develop skills out of the usual sequence.
- *Developmental dissociation* occurs when developmental spheres are achieved at different rates.
  — Children with cerebral palsy show motor delay and normal language.
  — Children with autism show normal motor and language delay.
- *Milestone regression*, loss of developmental skills, is a serious developmental problem suggesting an active, ongoing neurologic condition.

- Musculoskeletal growth and gross motor development are intricately related such that an abnormality in one can result in delayed or abnormal development of the other.
  - Toe walking is often seen in children with autism, cerebral palsy, or other developmental delay.
  - Temporary joint and muscle contractures can be caused by in utero positioning. Full-term newborns have 20- to 30-degree flexion contractures at the hip and knee that usually resolve by 6 months of age.

EARLY DETECTION AND EARLY INTERVENTION

- The goal of developmental surveillance and screening is to identify children with developmental problems early to ensure they receive the benefits of early intervention (EI).
- Early detection of motor problems and EI can eliminate or minimize many physical and related emotional problems.
  - Interventions for motor disorders have been shown to be effective at 18 months of age and there is strong evidence that EI can result in significant improvements in cognitive and emotional development and that later interventions in children with more established disabilities show more modest gains.
- Developmental surveillance is the process of identifying children who may be at risk of developmental delays (http://pathwaysawareness.org).
- Developmental surveillance should be incorporated into every well-child visit with additional developmental screening tests administered at the 9-, 18-, and 24- or 30-month visits or anytime concerns are raised by parents, clinicians, or others involved in the care of the child.
- Parental concerns about development are often appropriate and should be appropriately addressed, but lack of parental concern does not necessarily indicate normal development.
- Mild motor delays that were undetectable at 9-month screening may be more apparent at 18 months, and by 30 months of age, most motor delays may be identified with screening instruments.
- Surveillance should continue throughout childhood, and developmental concerns should be addressed at every pediatric health supervision visit for the first 5 years of life (Box 2-1).

Box 2-1. Normal Ages When Primitive Reflexes Extinguish

Reflex	Normal Age When Reflex Extinguishes
Rooting	4 mo
Moro	4–6 mo
Tonic labyrinthine	4–6 mo
Galant	4–6 mo
Palmar grasp	5–6 mo
Asymmetric and symmetric tonic neck reflexes	6–7 mo
Foot placement (stepping)	Before 12 mo
Babinski	12 mo

- Children identified as at risk for delayed or disordered development should receive further detailed diagnostic developmental evaluation including a thorough history, physical examination, vision and hearing assessment, family history, prenatal and postnatal history, review of newborn metabolic screening and growth charts, laboratory tests such as chromosome testing, and assessment of other environmental and social risk factors.
  — If a disorder is not identified, the child should be followed with more frequent visits to reevaluate the areas of concern.
- An underlying etiology will be identified in approximately 25% of children with delayed development, with higher rates (>50%) in children with global developmental delays and motor delays.
- Observations made over a period are most informative, and developmental screening tests should be used periodically.

EVALUATION TOOLS

- Developmental screening is the administration of a brief standardized tool that aids the identification of children at risk for a developmental disorder.
- Pediatrician assessment of a child's developmental status is less accurate without the use of a standardized screening tool (Table 2-1).
- Many screening tools are available but there is no universally accepted screening tool appropriate for all populations and ages.
- Sensitivity and specificity levels of 70% to 80% (moderate) are considered acceptable for developmental screening tests.
- Most tools can be completed by parents, scored by nonphysicians, and interpreted by physicians. See Table 2-1 for a list of common developmental screening tools.

Table 2-1. Developmental Screening Tools

Tool	Description	Testing Age Range
Parents' Evaluation of Developmental Status (PEDS)	Suitable for eliciting and addressing parental concerns. Indicates when to refer, screen further, or reassure (sensitivity 0.74, specificity 0.7–0.8).	0–8 y
Parents' Evaluation of Developmental Status: Developmental Milestone (PEDS:DM)	Useful for periodic evaluation of milestones. One question per each domain: fine motor, gross motor, social-emotional, self-help, expressive language, receptive language, reading, and math (sensitivity 0.83, specificity 0.84).	0–8 y
Denver Developmental II	125 items test 4 domains: personal-social, fine motor-adaptive, expressive and receptive language, and gross motor skills.	0–6 y
Early Screening Inventory (ESI)	Brief parent questionnaires based on the Denver milestones. Has increased sensitivity to detect subtle delays (sensitivity 0.56–0.83, specificity 0.43–0.80).	3–6 y

Table 2-1. Developmental Screening Tools, continued

Tool	Description	Testing Age Range
Ages and Stages Questionnaire (ASQ)	At-home screening test used between health supervision visits to assess communication, gross motor, fine motor, problem-solving, personal adaptive skills (sensitivity 0.70–0.90, specificity 0.76–0.91).	4–48 mo
Child Development Inventory (CDI)	300 items that measure social, self-help, motor, language, and general developmental skills. Suitable for more in-depth evaluation (sensitivity 0.8–1.0, specificity 0.94–0.96)	18 mo–6 y
Early Motor Pattern Profile (EMPP)	15 items, administered by a physician to examine movement, tone, and reflex development for ages 6–12 mo (sensitivity 0.87–0.92, specificity 0.98).	6–12 mo
Motor Quotient (MQ)	Assesses 11 milestones per visit and uses a simple ratio quotient with gross motor milestones to detect delayed motor development (sensitivity 0.87, specificity 0.89).	8–18 mo
Test of Infant Motor Performance (TIMP)	42 items with picture references that assess motor tone, axis symmetry, and movement. Administered by physician or physical/occupational therapist (sensitivity 0.92, specificity 0.76).	Preterm infants >34 wk post-conceptional age to 4 mo adjusted age

Bibliography

American Academy of Pediatrics Council on Children With Disabilities, Section on Developmental Behavioral Pediatrics, Bright Futures Steering Committee, Medical Home Initiatives for Children With Special Needs Project Advisory Committee. Identifying infants and young children with developmental disorders in the medical home: an algorithm for developmental surveillance and screening. *Pediatrics.* 2006;118:405–420

Behrman RE, Kliegman RM, Jenson HB, eds. *Nelson Textbook of Pediatrics.* 18th ed. Philadelphia, PA: WB Saunders Co; 2007

Beunen G, Malina RM. Growth and physical performance relative to the timing of the adolescent spurt. *Exerc Sport Sci Rev.* 1988;16:503–540

Beunen GP, Rogol AD, Malina RM. Indicators of biological maturation and secular changes in biological maturation. *Food Nutr Bull.* 2006;27(4 Suppl):S244–S256

Branta C, Haubenstricker J, Seefeldt V. Age changes in motor skills during childhood and adolescence. *Exerc Sport Sci Rev.* 1984;12:467–520

Burton WA. *Movement Skill Assessment.* Champaign, IL: Human Kinetics; 1998

Greulich WW, Pyle SI. *Radiographic Atlas of Skeletal Development of the Hand and Wrist.* 2nd ed. Palo Alto, CA: Stanford University Press; 1999

Harris SS, Anderson SJ, eds. *Care of the Young Athlete.* 2nd ed. Elk Grove Village, IL: American Academy of Pediatrics; 2010

Jürimäe T, Jürimäe J. *Growth, Physical Activity and Motor Development in Prepubertal Children.* Boca Raton, FL: CRC Press LLC; 2000

Katchadourian H. *The Biology of Adolescence.* San Francisco, CA: WH Freeman and Co; 1977

Kuczmarski RJ, Ogden CL, Grummer-Strawn LM, et al. CDC growth charts: United States. *Adv Data.* 2000;314:1–27

Landry GL, Bernhardt DT. *Essentials of Primary Care Sports Medicine.* Champaign, IL: Human Kinetics; 2003

Malina RM. Growth and maturation in sport. In: Birrer RB, Griesemzer BA, Cataletto MB, eds. *Pediatric Sports Medicine for Primary Care.* Philadelphia, PA: Lippincott Williams & Wilkins; 2002:39–58

Malina RM. Physical growth and biological maturation of young athletes. *Exerc Sport Sci Rev.* 1994;22:389–433

Malina RM, Bouchard C, Bar-Or O. *Growth, Maturation, and Physical Activity.* 2nd ed. Champaign, IL: Human Kinetics; 2004

Paley D, Bhave A, Herzenberg JE, Bowen JR. Multiplier method for predicting limb-length discrepancy. *J Bone Joint Surg Am.* 2000;82:1432–1446

Roberton M. Longitudinal evidence of developmental stages in the forceful overarm throw. *J Hum Movement Stud.* 1978;4:167–175

Rogol AD, Roemmich JN, Clark PA. Growth at puberty. *J Adolesc Health.* 2002;31(6 Suppl):192–200

Root AW. Endocrinology of puberty. I. Normal sexual maturation. *J Pediatr.* 1973;83:1–19

Seefeldt V HJ. Patterns, phases, and stages: an analytical model for the study of developmental movement. In: Kelso JA Scott, Clark JE, eds. *The Development of Movement Control and Coordination.* New York, NY: John Wiley & Sons; 1982

Slap GB. Normal physiological and psychosocial growth in the adolescent. *J Adolesc Health Care.* 1986; 7(6 Suppl):13S–23S

Staheli L. *Fundamentals of Pediatric Orthopedics.* Philadelphia, PA: Lippincott Williams & Wilkins; 2008

Tanner JM. *Growth at Adolescence.* 2nd ed. Oxford, England: Blackwell Scientific Publications; 1978

Tanner JM, Davies PS. Clinical longitudinal standards for height and weight velocity for North American children. *J Pediatr.* 1985;107:317–329

Tanner JM, Whitehouse RH, Marshall WA, et al. *Assessment of Skeletal Maturity and Prediction of Adult Height (TW2 Method).* London, England: Academic Press; 1983

Thomas JR, French KE. Gender differences across age in motor performance a meta-analysis. *Psychol Bull.* 1985;98:260–282

Part 2: Musculoskeletal Evaluation

TOPICS COVERED

CHAPTER 3

History

- Musculoskeletal complaints may result from a wide range of possible etiologies (Table 3-1).
- History is an important aspect of the musculoskeletal evaluation.
- History alone may provide the diagnosis in 75% of cases.
- The most common musculoskeletal complaints are injury, pain, deformity, and change in function.

Table 3-1. Categories of Etiologies of Musculoskeletal Complaints

Etiology	Examples
Trauma	
Acute	Fracture, tendon rupture
Chronic	Stress fracture, tendinopathy
Inflammation	Arthritis
Infection	Osteomyelitis
Neoplasm	
Malignant	Osteosarcoma, leukemia
Benign	Unicameral bone cyst, fibrous cortical defect
Congenital abnormality	Clubfoot, amniotic band syndrome
Neuro-developmental disorder	Cerebral palsy, hereditary motor sensory neuropathy
Endocrine disorder	Rickets
Hematologic disorder	Avascular necrosis
Genetic disorder	Osteogenesis imperfecta, trisomy 21

Mechanism of Injury

- Ask the child and family to provide a detailed account of how the injury occurred.
- The mechanism of injury is very important—it may identify injured structures and injury types.
  - An inversion injury to the ankle commonly results in sprain of the lateral ligaments.
  - Fall on an outstretched arm commonly results in a clavicle or distal radius fracture.
- If the trauma was not witnessed, knowing what the patient was doing at the time of the suspected injury may suggest a mechanism.

- Trauma is common in active children, but may not always be the cause of the symptoms.
- When the mechanism does not match the symptoms, or when the timing of the trauma does not coincide closely with the onset of symptoms, consider a coincidental condition such as neoplasm or infection.

Pain

Several factors are considered in assessing pain complaints.

- *Pain expression* depends on patient's age.
  - Infants usually refuse to move the painful area, cry, or are fussy.
  - Children will avoid using the painful part, alter its function, or complain of pain.
  - Adolescents will complain of pain.
- *Pain location* can be determined by asking the patient to point with one finger "where you feel the pain," or by asking the patient to indicate where he or she hurts on a corresponding drawing of a human figure (Figure 3-1).

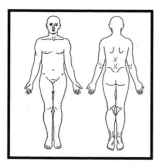

Figure 3-1. Human figure marked by patient to indicate location of pain.

- *Severity* can be rated using a numeric scale (1 to 10) or by using a pain face scale such as the Wong-Baker scale (Figure 3-2).
- *Quality* (eg, sharp, dull, aching, throbbing, burning), onset, frequency, and duration can be assessed using open-ended questions.
- *Factors that aggravate or relieve the pain* may assist in diagnosis and guide treatment.
  - Mechanical causes are worse with activity.
  - Inflammatory causes are worse after rest.
- *Progression over time* can indicate whether the condition is static, episodic, improving, or worsening.
- *Presence of associated symptoms* may suggest involvement of specific systems (Box 3-1).

Deformity

- Variants of normal musculoskeletal development, such as knock-knees, flatfeet, and in-toeing, are common and inconsequential. These should be differentiated from significant congenital and neuromuscular deformities.
- Determine the onset, progression over time, and whether the deformity causes pain or limits the child's functional abilities or motor development.

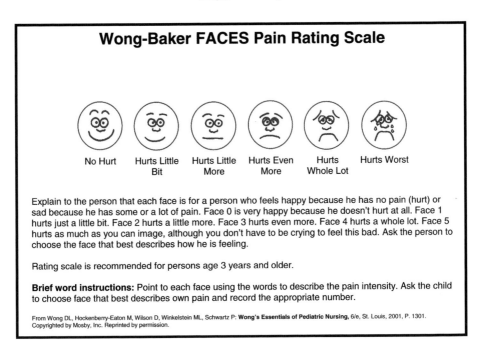

Figure 3-2. Wong-Baker scale.

Box 3-1. Symptoms Suggestive of Specific System Involvement

Neurologic: Numbness, tingling, and weakness

Musculoskeletal: Mechanical symptoms of clicking, locking, or instability

Infectious or inflammatory: Redness, warmth, swelling, and stiffness

Vascular: Changes in skin color and temperature

Systemic etiology: Fever, fatigue, or involvement of other joints

Change in Function

- May be caused by pain, injury, deformity, or weakness.

Previous Management

- Ask about the effects (beneficial and adverse) of prior treatments (eg, physical therapy, braces, orthotics, anti-inflammatory medications).
  — This may narrow the differential diagnosis and suggest treatments to continue, discontinue, or modify.
- Note duration and compliance, which may suggest reasons for lack of effect.

Sports and Physical Activity History (Box 3-2)

- Severity of symptoms may be estimated by the degree to which they limit the child's usual activities.
- May identify reasons for overuse injury or nonspecific complaints due to overtraining and burnout.
- Helps with diagnosis and guides rehabilitation and return to play.

Box 3-2. Sports and Physical Activity History Questions

What physical activities (eg, sports, dance, music, drama) does the child enjoy?
Are the symptoms limiting participation in these activities?
What is the child's position/role, level of competition, and hand/leg dominance?
How many hours per week are spent in practice and competition and how many days rest per week and per year?

Past Medical and Surgical History

- Systemic diseases may have musculoskeletal manifestations (Table 3-2).
- History of recent infection
  - Raises suspicion for post-infectious phenomena such as rheumatic fever (pharyngitis), reactive arthritis (gastrointestinal infection), and transient synovitis of the hip.
  - Provides clues to identifying the source and pathogen in the case of a septic joint.
- History of frequent fractures
  - May suggest inflicted trauma.
  - May be a sign of underlying metabolic bone disease.

Pregnancy and Birth History

- May identify risk factors for neonatal cardiorespiratory depression, neonatal fractures, or congenital abnormalities.

Medications and Allergies

- Some medications can have musculoskeletal side effects.
- Note any allergies to medications commonly used to treat musculoskeletal pain or injury (eg, anti-inflammatory medications).

Diet

- A diet history will identify potential nutritional deficiencies that have musculoskeletal manifestations. (See Box 6-1 on page 72.)

Table 3-2. Examples of Systemic Diseases With Musculoskeletal Manifestations

System	Condition	Musculoskeletal Manifestations
Neuromuscular	Cerebral palsy	Gait abnormalities
	Muscular dystrophy	Hip dislocations, scoliosis
	Spinal muscular atrophy	
Renal	X-linked hypophosphatemic rickets	Bony deformities, alignment abnormalities
Endocrine	Growth hormone deficiency	SCFE
	Hypothyroidism	
Genetic/ development syndromes	Marfan syndrome	Scoliosis
	VATER association	Skeletal anomalies
	Prader-Willi syndrome	Hip dysplasia, scoliosis, alignment abnormalities

SCFE, slipped capital femoral epiphysis; VATER, vertebrae, anus, trachea esophagus, renal.

Growth and Developmental History

- Systemic diseases with musculoskeletal manifestations may cause abnormal growth (Table 3-3).
- If developmental delay is present, the pattern may suggest the underlying diagnosis (see Chapter 1).
- Early preferential handedness may suggest an abnormality such as hemiplegia of the nondominant side.

Table 3-3. Examples of Systemic Diseases Associated With Poor Growth or Weight Loss

Condition	Musculoskeletal Manifestations
Eating disorder	Stress fractures
Inflammatory bowel disease, SLE, juvenile chronic arthritis	Arthritis
Renal osteodystrophy	SCFE
Trisomy 21	Hypotonia, scoliosis, cervical instability
Gaucher	Vertebral collapse, osteonecrosis, pathologic fracture caused by osteopenia, cervical instability
Mucopolysaccharidoses	Vertebral anomalies, scoliosis
GH deficiency	SCFE

SLE, systemic lupus erythematosus; SCFE, slipped capital femoral epiphysis; GH, growth hormone.

- Level of skeletal maturity can determine the potential for progression of growth-related deformities, such as scoliosis.
- In the absence of a radiographic bone age, skeletal maturity can be estimated from the stage of pubertal maturation.

Social History

- Ask about resources for treatment and social support at home and in the community (eg, county programs, school athletic trainer, nearby physical therapists).
- Travel or area of residence may increase concern for endemic disease (eg, Lyme disease, tuberculosis). For some infectious diseases, there may be a long delay between exposure and symptom onset.
- Note risk factors for social or emotional abuse and inflicted trauma (see Chapter 40).
- Environmental history may identify toxic exposures (eg, lead poisoning can cause musculoskeletal pain).

Family History

- Many musculoskeletal conditions have a hereditary basis; ask whether any blood relatives have orthopaedic, neurologic, dermatologic, or rheumatologic conditions. Provide examples (eg, psoriasis, Crohn disease), because many people may be unaware of the musculoskeletal manifestations of some diseases.
- Because inflammatory arthritis can be associated with inflammatory bowel disease and urethritis, patients with joint pain should be asked about abdominal pain, diarrhea, nausea, and dysuria.
- Sleep disturbance, specifically pain that wakes the child at night, suggests bone pain from malignant neoplasms or infection, whereas night pain relieved by nonsteroidal anti-inflammatory medication is classic for osteoid osteoma.

Review of Symptoms

- Box 3-3 lists a review of systems appropriate during a musculoskeletal examination.

Box 3-3. Review of Systems in a Musculoskeletal Evaluation

Fevers, night sweats, and changes in activity level or appetite raise concern for infection, neoplasm, or inflammatory conditions.

Multiple affected joints suggest inflammatory arthritis or systemic infection.

Mucocutaneous and ocular symptoms may be associated with inflammatory conditions.

A child with a spinal cord abnormality may have enuresis, encopresis, or constipation.

Recurrent headaches and paresthesias may signal neurologic disease.

CHAPTER 4

Physical Examination

General Principles of the Physical Examination

- Musculoskeletal examination should include
  — Inspection
  — Range of motion (active and passive)
  — Palpation
  — Evaluation of muscle strength, flexibility
  — Joint stability
  — Neurologic examination
- Special tests may elicit findings unique to specific diagnoses.
- Height, weight, and body mass index (BMI) should be plotted.

> BMI = weight (kg)/(height [m])^2
> BMI = 703 * weight (lb)/(height [in])^2

- Assist the child and family with keeping the child as calm and comfortable as possible during the examination.
- Ask parents to console or help the child actively perform specific motions; this may elicit better cooperation from the child. For example, parents can undress a toddler to a diaper and T-shirt and take him for a walk in the hallway while the physician observes his gait.
- Children may be more comfortable being examined on a parent's lap; the child can be transitioned to the examination table once she becomes more at ease with the practitioner.
- Inspection and active range of motion should be assessed before palpation and passive range of motion, lest the child become upset and resist examination altogether.
- Children often have difficulty localizing pain, and pain may be referred from an adjacent joint, so examine the joint above and the joint below the location of symptoms.
- To gain the child's trust, begin by examining areas farthest from the region of concern.
- Hip, spine, and gait evaluation should be a standard part of the routine well-child visit.
  — Evaluate the hips until the child walks and a normal gait is present.
  — Evaluate the spine for scoliosis and cutaneous abnormalities.
- Any child with skeletal anomalies requires examination for associated congenital or systemic abnormalities (see tables 3-2 and 3-3 for examples).
- Document the examination using standard orthopaedic terminology.

Inspection

- Inspect areas that are less directly related to the patient's chief complaint first to make sure they are not overlooked.
- Note surface landmarks, posture, and symmetry.
- Inspect for deformities such as abnormal alignment, joint effusions, skin changes, and unusual prominences.

Palpation

- Identifying the point of maximal tenderness (PMT) is the most valuable aspect of the physical examination because it locates the anatomic source of the pain or injury.
- When combined with the history or mechanism of injury, PMT can usually determine the diagnosis.
- Begin with the unaffected limb to put the child at ease and establish baseline range of motion, strength, and stability.
- For the affected limb, start distally and move proximally, which generates less distress and increases the likelihood of localizing the pain.
- While palpating, watch the child's face for grimacing or other signs of discomfort.
- Evaluate skin temperature, pulses, and capillary refill.

Range of Motion

- Passive and active range of motion is best measured with a goniometer (Figure 4-1), which allows for comparison to normal ranges (Table 4-1) and provides baselines for comparison to follow-up examinations. Measurements should include the opposite limb for comparison.

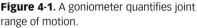

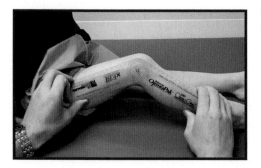

Figure 4-1. A goniometer quantifies joint range of motion.

- When a goniometer is unavailable, range of motion should be described by comparing with the opposite limb (eg, "symmetrical," "right is decreased by approximately 20 degrees compared to left").
- Very young or uncooperative children should be prompted to reach for or move toward a desired object, such as a toy or sticker, or have the parent perform passive range of motion.

Table 4-1. Normal Joint Range of Motion for Children[a]

Joint	Direction	Normal Degree of Motion
Cervical spine	Flexion	65
	Extension	85
	Lateral rotation	75
	Lateral bending	45
Shoulder	Abduction	180
	Forward flexion	180
	Extension	45
	Internal rotation	55
	External rotation	45
Elbow/forearm	Flexion	140–150
	Extension	0
	Supination	90
	Pronation	90
Wrist	Extension	80
	Flexion	70
	Ulnar deviation	30
	Radial deviation	20
Hip	Flexion	120–145
	Extension	20–25
	Abduction	45–70
	Internal rotation	35–50
	External rotation	45–55
Knee	Flexion	150
	Extension	0
Ankle	Dorsiflexion—knee flexed	20–25
	Dorsiflexion—knee extended	10–20
	Plantarflexion	50

[a]Normal for range of motion varies with age and sex, with females and younger children demonstrating greater joint mobility.

- The degree of ligamentous laxity or joint range of motion tends to be hereditary and is highly variable among individuals.
- A Beighton score (Figure 4-2a-c) greater than 4 indicates generalized ligamentous laxity or widespread joint hypermobility.
  — Approximately 7% of the population demonstrates generalized ligamentous laxity, most of whom have benign joint hypermobility.
  — A smaller proportion (usually those with Beighton scores of 8 or 9) have connective tissue disorders such as Marfan or Ehlers-Danlos syndrome.
  — Generalized ligamentous laxity has been associated with hip dysplasia and pes planus and increased risk for recurrent patellar and shoulder dislocations and other ligament sprains.

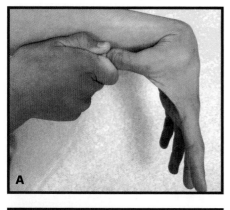
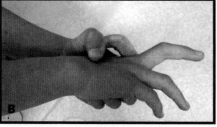
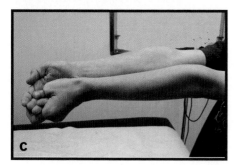

Figure 4-2. The Beighton 9-point score screens for widespread joint hypermobility as seen in this patient with Ehlers-Danlos syndrome. Score one point for each thumb that can touch palmar aspect of wrist (A), one point for each index finger than extends past 90 degrees at the metacarpophalangeal joint (B), one point for each elbow that hyperextends (C), one point for each knee that hyperextends (not shown), and one point for placing palms flat on floor without bending knees (not shown). While there is no established diagnostic cutoff, most rheumatologists consider scores of 4 and above indicative of hypermobility.

Muscle Tone

- Tone is resting muscle tension.
  - *Normal tone* is some degree of resistance to passive joint range of motion.
  - *Hypotonia* is decreased resistance to passive joint range of motion.
    - An infant who "slips through" the examiner's hands when being held underneath the arms has hypotonia.
    - Mild hypotonia is not uncommon in infants.
  - *Hypertonia* is increased resistance to passive joint range of motion.
    - Indicates an upper motor neuron lesion, such as spastic cerebral palsy. In these patients, tone will be greatest with the initiation of passive movement and then decrease somewhat with continued movement.

- Normally, during abrupt ankle dorsiflexion, there is a "catching sensation" followed by a relaxation. This catch is often absent in patients with hypotonia. When this catch repeats itself rhythmically, *clonus* is present.
  - The number of beats determines whether clonus is pathologic.
  - Normal infants may exhibit up to 5 beats of clonus, while adults should have fewer than 2.
  - Sustained clonus usually represents upper motor neuron pathology and related hypertonia.

Muscle Strength

- Evaluate strength in infants by noting grasp strength, head control, ability to bear weight on legs, and muscle tone.
- In children and teens, manual muscle testing is commonly used to grade strength of individual muscles or functional movements (eg, elbow flexion) by asking the patient to actively contract the muscle as the examiner provides resistance (Table 4-2). The pattern of weakness can locate the deficit to a specific muscle, nerve, or spinal cord level (Table 4-3).
- Assess proximal lower extremity strength by watching the child rise from a seated position on the floor. A child with proximal lower extremity weakness (eg, muscular dystrophy) will use Gowers sign (Figure 4-3) to rise by walking his hands up his thighs.

Table 4-2. Grading Muscle Strength

Muscle Strength Grades	
Grade 1	Patient has muscle contraction that can be seen or felt but which does not result in movement.
Grade 2	Movements can only be made when the force of gravity is counteracted by changing a patient's position.
Grade 3	Patient can resist gravity but no additional force.
Grade 4	Patient has only some ability to resist the examiner.
Grade 5	Patient has full ability to resist the examiner.

Table 4-3. Reflexes and Motor Function of Specific Spinal Cord Levels

Nerve Root	Motor Function	Reflex	Sensory Distribution
C4			Lateral aspect of lower half of neck
C5	Shoulder abduction (deltoid)	Biceps	Sensation over lateral aspect of shoulder
C6	Elbow flexion (biceps), wrist extension (extensor carpi radialis longus and brevis)	Brachioradialis	Sensation over radial aspect of forearm

Table 4-3. Reflexes and Motor Function of Specific Spinal Cord Levels, continued

Nerve Root	Motor Function	Reflex	Sensory Distribution
C7	Elbow extension (triceps), wrist flexion (flexor carpi radialis)	Triceps	Sensation over digits 2 and 3
C8	Finger flexion (lumbricals of digits 4 and 5)		Sensation over ulnar aspect of forearm, digits 4 and 5
T1	Finger abduction (intraossei)		Sensation over middle of forearm on palmar side
T8–T11		Umbilical reflexes	Periumbilical sensation
L1	Seated hip flexion (iliopsoas)	Cremasteric reflex	Medial aspect of upper thigh, inguinal region
L2	Seated hip flexion (iliopsoas), knee extension, hip adduction	Cremasteric reflex	Medial aspect of middle of thigh
L3	Knee extension, hip adduction		Medial aspect of lower thigh and knee
L4	Ankle dorsiflexion (tibialis anterior)	Patellar	Medial aspect of great toe
L5	Hip abduction (gluteus medius), great toe extension		Lateral aspect of calf
S1	Ankle plantarflexion and eversion	Achilles	Lateral aspect of ankle and foot
S2	Anal wink		Posteromedial thigh and calf
S3–S5	Anal wink		Perianal sensation

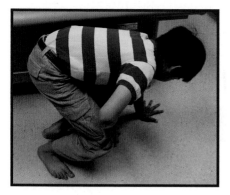

Figure 4-3. Gowers maneuver. Child rises from seated position on the floor by using hands to walk his hands up his thighs, indicating proximal lower extremity weakness as seen in muscular dystrophy.

Muscle Flexibility

- Because bones grow faster than muscles, children often have symmetrical tightness in the lower extremity muscles during growth spurts. This tightness increases traction on growth centers, increasing the risk for some overuse syndromes (see Chapter 29). The most commonly affected muscles are those that cross 2 joints—gastrocnemius (Figure 4-4 a, b), hamstring (Figure 4-5), rectus femoris (Figure 4-6), and tensor fascia lata or iliotibial band (Figure 4-7).

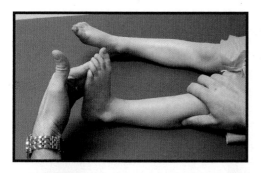

Figure 4-4a. With gastrocnemius tightness or contracture, passive ankle dorsiflexion will be less than 10 degrees while the knee is fully extended.

Figure 4-4b. The degree of ankle dorsiflexion should increase when the knee is flexed; if it does not, the soleus muscle is also tight.

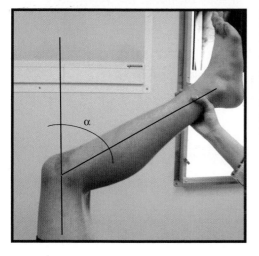

Figure 4-5. Popliteal angle to measure hamstring flexibility. Patient is supine with the contralateral leg flat on the exam table. Hold the ipsilateral hip at 90 degrees and possibly extend the knee to its natural limit. Generally, the complement of the angle formed by the thigh and lower leg is recorded. Popliteal angle (α) greater than 30 degrees indicates hamstring tightness.

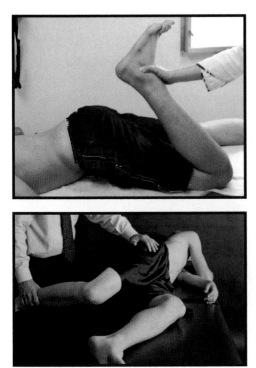

Figure 4-6. Ely test for rectus femoris contracture: with patient prone, passively flex the knee; in the presence of a rectus femoris contracture, the pelvis will rise off the examination table as shown.

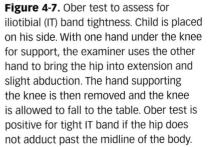

Figure 4-7. Ober test to assess for iliotibial (IT) band tightness. Child is placed on his side. With one hand under the knee for support, the examiner uses the other hand to bring the hip into extension and slight abduction. The hand supporting the knee is then removed and the knee is allowed to fall to the table. Ober test is positive for tight IT band if the hip does not adduct past the midline of the body.

Reflexes

- Each reflex represents a specific level of spinal cord function (Table 4-3).
- Deep tendon reflexes are graded on a 0 to 4 scale (Table 4-4) or characterized as normal, increased, or decreased.
- Children with upper motor neuron pathology often have increased reflexes, while children with lower motor neuron disease tend to have decreased reflexes.
- Superficial reflexes including umbilical, cremasteric, and plantar reflexes may yield information about spinal cord pathology.
- Distraction techniques reduce inhibition so reflexes can be more easily elicited.
  — Ask the child about her interests or activities or ask her to interlock her hands and pull while reflexes are checked (Figure 4-8).
- When neonatal reflexes persist beyond the age when they normally extinguish, suspect a neurodevelopmental problem.

Table 4-4. Grading Reflexes

Grade	Response
Grade 0	No response
Grade 1	Minimal response
Grade 2	Normal response
Grade 3	Slightly hyperactive
Grade 4	Very hyperactive with clonus present

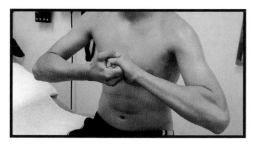

Figure 4-8. Distraction technique to elicit deep tendon reflexes. Ask patient to clasp hands and pull outward.

Sensation

- Older children and adolescents can participate in a thorough sensory examination.
- Sensation to light touch is tested first.
- When a sensory deficit is present, determining which dermatomes or nerve distributions are affected can point to the location of the pathology (nerve distributions) (Table 4-3).
- If the history suggests a neurologic etiology, evaluate vibration and temperature sensation, pain, stereognosis, and two-point discrimination.
- In general, peripheral nerve lesions affect all aspects of sensation while spinal cord lesions affect only some aspects, depending on the spinal cord tracts involved.

Joint-Specific Evaluations

- General examination techniques for specific joints are described in this section.
- Special tests to identify specific injuries and diagnoses are described in corresponding chapters.

SPINE

Inspection

- Inspect the spine from the front, back, and side with the patient standing.
- Note posture, head position, and skin abnormalities.
- A tilted and rotated head position suggests torticollis, which is frequently associated with abnormalities in skull shape (plagiocephaly).
- If torticollis is present, palpate the sternocleidomastoid muscle for a mass.
- Loss of the normal cervical or lumbar lordosis (concave curve) suggests muscle strain and spasm as a primary diagnosis or secondary to a bone, ligament, or disc injury.
- Exaggeration of the normal thoracic kyphosis (convex curve) is seen with Scheuermann disease, a condition in adolescence that involves anterior wedging of 3 consecutive vertebrae, most commonly in the thoracic spine.
- Asymmetric shoulder or hip height may indicate spinal asymmetry or scoliosis, which can be estimated with the Adam forward bending test (Figure 4-9) and a scoliometer.
  — If the *angle of trunk rotation* (ATR) is greater than 5 degrees, radiographs should be obtained to more precisely measure the curvature and identify any vertebral body defects.
- Midline cutaneous lesions, such as vascular lesions, tufts of hair, or sacral dimples, may be associated with underlying spinal dysraphism.

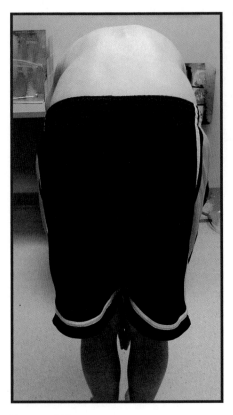

Figure 4-9. Adam forward bending test. Ask patient to put palms together and bend forward. Note any asymmetry. This young man has slight right thoracic prominence. Location of prominence often indicates location of the curve apex. Scoliometer placed at point of maximal asymmetry measures angle of trunk rotation.

Range of Motion

- Evaluate cervical and lumbar motion in flexion, extension, lateral bending, and rotation.

Palpation

- Palpate vertebral spinous processes and paraspinal muscles for tenderness or spasm.
- Palpate the sternocleidomastoid muscles if torticollis is present.
- Palpate the level of the iliac crests to identify a leg-length discrepancy that may be causing a compensatory curve to the spine.

Neurologic Examination

- Evaluate sensory and motor function, including deep tendon reflexes to evaluate spinal cord integrity.

Special Tests

- Pain with the *single leg lumbar hyperextension test* (stork test) (Figure 4-9) suggests spondylolysis (defect of the pars interarticularis).
- Pain due to pathology in the posterior elements of the spinal column (facet joints, pars interarticularis, spinous processes) is typically relieved with flexion and exacerbated by extension. The converse is true for pathology in the anterior elements (vertebral bodies, intervertebral discs).

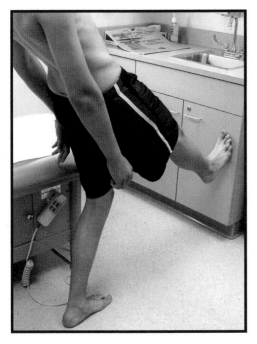

Figure 4-10. Single leg lumbar hyperextension test (stork test): ask patient to stand on one leg and extend at the lumbar spine (examiner can provides some support to hips for balance). If painful, this suggests spondylolysis on the side of the supporting leg.

- Pain that is exacerbated by a *straight leg raise test*, causing radiation of the pain into the leg, suggests radiculopathy, such as from a herniated disc.

SHOULDER

Inspection

- Inspect from front and back.
- Inspect males without a shirt and females in a tank top or halter that allows maximal visualization of shoulders and spine.
- Asymmetric shoulder height can be caused by
  - Spinal curvature
  - Spasm in the upper trapezius muscle that elevates the ipsilateral shoulder
  - Repetitive unilateral overhead activity (eg, baseball, tennis) that leads to stronger rotator cuff muscles on the dominant side, depressing that shoulder
- In patients with Erb palsy, the affected arm will be held in internal rotation and adduction.
- Sprengel deformity is a congenital failure of the scapula to descend; this can result in limited shoulder range of motion and asymmetric appearance of the upper back and neck.
- Patients with long thoracic nerve palsy exhibit winging of the scapula on the affected side, which can be elicited by having the patient perform a push-up against a wall (Figure 4-11).
- In patients with a shoulder dislocation, the acromion will be especially prominent.

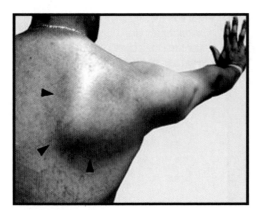

Figure 4-11. A long thoracic palsy causing scapular winging when the arm is protracted.

Range of Motion

- Evaluate for symmetry of motion with Apley scratch tests (Figure 4-12 a, b).
- Athletes in sports that involve repetitive overhead motion (eg, baseball pitchers) usually develop more external rotation and less internal rotation in the dominant arm compared with the nondominant arm.

Palpation

- May be easiest to perform while standing behind the patient.
- The PMT may suggest the diagnosis (Figure 4-13).

Strength

- Evaluate for symmetry of strength of the rotator cuff muscles (Figure 4-14).

Special Tests

- Glenohumeral joint laxity is evaluated with the *load and shift test, sulcus sign, apprehension test,* and *relocation test* (figures 4-15–4-18).
- Patients with multidirectional instability may be able to voluntarily sublux or dislocate their shoulders.
- A positive *impingement test* suggests rotator cuff tendinopathy, which is uncommon in children but may occur in adolescent athletes.
  — Impingement tests reproduce the pain of rotator cuff tendonitis and subacromial bursitis by passively moving the shoulder into positions that pinch the rotator cuff tendons and bursa between the acromion and humeral head (Figure 4-19).

ELBOW, FOREARM, WRIST, AND HAND

Inspection

- The normal *carrying angle* of the elbow is 5 to 15 degrees of valgus angulation (Figure 4-20).
- Malunion of a supracondylar humerus fracture may lead to a varus angulation of the elbow, also called a *gunstock deformity* (Figure 4-21).

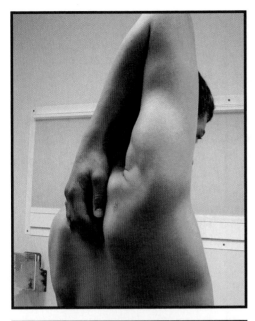

Figure 4-12a. Superior Apley scratch test to assess shoulder external rotation and abduction, measured by the spinal level reached with the tip of the middle finger and compared to uninjured arm.

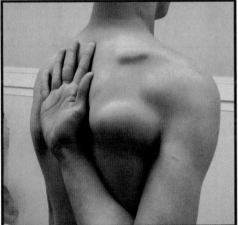

Figure 4-12b. Inferior Apley scratch test to assess shoulder internal rotation and adduction, measured by the spinal level reached with the tip of the middle finger compared to uninjured arm.

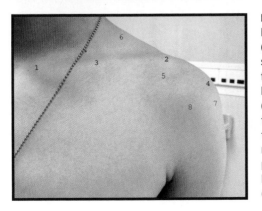

Figure 4-13. Anterior shoulder palpation landmarks. (1) Sternoclavicular joint; (2) Acromioclavicular joint: shoulder separation (AC joint sprain); (3) Clavicle: fracture; (4) Supraspinatus insertion onto humeral head: supraspinatus tendonitis; (5) Subacromial space: impingement due to subacromial bursitis or rotator cuff tendonitis; (6) Upper trapezius: trapezius muscle strain/spasm; (7) Proximal humeral physis: Salter-Harris I fracture proximal humerus ("Little League shoulder"); (8) Bicipetal groove: biceps tendonitis.

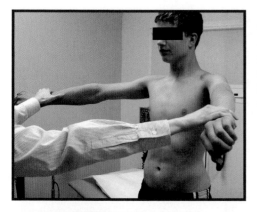

Figure 4-14. Jobe test ("empty can" test) for supraspinatus pathology. Shoulders are internally rotated with thumbs pointing down and abducted to 90 degrees as shown. Inabilty to resist downward pressure indicates weakness. Pain suggests tendinitis.

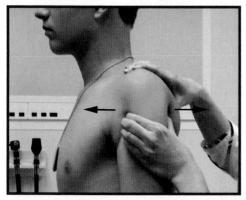

Figure 4-15. Load and shift test: while stabilizinge the scapula with one hand, use the other hand to shift the humeral head anteriorly then posteriorly. Grade degree of translation in each direction on a scale of 1–3: (1) minimal translation; (2) moderate translation to edge of glenoid; (3) translation past glenoid rim (dislocated).

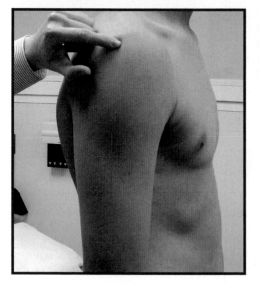

Figure 4-16. Sulcus sign. Pull forearm downward while stabilizing the clavicle and acromion; if a gap or depression appears below the acromion, sulcus sign is positive, indicating inferior shoulder laxity.

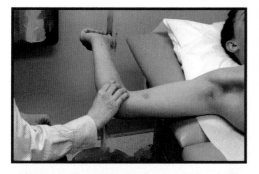

Figure 4-17. Shoulder apprehension test. With passive external rotation of the shoulder in 90 degrees of abduction, patients with anterior shoulder instability will report apprehension that the shoulder will dislocate.

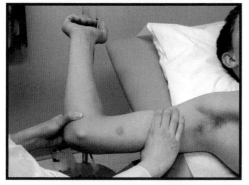

Figure 4-18. Relocation test. Following a positive apprehension test, posterior pressure on the upper arm alleviates the sensation that the shoulder is about to dislocate, indicating positive relocation test.

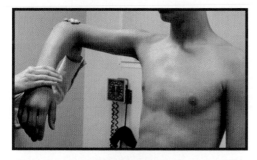

Figure 4-19. Hawkins impingement test. Pain with passive internal rotation of the shoulder with the shoulder and elbow in 90 degrees of flexion is positive, indicating impingement due to rotator cuff tendonitis or subacromial bursitis.

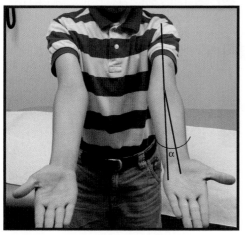

Figure 4-20. Elbow carrying angle (α).

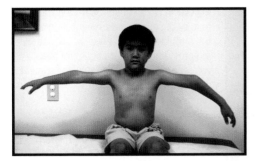

Figure 4-21. Cubitus varus ("gunstock deformity") of left elbow; sequela of malunion of supracondylar humerus fracture.

Range of Motion

- Range of motion examination for the elbow includes flexion, extension, pronation, and supination.
- Children with elbow injuries almost always have some loss of motion.
- An efficient way to test motor function of the forearm is to have the child make a thumbs-up sign and an OK sign. These motions test the radial nerve (wrist and thumb extension), median nerve (flexion of digits), ulnar nerve (digits 3, 4, and 5 abduction), and anterior interosseous nerve (digits 1 and 2 flexion).

Palpation

- The PMT often suggests the diagnosis (Figure 4-22a, b).

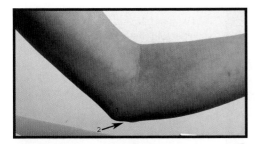

Figure 4-22a. Medial elbow palpation landmarks. (1) Medial epicondyle: "Little League elbow" (medial epicondyle apophysitis); (2) olecranon: olecranon apophysitis can be seen in weight lifters.

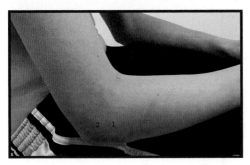

Figure 4-22b. Lateral elbow palpation landmarks. (1) Capitellum: Panner disease or osteochondritis dissecans; (2) lateral epicondyle: "tennis elbow" (lateral epicondylitis).

HIPS/PELVIS

Inspection

- In infants, examination of the hip should include inspection of the subgluteal creases for symmetry as well as the levels of the knees with the patient supine and the knees and hips flexed to 90 degrees. A difference in the heights of the knees is a positive Galeazzi sign (Figure 4-23) and suggests a true or functional (eg, hip dislocation) difference in femur lengths.

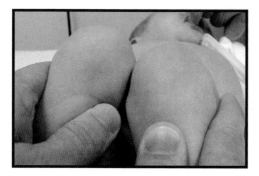

Figure 4-23. Galeazzi sign. Infants with a hip dislocation will have apparent femur shortening on the affected side.

Range of Motion

- Hip joint pathology frequently causes a loss of internal rotation and abduction.
- To prevent measurement errors, the hip range of motion examination should be performed with one hand used to stabilize the pelvis.

Special Tests

- *Barlow and Ortolani maneuvers* are used to screen for hip dislocation in infants (see Chapter 18).
- In an older child, the *Trendelenburg test* can be performed to assess for hip abductor muscle weakness (Figure 4-24).
- Tests for sacroiliac pathology include Patrick test (also called flexion, abduction, and external rotation [FABER] test) (Figure 4-25).

KNEE

Inspection

- Note patellar position. Figure 4-26 has an illustration of normal knee anatomy.
  - Patella alta, anatomic upward positioning of the patella, may increase the risk for patellofemoral pain, Osgood-Schlatter disease, Sinding-Larsen-Johanssen syndrome, and patellar tendonitis.
  - Squinting (kissing) patellae (Figure 4-27) are frequently seen with femoral anteversion.
  - Bipartite patella is seen in at least 1% of the population. The smaller piece is almost always in the superior lateral quadrant. It can become painful after a direct blow or repetitive overuse.

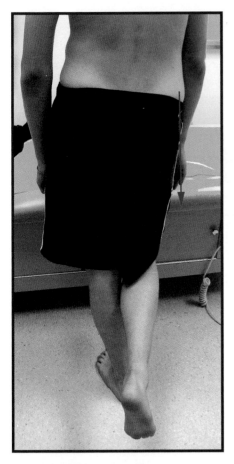

Figure 4-24. Trendelenberg test for hip abductor weakness. Ask patient to stand on one leg while observing from behind. If the iliac crest of the elevated leg drops, this indicates the hip abductors (primarily gluteus medius) of the standing leg are weak.

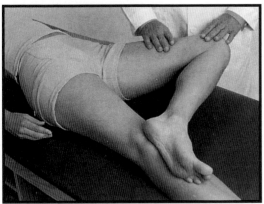

Figure 4-25. Patrick or FABER test for sacroiliac pathology. Pain in area of sacroiliac is a postive test.

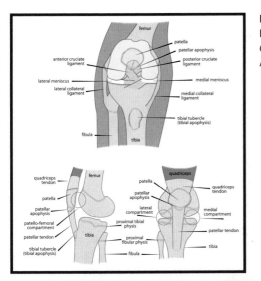

Figure 4-26. Normal knee anatomy. From Metzel JD. *Sports Medicine in the Pediatric Office.* Elk Grove Village, IL: American Academy of Pediatrics; 2008.

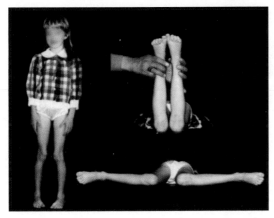

Figure 4-27. Young girl with femoral anteversion. Note squinting (kissing) patellae and severe femoral torsion. From Staheli LT. *Practice of Pediatric Orthopedics.* Philadelphia, PA: Lippincott Williams & Wilkins; 2001. Reprinted by permission.

Palpation

- To detect a small effusion, the examiner can attempt to "milk" the fluid to the inferomedial or inferolateral aspect of the knee and push it to the opposite side to determine if a visible fluid wave is present. For extra-articular swelling, such as with a prepatellar or infrapatellar bursitis, there will be no fluid wave.
- The PMT will often suggest the diagnosis (Figure 4-28 a, b, c).

Special Tests

- The *Lachman test, posterior drawer test,* and *valgus and varus stress tests* should be performed if a ligamentous injury is suspected (figures 4-29–4-32).
- The *McMurray test* and *Apley compression test* are used to detect meniscal injury (figures 4-33, 4-34).
- Patients with recent or recurrent patellar dislocation will have excessive patellar mobility and may also have a positive *patellar apprehension test* (Figure 4-35).

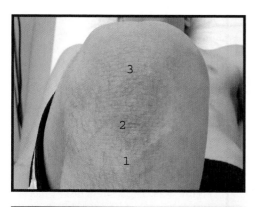

Figure 4-28a. Anterior knee palpation landmarks: (1) Tibial tubercle: Osgood-Schlatter disease; (2) Patellar tendon: patellar tendonitis; (3) Inferior pole of patella: Sindig-Larsen-Johanssen disease.

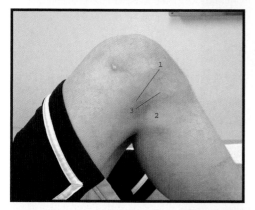

Figure 4-28b. Medial knee palpation landmarks: (1) Medial joint line: medial meniscus injury; (2) medial collateral ligament (MCL): MCL sprain.

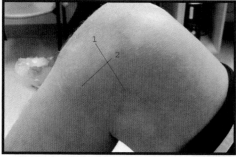

Figure 4-28c. Lateral knee palpation landmarks: (1) Lateral joint line: meniscus injury or discoid meniscus; (2) Head of fibula: fracture; (3) Iliotibial band: iliotibial band friction syndrome.

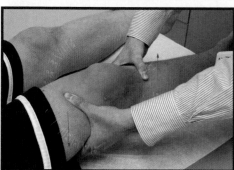

Figure 4-29. Lachman test for anterior cruciate ligament (ACL) injury. With the knee in 20 degrees of flexion, stabilize the thigh with one hand and use the other hand to briskly pull the lower leg anteriorly. Increased movement compared with the uninjured knee or lack of a firm endpoint indicate ACL injury.

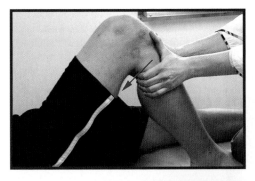

Figure 4-30. Posterior drawer test for posterior cruciate ligament (PCL) injury. With patient supine and knee flexed 90 degrees, stabilize the foot as shown and use both hands to push posteriorly on the proximal tibia. Increased posterior translation compared with the uninjured knee indicates PCL injury.

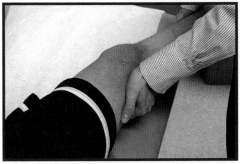

Figure 4-31. Valgus stress test for medial collateral ligament (MCL) injury. With the knee in 30 degrees of flexion, stabilize lower leg with one hand and use heel of other hand to apply valgus stress. Laxity or lack of firm endpoint compared with uninjured knee indicates MCL injury.

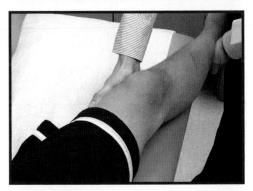

Figure 4-32. Varus stress test for lateral collateral ligament (LCL) injury. With the knee in 30 degrees of flexion, stabilize lower leg with one hand and use heel of other hand to apply varus stress. Laxity or lack of firm endpoint compared with uninjured knee indicates LCL injury.

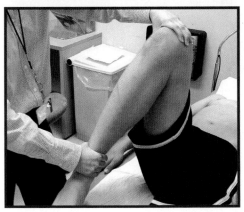

Figure 4-33. McMurray test for meniscus injury. With thumb on one joint line and finger on the other, use other hand to flex the knee while rotating the tibia. A painful click at either joint line is considered a positive test suggesting meniscus injury.

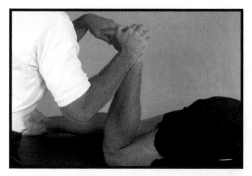

Figure 4-34. Apley compression test for meniscus injury. Apply downward pressure on heel and twist lower leg to load meniscus. Pain indicates a positive test. Available at: www.mhhe.com/hper/physed/athletictraining/illustrations/ch20/20-25.jpg. Reprinted by permission of The McGraw-Hill Companies, Inc.

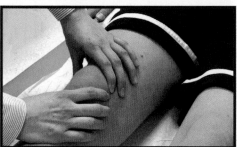

Figure 4-35. Patellar apprehension test. Gently move patella medially and laterally. More than 1 cm of motion in either direction is considered excessive mobility. Patients with a history of patellar subluxation/dislocation will often report apprehension that patella will dislocate with lateral movement. This is a positive patellar apprehension test.

FOOT AND ANKLE

Inspection

- Calluses in unusual locations may be caused by abnormalities of foot position and gait.
- Pes cavus, or high arch, can be caused by central or peripheral nerve disorders and should prompt neurologic evaluation.
- Pes planus (flatfoot deformity) is usually flexible (Figure 4-36a), and may be associated with hindfoot valgus (subtalar joint pronation) (Figure 4-36b).
- A flexible flatfoot, unlike a rigid flatfoot, regains an arch when the patient is non–weight-bearing, standing on his toes, or performing active great toe extension (Jack test) (Figure 4-37).
- A rigid flatfoot should raise suspicion for tarsal coalition.

Range of Motion

- Ankle dorsiflexion and plantarflexion are be measured with the knee in extension and flexion, keeping the subtalar joint in a neutral position and the forefoot slightly supinated.
- Subtalar joint range of motion is assessed by examining eversion and inversion of the ankle.

Palpation

- The PMT often suggests the diagnosis (Figure 4-38 a, b).

Special Tests

- The *anterior drawer test* assesses the integrity of the anterior talofibular ligament, the most commonly sprained ligament in the ankle (Figure 4-39).

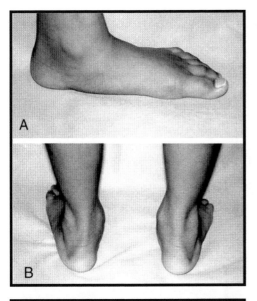

Figure 4-36. Flatfoot, medial (A) and posterior (B) views with hindfoot valgus. Reproduced with permission from Griffin LY (ed): *Essentials of Musculoskeletal Care,* 3rd edition. Rosemont, IL: American Acadmey of Orthopaedic Surgeons; 2005.

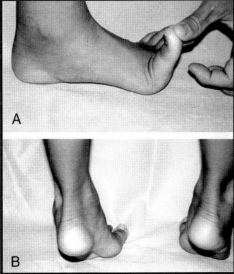

Figure 4-37. Elevation of the arches in flexible flatfeet by Jack toe extension test (A) and standing on toes (B). Reproduced with permission from Griffin LY (ed): *Essentials of Musculoskeletal Care,* 3rd edition. Rosemont, IL: American Acadmey of Orthopaedic Surgeons; 2005.

Lower Extremity Rotation and Alignment

- The first step in evaluating a child's lower extremity rotation is observation of the foot progression angle (FPA) when walking (see "Gait Evaluation" on page 55).
- In-toeing (internal FPA) can be caused by (1) metatarsus adductus, a congenital deformity of the forefoot due to in utero positioning; (2) internal tibial torsion; or (3) femoral anteversion, 2 common variants of normal anatomy.
  — Tibial torsion is assessed by measuring the thigh-foot angle.
  — Hip internal rotation significantly greater than external rotation suggests femoral anteversion (see Figure 4-27).

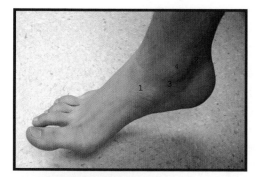

Figure 4-38a. Medial ankle palpation landmarks: (1) Navicular: irritation of accessory navicular bone or navicalar stress fracture; (2) Posterior tibialis tendon: tendonitis common in dancers; (3) Deltoid ligament: medial ankle sprain; (4) Distal tibial physis: Salter-Harris fracture.

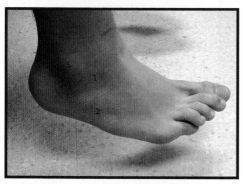

Figure 4-38b. Lateral ankle palpation landmarks: (1) anterior talofibular ligament: ankle sprain; (2) Base of fifth metatarsal: Iselin syndrome or avulsion fracture; (3) Calcaneus/achilles tendon insertion: Sever disease; (4) calcaneofibular ligament: ankle sprain; (5) Distal fibular physis: Salter-Harris fracture.

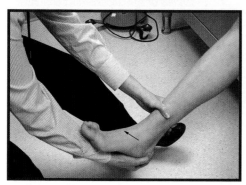

Figure 4-39. Anterior drawer test for anterior talofibular ligament (ATFL) injury. With patient seated with knee flexed and ankle relaxed in about 10 degrees of plantarflexion, stabilize the lower leg with the one hand and use the other hand to cup the heel and pull it briskly anteriorly. More anterior displacement or lack of firm endpoint compared with the uninjured ankle indicates injury to the ATFL.

- Angular deformities should be evaluated with the child standing and patellae pointing straight ahead.
  — Infants and toddlers generally have some degree of genu varum (Figure 4-40) that progresses to accentuated valgus at about 4 years of age, then gradually regresses to the normal adult range of about 5 degrees of valgus by the age of 6 or 7 years.
- Pelvic obliquity indicates a leg-length discrepancy.
  — A functional leg-length discrepancy can result from scoliosis, hip muscle contractures, and pelvic abnormalities. These patients will have asymmetric measurements from the umbilicus to the medial malleolus (Figure 4-41a, b) of each ankle, but equal tibia and femur lengths.

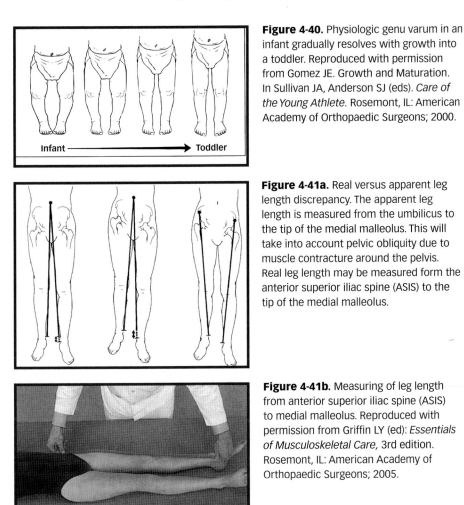

Figure 4-40. Physiologic genu varum in an infant gradually resolves with growth into a toddler. Reproduced with permission from Gomez JE. Growth and Maturation. In Sullivan JA, Anderson SJ (eds). *Care of the Young Athlete.* Rosemont, IL: American Academy of Orthopaedic Surgeons; 2000.

Infant ⟶ Toddler

Figure 4-41a. Real versus apparent leg length discrepancy. The apparent leg length is measured from the umbilicus to the tip of the medial malleolus. This will take into account pelvic obliquity due to muscle contracture around the pelvis. Real leg length may be measured form the anterior superior iliac spine (ASIS) to the tip of the medial malleolus.

Figure 4-41b. Measuring of leg length from anterior superior iliac spine (ASIS) to medial malleolus. Reproduced with permission from Griffin LY (ed): *Essentials of Musculoskeletal Care,* 3rd edition. Rosemont, IL: American Academy of Orthopaedic Surgeons; 2005.

— A true leg-length discrepancy results from asymmetric growth of the tibia or femur. This can be congenital or acquired (eg, growth disturbance caused by previous growth plate fracture), and is suggested by unequal femur or tibia lengths in the hook-lying position. Radiographs (standing anteroposterior view of lower extremities) confirm the diagnosis.

Gait Evaluation

- Visual assessment of a child's walking pattern is an integral part of the pediatric physical examination that may provide clues to the underlying diagnosis.
- Parental concern about how a child walks or runs is a common presenting complaint in the pediatric clinic.
- An acute change in gait pattern may indicate a significant musculoskeletal condition requiring urgent treatment.

NORMAL GAIT (TABLE 4-5)

- Cyclic, reciprocal, heel-toe, and energy efficient
- Requires proper functioning and coordination of the musculoskeletal and nervous systems.
- The gait cycle is divided into 2 phases (Figure 4-42).
  — *Stance phase* begins at heel strike and ends with toe-off.
    ▪ Constitutes 63% of the cycle.
  — *Swing phase* begins at toe-off and ends with heel strike.
    ▪ Constitutes 37% of the gait cycle.
- Criteria for an effective and efficient gait
  — Stability of the limb during stance phase
  — Clearance of the limb during swing phase
  — Energy conservation
- Abnormal gait patterns are listed in Table 4-6.

Table 4-5. Observations of a Normal Gait

Body Segment	Normal Position and Movement
Ankle in the sagittal plane[a]	Heel strike at initial contact Flat foot in midstance Heel rise occurs just before the opposite swing limb contacting the floor.
Knee in the sagittal plane	Extended at initial contact A small flexion wave during loading response A large flexion wave during swing phase
Hip	Fully flexed at the beginning of stance phase and fully extended at the end of stance phase
Pelvis	Should exhibit minimal dynamic deviations in all planes.
Trunk	Should be stable throughout the gait cycle.
Upper extremities	Should exhibit a reciprocal swinging pattern that is out of phase with the ipsilateral lower extremity.

[a]Foot-progression angle and hindfoot alignment are observed in the coronal plane. Foot-progression angle is the degree of in-toeing or out-toeing. The normal range for young children is from -5 to 15 to 20 degrees; average is 5 to 10 degrees. Hindfoot alignment is the degree of subtalar pronation or supination.

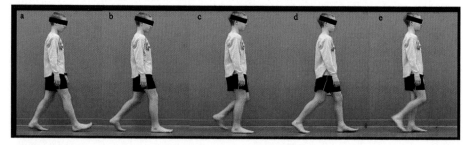

Figure 4-42. (a) Stance phase begins when the heel (right leg) hits the floor (heel strike). (b) During loading response, the stance foot is flat and the knee slightly flexed. (c) At midstance, the opposite limb is in swing phase. (d) Heel rise occurs at the end of stance phase while the opposite swing limb contacts the floor and begins heel strike. (e) In mid-swing, the knee is flexed to promote clearance while the opposite limb is in stance phase.

Table 4-6. Common Abnormal Gait Patterns

Gait	Pattern and Causes	Associated Conditions
Antalgic gait	Limping because of pain in the lower extremity or back Characterized by shortened stance phase duration on the affected limb When caused by back pain, the gait is not asymmetrical, but rather slow and cautious with short steps to avoid jarring the back.	Most commonly, trauma or infection Physical examination should focus on inspection, palpation, and range of motion testing, which can usually localize the pain source.
Trendelenburg gait (abductor lurch)	Results from weak hip abductors. Hip abductors are responsible for maintaining a level pelvis during single limb stance. Weakness causes the unsupported (contralateral) hip to drop during single limb stance (positive Trendelenburg sign). To compensate, body weight is shifted over the weak hip during stance phase to lateralize the center of gravity (lurch).	Commonly seen in hip disorders or neuromuscular disease (eg, Legg-Calve-Perthes disease, developmental hip dysplasia, congenital coxa vara, slipped capital femoral epiphysis).
Circumduction gait	During swing phase, the longer limb circumducts (swings around and to the side) to clear the ground and move forward. May be accompanied by vaulting of the short extremity, which involves early heel rise during stance phase to assist with clearance of the long side in swing phase.	Most commonly results from a structural or functional limb-length inequality, but may also be seen as a pain avoidance pattern (ie, foot pain).
Steppage gait	Increased hip and knee flexion during swing phase to help promote adequate clearance of the foot and ankle	May be seen with limb-length inequality or weakness of the ankle dorsiflexors.
Equinus gait (toe walking)	Initial contact occurs at forefoot instead of heel. Caused by heel cord contracture or muscle imbalance about the ankle.	Commonly seen in cerebral palsy, clubfoot deformity, and idiopathic heel cord contracture
Stiff knee gait	Characterized by diminished and delayed peak knee flexion during swing phase, which inhibits toe clearance, causing patients to trip or adopt energy-inefficient compensatory movements. Commonly caused by inappropriate overactivity of the quadriceps or rectus femoris muscle	Seen in patients with cerebral palsy who have quadriceps spasticity and contracture May also be an antalgic pattern in patients with knee pain.
Scissoring gait	Excessive hip adduction in swing phase causes knees and thighs to hit or cross.	Seen in patients with cerebral palsy who have spasticity and contracture of hip adductors
Crouch gait	Increased knee flexion and ankle dorsiflexion during stance phase Causes include weak ankle plantar flexors, hamstring spasticity and contracture.	Overzealous surgical lengthening of the Achilles tendon in children with cerebral palsy

HOW NORMAL GAIT CHANGES WITH DEVELOPMENT

- Twelve to 18 months of age (or first few months of walking)
  — Wide base of support
  — Reduced duration of single limb stance
  — Higher step frequency
  — Lack of reciprocal arm swing
  — Arms are held in the "high-guard" position to facilitate balance and provide protection during frequent falls.
  — Hips may be externally rotated.
  — Knees tend to remain flexed.
  — Ankles have plantarflexion at initial contact in some children exhibiting plantarflexion (toe-strike) throughout the gait cycle.
  — Mild genu varum and in-toeing is normal in the first few months of walking.
  — Neutral knee alignment is usually acquired by 18 months of age.
- Typically by age 2 years, the early deviations minimize.
  — Base of support narrows but remains wider than seen with a mature gait pattern.
  — Hips have less external rotation.
  — Eighty percent exhibit normal reciprocal arm swing.
- Mature gait pattern is established by 3 to 7 years of age.
  — Narrow base of support
  — Smooth movements with minimal oscillations of the center of gravity
  — Reciprocal arm swing
  — By age 3 years, increased genu valgum develops followed by resolution to the normal 5 to 10 degrees of knee valgus by age 5 years.

OBSERVATION OF GAIT

- The child should be dressed in the least amount of clothing.
- Observe the child walk in a long hallway in the coronal (ie, walking toward and away from the observer) and sagittal (ie, walking past the observer in both directions) planes.
- Global assessment should focus on speed, stability, balance, and symmetry.
- The 6-point gait examination quick check
  — Regular walking
  — Walking on the toes
  — Walking on the heels
  — Running
  — Tandem walking
  — Rising from seated position on the floor to assess for Gowers sign

QUANTITATIVE GAIT ANALYSIS

- With specialized computer software, cameras, reflective markers, in-floor force plates, dynamic electromyograms, and pedobarographs, movement can be analyzed in multiple planes, while muscle firing patterns, ground reaction forces, and oxygen consumption are recorded simultaneously.
- Important research tool
- May be used for surgical planning and assessment of surgical interventions.

CHAPTER 5

Musculoskeletal Imaging Studies

- Imaging studies are sometimes necessary in the diagnosis and management of musculo-skeletal injuries and conditions.
- Because most imaging studies involve exposure to radiation, time, and financial expense, they are used only when essential in making a diagnosis or determining proper treatment.
- Consult with a radiologist or orthopaedic specialist if there is uncertainty as to which study or views are appropriate.
- Box 5-1 lists strategies for minimizing radiation exposure.

Effective Radiation Doses

- Absorption of radiation by the tissues depends on the technology employed, technique used, and density of the tissues imaged (Table 5-1).
  — Because computed tomography (CT) includes a large number of images, it exposes the patient to significantly higher effective radiation doses compared with plain radiographs; CT scans with narrower cuts and higher resolution result in even greater radiation exposure.
  — Because of differences in tissue properties, radiographs of the extremities are associated with a lower effective radiation dose than radiographs of the torso.

Box 5-1. Strategies for Minimizing Radiation Exposure

Order imaging studies only when the information is likely to affect patient management.

Whenever possible, try to use imaging modalities that do not involve radiation exposure.

Communicate with the radiologist to make certain the most appropriate imaging study is performed.

Shield the gonads at all times except for the initial pelvic image.

Request that parents obtain copies of outside films to avoid duplicating examinations and advise them to carry these to the appointment with the orthopaedic consultant.

Limit follow-up images.

Avoid routinely ordering comparison views of the opposite limb.

Table 5-1. Effective Radiation Doses

Examination	Effective Dose (mSv)	Equivalent Number of Chest Radiographs	Equivalent Dose of Natural Background Radiation
Background radiation	3.0	150	—
Transatlantic airline flight (New York to London)	3.6	180	1 y, 85 d
Skull radiograph	0.07	3.5	9 d
2-view chest radiograph	0.02	—	3 d
Abdomen radiograph	1.0	50	125 d
Pelvic radiograph	0.7	35	86 d
Barium swallow	1.5	75	188 d
Barium enema	7	350	2 y, 145 d
Head CT	2	100	250 d
Chest CT (pediatric parameters)	Up to 3	150	1 y, 10 d
Chest CT (adult parameters)	8	400	2 y, 270 d
Abdomen/pelvis CT (pediatric parameters)	Up to 5	250	1 y, 260 d
Abdomen/pelvis CT (adult parameters)	15 to 20	750 to 1,000	5.1 to 6.8 y
Radionuclide renal scan (99m-Tc)	1	50	125 d
Radionuclide bone scan (99m-Tc)	4	200	1 y, 135 d

CT, computed tomography.
From Donaldson JS. Radiology. *Pediatr Ann.* 2008;37:370–371. Reprinted by permission of Slack, Inc.

Radiography

- When evaluating for bone injury or pathology, plain radiographs are always performed before considering advanced imaging studies.
- It is the physician's responsibility to ensure the most appropriate views are ordered.
  - The number and type of views recommended depends on the anatomic location and suspected diagnosis (Table 5-2). Generally, at least 2 views are recommended, but in some cases a single radiograph may suffice (eg, anteroposterior pelvis to evaluate for hip dysplasia).
  - The area of interest (point of maximal tenderness) should be in the center of the film, as x-ray beams are most concentrated at the center. Images at the edge are often less focused.
  - When evaluating a growth plate, comparison views of the uninjured limb are sometimes helpful.

Table 5-2. Common Radiograph Views

	Standard Views[a]	Common Special Views
Shoulder	AP in ER AP in IR Axillary view (best true lateral view of shoulder to assess humeral head location in glenoid) Scapular Y view (another lateral view to assess humeral head position in patients who cannot abduct the arm for axillary view)	Clavicle view Scapular outlet view to assess subacromial space and supraspinatus outlet for bony causes of impingement Stryker notch view to assess for Hill-Sachs lesion after a dislocation
Elbow	AP, lateral	Radial head Oblique views: (1) Medial rotation to assess medial condyle; (2) Lateral rotation to assess lateral condyle
Hand/wrist	AP, lateral 45° PA oblique	AP view in ulnar deviation to assess scaphoid
Hips/pelvis	AP and frog pelvis	Cross table lateral if patient cannot abduct hips for frog view Judet views to assess for acetabular fractures
Knee	AP, lateral Tunnel view (AP weight-bearing with knees flexed to 30°) to assess for osteochondritis dissecans Merchant or sunrise views to assess patellofemoral joint	Oblique views if articular cartilage fractures are suspected
Ankle	AP, lateral Mortise (AP with 15° of internal rotation)	Stress views to assess ligamentous instability:(1) AP talar tilt view; (2) Anterior drawer stress view Broden views: non–weight-bearing view to assess subtalar joint
Foot	AP, lateral 45° oblique	Harris view to evaluate calcaneus
Spine	AP, lateral	Scoliosis AP/lateral Spot lateral to follow spondylolisthesis Obliques to assess for spondylolysis/spondylolisthesis
Cervical spine		Open-mouth odontoid view to assess C1–C2 Flexion/extension views to evaluate for instability due to ligamentous injury Oblique views to evaluate for foraminal narrowing Swimmer view to assess lower cervical spine Lateral view of skull to assess patients with torticollis for craniosynostosis

AP, anteroposterior; ER, external rotation; IR, internal rotation; PA, posteroanterior.
[a]Anteroposterior and lateral projections are part of standard views. For anteroposterior views, the x-ray beam passes through the body part from anterior to posterior. For posteroanterior views, the x-ray beam passes from posterior to anterior.

- A systematic approach should be applied when reading films to avoid errors.
  — Examine the soft tissues and the outer edge of the film first before focusing on the area of concern.
  — Correlate radiographic findings with the history and physical examination findings. For example, accessory ossicles in the foot and ankle are common variants of ossification that can be mistaken for fractures.
- Specific radiographic studies
  — A *bone age* film is a plain radiograph consisting of a single posteroanterior projection view of the left hand and wrist that is compared to an atlas of standards to estimate a child's skeletal maturity.
  — Rotational and angular deformities of the lower extremities are evaluated using transient visual obscuration (lowers view) (Figure 5-1).
  — A *scanogram* is a single anteroposterior radiograph that includes the hips, knees, and ankles, with a radiopaque ruler between the extremities for direct measurement of bone length (Figure 5-2).
  — *Scoliosis films* consist of 2 images of the entire spine from the cervical vertebrae to the sacral spines, a posteroanterior projection view (which minimizes radiation exposure to the thyroid and breast) to evaluate coronal alignment, and a lateral view to evaluate sagittal alignment.
- Advantages of plain radiographs
  — Usually easiest of all imaging modalities to obtain
  — Require the least amount of time and expense.
  — Least likely of all the imaging studies to be misread
  — Good sensitivity for bony abnormalities
- Disadvantages of plain radiographs
  — Low sensitivity for soft tissue abnormalities—radiolucent tissues, such as fat- and air-filled structures, allow x-rays to pass through to varying degrees, but seldom with enough variation to differentiate between these tissues.

Computed Tomography

- With conventional CT, an x-ray tube rotates around the patient as she is moved every few seconds through an opening in the scanner.
- Provides the most detailed view of bony architecture because of multiple "slices" or "cuts" in each of 3 planes—sagittal, coronal, and axial (Figure 5-3).
- Because there are many different CT protocols, it is prudent to consult a radiologist prior to ordering a CT scan for a musculoskeletal problem.
- Advantages of CT
  — Can identify subtle fractures.
  — Can examine complicated fractures in further detail, which has been enhanced by the development of 3-D reconstructions.
  — Excellent modality for evaluating bony lesions, such as fibrous dysplasia

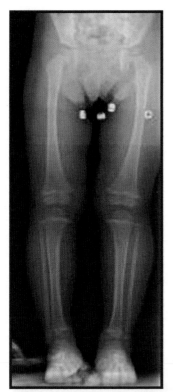

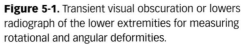

Figure 5-1. Transient visual obscuration or lowers radiograph of the lower extremities for measuring rotational and angular deformities.

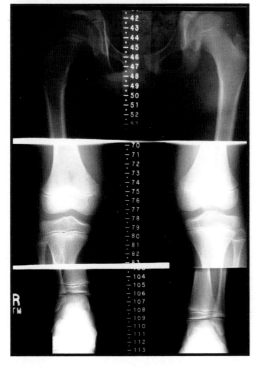

Figure 5-2. Scanogram. Anteroposterior radiographs of the hips, knees, and ankles taken on the same cassette with a radiopaque ruler included to measure differences in leg length.

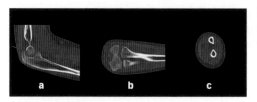

Figure 5-3. Computed tomography scan: sagittal (a), coronal (b), and axial views (c) of the left forearm/elbow.

- Disadvantages of CT
  — Effective radiation doses are generally higher for CT than for plain radiographs.
  — Radiation dose depends on the anatomic location being studied, number of cuts, and type of technology being used.
  — More expensive than plain radiographs
  — May be inaccessible in some locales.
  — Potential need for sedation

Magnetic Resonance Imaging

- Like CT, magnetic resonance imaging (MRI) yields images in 3 planes.
- Procedure
  — When the patient is placed in the magnetic field, the protons in the tissues align themselves parallel to the field. A radio frequency pulse is delivered, which causes the protons to change direction and then relax and realign parallel to the magnetic field. During realignment, there is a radio frequency emission that is picked up by the scanner. The rate at which the protons relax is specific to different types of tissue and can be analyzed by the computer.
  — On *T1-weighted images*, fat has high signal intensity and shows up bright white. T1-weighted images are helpful for delineating anatomy.
  — On *T2-weighted images*, fluid appears bright white, highlighting inflammation, tumors, and infections.
  — *Fat suppression* is a generic term for a variety of techniques that improve contrast and decrease artifact from the high signal intensity of adipose tissue (Figure 5-4).
  — *Intravenous gadolinium* is the most commonly used contrast for MRI scans; contrast enhances the appearance of lesions with increased blood flow such as infections, tumors, and vascular malformations.
  — Gadolinium can also be injected directly into the joint to obtain a *magnetic resonance arthrogram*, useful for identifying articular surface lesions and hip and shoulder labral injuries.

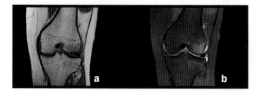

Figure 5-4. Magnetic resonance imaging scan: T1 image (a) and T2 image with fat suppression (b) of the knee. T2 image shows edema at the lateral femoral condyle, indicative of a bone bruise or fracture.

— Because of the many factors to consider when determining the most appropriate magnetic resonance protocol, consultation with a radiologist or orthopaedic specialist is recommended before ordering an MRI study.

- Advantages of MRI
  — Excellent soft tissue resolution
  — Can identify tumors, infection, avascular necrosis, and cartilage, ligament and tendon, and growth plate pathology.
  — No exposure to radiation
- Disadvantages of MRI
  — Provides poor imaging of bone.
  — Potential for "over-reading"
    - Interpretation in children can be difficult because of limited experience and difficulty distinguishing pathology from normal variants.
  — Sedation is often required for young children due to the length of most scans.
  — Some patients may feel claustrophobic inside the scanner.
  — The noise generated by the scanner may be unsettling.
  — Because a strong magnetic field is applied, patients with certain types of metal implants or foreign bodies cannot safely have magnetic resonance scans performed.
  — Generally more expensive than other imaging modalities
  — Access may be limited in many locales.

Ultrasonography

- Ultrasonography is a safe, painless, and relatively inexpensive method of obtaining anatomic images in multiple planes.
- Prenatal ultrasound is increasingly being used for identifying musculoskeletal abnormalities, such as clubfoot, allowing for early parental education and preparation.
- Procedure
  — A technician or radiologist moves a transducer, which emits sound waves that are refracted back at different levels depending on the type of tissue encountered. A computer interprets the deflected sound waves and constructs an image.
- Advantages of ultrasonography
  — Delineates muscle, tendon, and ligament architecture well.
  — Excellent tool for evaluating hip and spine pathology in infants, especially developmental dysplasia of the hip
  — Dynamic studies can be obtained while an examiner manipulates the hips.
  — Can identify hip effusion and guide aspiration in older children.
  — Optimal study for evaluating cystic structures and vascular anomalies, as blood flow can be assessed simultaneously with Doppler
  — Localization of abscesses, effusions, and foreign bodies
  — Well-tolerated by children
  — Parents can stay with their children during the study.
  — Usually less expensive than magnetic resonance and CT

- Disadvantages of ultrasonography
  - Air-filled structures can distort ultrasonography pictures and the sound waves cannot effectively penetrate through dense tissues (bone or large amounts of adipose tissue).
  - Quality is very operator-dependent. Smaller medical centers may lack highly skilled personnel and appropriate equipment, limiting the availability of high-quality ultrasound studies.

Nuclear Medicine

- Nuclear medicine studies provide information about the metabolic activity of various tissues.
- Procedure
  - The patient receives an intravenous injection of a radioactive-labeled isotope (radionuclide).
  - The isotope is taken up by the tissue being studied and emits gamma rays, which are measured by a special camera.
  - Several isotopes are available, each with an affinity for a specific tissue.
  - Technetium 99m bone scan
    - Most commonly used nuclear medicine study in pediatric orthopaedics
    - Typically used to screen for infection, neoplasm, or stress fracture
    - Technetium incorporates into metabolically active bone.
    - Patients are scanned 2 or 3 hours after injection.
    - Technetium 99m bone scans can be performed with single photon emission CT (SPECT), which uses a gamma ray sensor that rotates around the patient and creates slices similar to those obtained with CT. SPECT images allow enhanced resolution of small anatomic areas, such as the lumbar spine in patients with suspected spondylolysis.
    - *Triple-phase bone scan* can more clearly distinguish bone from soft tissue uptake and may better demonstrate stress fractures by providing 3 sets of images—angiogram images immediately following contrast injection, blood pool images within several minutes of the injection, and delayed images after 3 hours.
    - *Complex regional pain syndrome* (formerly known as reflex sympathetic dystrophy) has a characteristic pattern of decreased uptake on delayed bone scan image.
  - Gallium 67 scan
    - Gallium has affinity for areas of inflammation and rapid cell division.
    - Useful for localizing osteomyelitis in the spine and tumors
  - Indium 111 scan
    - Injection of radiolabeled leukocytes
    - Useful for localizing osteomyelitis in the extremities
- Advantages of nuclear medicine scans
  - High sensitivity
    - Useful as a screening test to localize pathology in cases of limp, infection, or non-accidental trauma
    - Bone scans can identify stress fractures much earlier than radiographs.

- Disadvantages of nuclear medicine scans
  — Low specificity
  — Radiation exposure and cost are similar to CT.
  — Invasive because intravenous line placement is required.
  — Young patients may need sedation because of the duration of the study.

Dual Energy X-ray Absorptiometry

- Dual energy x-ray absorptiometry measures bone mineral density (BMD).
- In children, BMD is reported as a z-score.
  — Z-score represents the standard deviations from the mean for age and sex.
  — Standards vary by age, sex, scanner type, and institution.
  — In some cases, specific diseases may be considered to have different norms.
  — Unlike t-scores used for reporting adult BMD, z-scores do not have cutoff values that define osteopenia and osteoporosis.
  — Most experts consider a z-score more than 2 standard deviations below the mean to indicate low BMD; however, the correlation between z-score and fracture risk in children is not yet well understood. As a result, ordering bone density measurements is best left to the specialist interpreting the scans and managing the patient's bone disease.
- Advantages of duel energy x-ray absorptiometry
  — Most accurate method for assessing BMD
  — May assist in the diagnosis of disorders of bone mass acquisition and monitoring treatment.
  — Relatively inexpensive and accessible
- Disadvantages of duel energy x-ray absorptiometry
  — Radiation exposure (approximately one tenth that of a standard chest x-ray)
  — Quality varies widely and is very operator-dependent.
  — Bone mineral density obtained from 2 different machines are not comparable.

CHAPTER 6

Laboratory Studies

- Laboratory studies can help identify infection (eg, osteomyelitis, septic arthritis) or systemic disease.
- An elevated white blood cell (WBC) count with an increase in immature cells (bands) is highly suggestive of bacterial infection.
- *Lactate dehydrogenase* and *uric acid levels* may be elevated in patients with malignancies.
- Erythrocyte sedimentation rate (ESR) and C-reactive protein (CRP) are nonspecific inflammatory markers.
  — A slightly elevated ESR in the range of 20 to 30 mm/hour suggests an inflammatory condition such as juvenile arthritis.
  — In the presence of infection, neoplasm, or significant trauma, ESR is typically above 30 mm/hour.
  — Compared with ESR, CRP has higher sensitivity and specificity for infection.
  — C-reactive protein tends to rise early and decline early; conversely, ESR may be normal early in the course of infection and remain elevated for a prolonged period. As a result, CRP is a better marker than ESR for following the course of infection and response to treatment.
- *Cultures of blood, joint fluid, and bone* are crucial in evaluating for infection.
  — Because of the significant rate of false-negative cultures, multiple samples should be obtained when feasible.
- *Synovial fluid analysis* is an important tool in the diagnosis of monoarticular arthritis.
  — Greater than 2,000 WBCs per mL of synovial fluid suggests an inflammatory process.
  — Greater than 50,000 WBCs per mL is highly suggestive of septic arthritis, while greater than 100,000 WBCs per mL is virtually diagnostic of septic arthritis (Table 6-1).
- *Creatine phosphokinase* is used to screen for muscular dystrophy in a child with weakness and tight heel cords.
- *Serum calcium, phosphate,* and other markers of bone metabolism are ordered when a metabolic bone disease such as rickets is suspected.
- Laboratory studies have limited utility when screening for *inflammatory arthritides*, but they are helpful in supporting a suspected clinical diagnosis.
  — *Antinuclear antibody* is neither sensitive nor specific for juvenile inflammatory arthritis; it is sensitive but not specific for systemic lupus erythematosus.

— *Rheumatoid factor (RF) assay* is a sensitive test for rheumatoid arthritis in adults.
  ▪ In children, the sensitivity of RF in detecting juvenile inflammatory arthritis is about 5%; however, the test is approximately 98% specific.
  ▪ Older children, girls, and patients with a large number of affected joints are more likely to have positive rheumatoid factor assays.
— *HLA-B27 serotype* has a strong association with juvenile ankylosing spondylitis, Reiter syndrome, arthritis associated with inflammatory bowel disease, and juvenile psoriatic arthritis.
  ▪ The presence of HLA-B27 is sensitive but not specific for these disorders; therefore, serotype testing is only done to support strong clinical suspicions.
— Arthritis can be a finding in late-stage Lyme disease.
  ▪ *Lyme titers* have 95% sensitivity when performed in patients with late-stage disease; however, specificity is only about 80%.
  ▪ Patients with suspected Lyme arthritis who have positive enzyme-linked immunosorbent assay serology testing should have confirmatory Western blot testing to decrease the rate of false positives.
- Dietary deficiencies and excesses may manifest as musculoskeletal disorders (Box 6-1).

Box 6-1. Musculoskeletal Manifestations of Dietary Deficiencies and Excesses

Vitamin A deficiency
- Excessive deposition of periosteal bone

Vitamin A excess (hypervitaminosis A)
- Bone pain, tenderness, and swelling
- Craniotabes (decreased mineralization of the skull)
- Hyperostosis of long bones (usually mid shaft)

Vitamin C deficiency (scurvy)
- Arthralgia, myalgia, hemarthrosis, muscular hematomas, osteonecrosis, osteopenia

Deficiency of vitamin D, calcium, or phosphorous (rickets)
- Musculoskeletal pain, osteomalacia, skeletal deformities (eg, genu varum or valgum, scoliosis), fractures

Iron deficiency
- Restless legs syndrome

Magnesium deficiency
- Sudden, involuntary muscle twitches or jerks (myoclonus)
- Muscle weakness

Copper deficiency
- Osteoporosis, arthritis

Table 6-1. Synovial Fluid Characteristics

Characteristic	Normal	Inflammatory Arthritis	Septic Arthritis
Quality	Clear, straw colored	May be slightly cloudy	Thick, purulent, white/yellow-green
White blood cells (per mm³)	<200	20,000–50,000	>50,000
Polymorphonuclear leukocytes (percentage)	<25%	>50%	>75%
Protein	1.8 g/dL	3–4 g/dL	4 g/dL
Glucose	20 mg/dL below serum	20 mg/dLbelow serum	30–50 mg/dL below serum

Bibliography

Aguero-Rosenfeld ME, Wang G, Schwartz I, Wormser GP. Diagnosis of lyme borreliosis. *Clin Microbiol Rev.* 2005;18:484–509

Barnes CJ, Van Steyn SJ, Fischer RA. The effects of age, sex, and shoulder dominance on range of motion of the shoulder. *J Shoulder Elbow Surg.* 2001;10:242–246

Bennell K, Khan KM, Matthews B, et al. Hip and ankle range of motion and hip muscle strength in young female ballet dancers and controls. *Br J Sports Med.* 1999;33:340–346

Brown SL, Hansen SL, Langone JJ. Role of serology in the diagnosis of Lyme disease. *JAMA.* 1999;282: 62–66

Eichenfield AH, Athreya BH, Doughty RA, Cebul RD. Utility of rheumatoid factor in the diagnosis of juvenile rheumatoid arthritis. *Pediatrics.* 1986;78:480–484

Fabry G, Cheng LX, Molenaers G. Normal and abnormal torsional development in children. *Clin Orthop Relat Res.* 1994;302:22–26

Fischer SU, Beattie TF. The limping child: epidemiology, assessment and outcome. *J Bone Joint Surg Br.* 1999;81:1029–1034

Forriol F, Pascual J. Footprint analysis between three and seventeen years of age. *Foot Ankle.* 1990;11:101–104

Goldberg SR, Ounpuu S, Delp SL. The importance of swing-phase initial conditions in stiff-knee gait. *J Biomech.* 2003;36:1111–1116

Heath CH, Staheli LT. Normal limits of knee angle in white children—genu varum and genu valgum. *J Pediatr Orthop.* 1993;13:259–262

Katz K, Rosenthal A, Yosipovitch Z. Normal ranges of popliteal angle in children. *J Pediatr Orthop.* 1992; 12:229–231

Kocher MS, Mandiga R, Zurakowski D, Barnewolt C, Kasser JR. Validation of a clinical prediction rule for the differentiation between septic arthritis and transient synovitis of the hip in children. *J Bone Joint Surg Am.* 2004;86-A:1629–1635

Kocher MS, Zurakowski D, Kasser JR. Differentiating between septic arthritis and transient synovitis of the hip in children: an evidence-based clinical prediction algorithm. *J Bone Joint Surg Am.* 1999;81:1662–1670

Ledue TB, Collins MF, Craig WY. New laboratory guidelines for serologic diagnosis of Lyme disease: evaluation of the two-test protocol. *J Clin Microbiol.* 1996;34:2343–2350

Malleson PN, Sailer M, Mackinnon MJ. Usefulness of antinuclear antibody testing to screen for rheumatic diseases. *Arch Dis Child.* 1997;77:299–304

Meyer B, Schaller K, Rohde V, Hassler W. The C-reactive protein for detection of early infections after lumbar microdiscectomy. *Acta Neurochir (Wien).* 1995;136:145–150

Mirovsky Y, Copeliovich L, Halperin N. Gowers' sign in children with discitis of the lumbar spine. *J Pediatr Orthop B.* 2005;14:68–70

Peltola H, Vahvanen V, Aalto K. Fever, C-reactive protein, and erythrocyte sedimentation rate in monitoring recovery from septic arthritis: a preliminary study. *J Pediatr Orthop.* 1984;4:170–174

Perry J. *Gait Analysis Normal and Pathological Function.* Thorofare, NJ: SLACK Inc; 1992:1–16

Rao KN, Joseph B. Value of measurement of hip movements in childhood hip disorders. *J Pediatr Orthop.* 2001;21:495–501

Staheli LT, Corbett M, Wyss C, King H. Lower-extremity rotational problems in children. Normal values to guide management. *J Bone Joint Surg Am.* 1985;67:39–47

Sutherland DH, Olshen R, Cooper L, Woo SL. The development of mature gait. *J Bone Joint Surg Am.* 1980;62:336–353

Wong DL, Baker CM. Pain in children: comparison of assessment scales. *Pediatr Nurs.* 1988;14:9–17

Youdas JW, Garrett TR, Suman VJ, Bogard CL, Hallman HO, Carey JR. Normal range of motion of the cervical spine: an initial goniometric study. *Phys Ther.* 1992;72:770–780

Part 3: Approach to Infection

TOPICS COVERED

CHAPTER 7

Osteomyelitis

General Principles

Bone, joint, and soft tissue infections are a significant cause of morbidity in pediatric populations. Clinical diagnoses may be especially challenging and even sometimes delayed when classic symptoms such as chills, fever, pain, and swelling are absent or subtle as is seen in the very young pediatric patient. While the principles of effective treatment are generally well understood, changing microbial sensitivity to medications has altered clinical decision-making about best treatment. Newer technologies including magnetic resonance imaging have also allowed for more accurate diagnosis.

Methicillin-resistant *Staphylococcus aureus* has led to an increased incidence of certain varieties of serious musculoskeletal infections in children. From 1982 to 2002, Gafur et al reported the incidence of osteomyelitis rose almost threefold, while the incidence of septic arthritis and pyomyositis was relatively unchanged. They identified increasing severity of illness based on a hierarchical pyramid of tissue involvement, with osteomyelitis being of greatest severity followed sequentially by septic arthritis, pyomyositis, and abscess. Methicillin-resistant *S aureus* was the most common causative organism found in these infectious cases. They recommended a comprehensive approach to the diagnosis and treatment of bone, joint, and soft tissue infections in children as is outlined in this chapter.

- Inflammation of bone caused by bacterial or fungal infection
- Classification into acute, subacute, and chronic categories is based on clinical course, histologic findings, and duration; yet these are poorly defined.
- Hematogenous spread from a distant site is the most common mechanism of infection in children.
- Distal metaphyses of growing bones (tibia and femur) are typically involved.
  — Hands, feet, and hips are also common sites of involvement.
  — Local spread from a traumatized contiguous site is a less common mechanism of infection in children.
  — Loss of skin integrity caused by penetrating trauma, open fractures, surgery, burns, skin ulcerations, or local soft tissue infections

Acute Hematogenous Osteomyelitis

INTRODUCTION/ETIOLOGY/EPIDEMIOLOGY

- Hematogenous spread of bacteria to the metaphyses of long bones is caused by slow, turbulent blood flow around areas of endochondral bone formation associated with less phagocytic activity and more bacterial growth (Figure 7-1).
- Acutely, the infection results in bone edema, vascular congestion, and small vessel thrombosis unique to pediatrics.
- Periosteal elevation may occur secondary to localized edema, and an *involucrum* of periosteal new bone may form to "wall" off the infection (Figure 7-2).
- Necrosis of bone may form a sequestrum (large area of necrosis).
- Fibrous, granulomatous tissue subsequently forms around dead bone, effectively containing the infection but also resulting in diminished blood flow and a decreased inflammatory response as is seen in chronic infections.
- In infants, damage to the physis can cause premature growth arrest with subsequent significant growth abnormalities.
- Incidence is 1 in 5,000 children younger than 13 years.
- Usually occurs in first decade of life (50% of cases are in children younger than 5 years).
- Males are more commonly affected than females.
- Age may influence or determine site of infection (Box 7-1).
- Risk factors for acute hematogenous osteomyelitis include sickle cell disease, granulomatous disease, and diabetes mellitus.
- Neonates are at increased risk for osteomyelitis because of immature immune system. Additional risk factors include prematurity, ventilator dependence, and indwelling lines and catheters.
- Until 18 months of age, metaphyseal capillaries supply the epiphyseal cap, so spread of infection to the epiphysis is possible (Figure 7-1).
- Spread into the joint can also occur and accounts for the increased frequency (up to 76%) of coexistent septic arthritis in children younger than 2 years.
- In children older than 2 years, the joint is usually spared unless the area of bone infected is intracapsular or epiphyseal (Figure 7-2).
- *Staphylococcus aureus* causes 70% to 90% of osteomyelitis in all age groups.
- Community-associated methicillin-resistant *S aureus* (CA-MRSA) is becoming more common.
  - Community-associated MRSA can carry the genes encoding Panton-Valentine leukocidin (PVL). Community-associated MRSA PVL+ isolates have been found to have multiple sites of infection approximately 15% of the time.
  - Myositis, pyomyositis, and intraosseous or subperiosteal abscesses are more common with PVL+ isolates.
  - Severe life-threatening complications such as septic pulmonary emboli and deep vein thromboses are more common with CA-MRSA osteomyelitis.

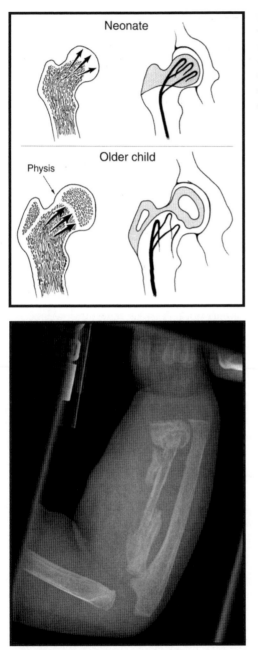

Figure 7-1. Relation of blood supply to the proximal femur and spread of infection (arrows). Reproduced from Dormans JP, Drummond DS: Pediatric hematogenous osteomyelitis: New trends in presentation, diagnosis, and treatment. *J Am Acad Orthop Surg.* 1994;2:333–341.

Figure 7-2. Radiographs of chronic osteomyelitis showing a necrosis in entire shaft of the bone (essentially the entire bone has become a sequestrum) and a developing involucrum.

- Group A streptococcus, *Streptococcus pneumoniae*, and *Kingella kingae* are next most common. *K kingae* is a gram-negative coccobacillus found in normal respiratory flora. Hematogenous spread from disrupted respiratory mucosa results in bone infection.
- In neonates, *S aureus* and coagulase-negative *Staphylococcus* are the most common cause, followed by group B streptococcus, gram-negative enteric bacteria, and *Candida*.

Box 7-1. Organisms Associated With Osteomyelitis and Septic Arthritis by Age Group

Age	Organism
0–2 mo	*Staphylococcus aureus* (methicillin-susceptible *S aureus* and methicillin-resistant *S aureus*) *Streptococcus agalactiae* Gram-negative enteric bacteria *Candida*
2 mo–5 y	*S aureus* *Streptococcus pyogenes* *Streptococcus pneumoniae* *Kingella kingae*
5–12 y	*S aureus* *S pyogenes*
Adolescence	*Neisseria gonorrhoeae*

- In patients with hemoglobinopathies, *Salmonella* is commonly associated with osteomyelitis, although overall *S aureus* is still the most common pathogen.
- See Box 7-2 for common clinical settings for microorganisms that cause osteomyelitis.

SIGNS AND SYMPTOMS

- Onset is usually sudden and may occur in conjunction with or as a complication of a non-musculoskeletal infection.
- Clinical presentation varies from vague, mild localized symptoms to concurrent, more severe systemic symptoms.
  — Localized symptoms include limb pain, swelling, erythema, induration, gait abnormalities, or local skin trauma.

Box 7-2. Common Clinical Settings for Microorganisms That Cause Osteomyelitis

Microorganism(s)	Clinical Setting
Staphylococcus aureus	Most common (70%–90%) of all infections Methicillin-sensitive *S aureus* and methicillin-resistant *S aureus* (health care–associated MRSA and community-associated MRSA) All types of osteomyelitis
Coagulase negative staphylococci	Foreign body infections or surgical instrumentation
Streptococci or anaerobes	Bites, diabetes mellitus, necrotic skin lesions
Pseudomonas aeruginosa	Puncture wounds through shoes and nosocomial infections
Salmonella	Sickle cell disease
Bartonella henselae, Pasteurella multocida, or *Eikenella corrodens*	HIV
Aspergillus, Mycobacterium avium complex, or *Candida albicans*	Immunocompromised patients

- A history of antecedent trauma is often reported.
- In neonates, predominant symptoms are decreased limb movement, poor feeding, and temperature instability; 40% of cases involve multiple sites.

DIFFERENTIAL DIAGNOSIS (BOX 7-3)

Box 7-3. Differential Diagnosis for Osteomyelitis

Trauma
Accidental and non-accidental

Neoplasms
Primary bone tumors: Ewing sarcoma, osteosarcoma
Non-primary bone tumor involvement: leukemia, neuroblastoma

Noninfectious Conditions
Chronic recurrent multifocal osteomyelitis, synovitis, inflammatory bowel disease, hyperostosis, osteitis syndrome, pustulosis, psoriasis, neutrophilic dermatosis, pyoderma gangrenosum, arthropathy

Infectious Conditions
Septic arthritis, synovitis

MAKING THE DIAGNOSIS

- *Radiographs* are the initial imaging study of choice.
  — Generally unremarkable for first 5 to 7 days in children and 10 to 14 days in skeletally mature individuals.
  — Earliest findings are soft tissue swelling with obliteration of tissue planes, periosteal thickening or elevation, and focal osteopenia.
  — Lytic changes are a later finding because at least 50% to 75% of the bone matrix must be destroyed to result in radiographic abnormalities (Figure 7-3).
  — Brodie abscess appears as an oval or round lesion walled off in a fibrous capsule with a sclerotic rim (Figure 7-4).
  — An involucrum, a periosteal sheath of new bone formation, is usually seen after about 3 weeks (see Figure 7-2).

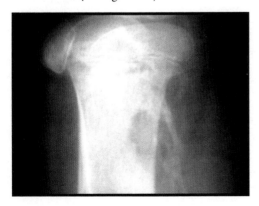

Figure 7-3. A lytic lesion of the proximal femoral diaphysis with adjacent periostitis secondary to chronic osteomyelitis due to *Staphylococcus aureus*.

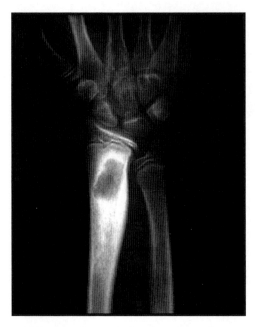

Figure 7-4. Anteroposterior radiograph of the distal radius. This image depicts a central metaphyseal lesion (ie, Brodie abscess). Reprinted with permission from eMedicine.com, 2008. Available at: emedicine.medscape.com/article/1248682-media.

- *Technetium 99m polyphosphate scan* is the most sensitive early diagnostic test—it may be positive as early as 48 hours into infection.
  — Accumulates in areas of inflammation, increased blood flow, and reactive new bone formation.
  — Sensitivity is good (70%–100%), but specificity is low (38%–96%).
  — Does not localize exact site of infection effectively.
  — Three- or 4-phase bone scans consist of angiographic phase (first minute after radionuclide injection), blood pool phase (5–15 minutes postinjection), delayed phase (2–3 hours postinjection), and static phase (24 hours postinjection—rarely used).
  — Delayed phase often distinguishes acute osteomyelitis from cellulitis and septic arthritis.
    - In acute osteomyelitis, the delayed phase usually has intensely positive uptake.
    - In cellulitis and septic arthritis, the delayed phase is usually negative (normal).
  — A negative or "cold" bone scan has 3 possible causes.
    - Osteomyelitis is not present.
    - The affected area may be falsely negative early in infection because of compression from intraosseous pus—this area is often "hot" a few hours later as the infection spreads.
    - Decreased blood flow caused by necrosis or cessation of metabolic activity.
- *Gallium citrate scan* is more specific than technetium 99m because it is not dependent on blood flow.
  — Uses gallium 67, which resembles iron and is rapidly bound to transferrin and lactoferrin.
  — Physiologic accumulation occurs in areas of active inflammation.

— Does *not* distinguish acute osteomyelitis from cellulitis or septic arthritis (disadvantage).

— Rarely used because of high radiation exposures, long examination times, and low spatial resolution.

- *Indium 111 labeled leukocyte scans* may be the most sensitive nuclear imaging study for acute osteomyelitis (88%–89% sensitivity, 85% specificity).

— White blood cells are labeled, so results are not dependent on blood flow.

— Infrequently used in children because of need for 40 to 60 mL of whole blood and long examination time.

- Magnetic resonance imaging (MRI)

— Very high sensitivity and specificity for diagnosing osteomyelitis

— Allows differentiation between bone and soft tissue infections.

— Localizes site of infection (ie, epiphysis vs physis).

— No ionizing radiation (major advantage to pediatric population)

— T1-weighted images demonstrate low marrow signal intensity, while T2-weighted images show high signal intensity (Figure 7-5).

— Intravenous gadolinium contrast on T1-weighted images with fat suppression will demonstrate abscesses in detail.

— The major disadvantage of MRI is that a localized examination is unable to evaluate for the presence of other affected areas seen on nuclear medicine whole body imaging studies.

- *Ultrasound* is not routinely used in the diagnosis of acute osteomyelitis, although it may serve as an important adjunct.

— Soft tissue abnormalities or periosteal elevation may be visible within 24 to 48 hours.

— May delineate an abscess and allow for fine needle aspiration to obtain material for cytology and culture.

— No radiation and often no sedation required

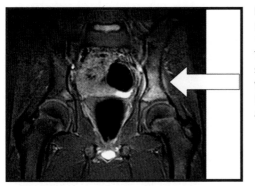

Figure 7-5. T2-weighted magnetic resonance imaging of the pelvis of a 10-year-old boy with fever and hip pain. The left iliac wing shows increased signal intensity (arrow), consistent with osteomyelitis of the left iliac wing. Note the pyomyositis of the iliopsoas and abductor muscles.

- *Laboratory tests*
  - No specific laboratory tests are diagnostic for osteomyelitis; most are adjunctive.
  - White blood cell count, C-reactive protein (CRP), and erythrocyte sedimentation rate (ESR) are typically elevated.
    - Erythrocyte sedimentation rate is elevated in 90%; rises slowly, and peaks at 3 to 5 days.
    - C-reactive protein is elevated in 98%; increases dramatically within 24 to 48 hours.
    - Erythrocyte sedimentation rate may be normal in setting of acute osteomyelitis in neonates, children on steroids, and those with sickle cell disease.
  - *Blood cultures* are essential to obtain prior to the initiation of antibiotic therapy and are positive for bacteremia in approximately 50% of cases.
  - *Aspiration of bone* for gram stain and culture under computed tomography or ultrasound guidance may reveal etiologic agent more frequently than blood cultures.
  - *Biopsies of soft tissues* may isolate bacterial pathogens in lieu of obtaining bone aspirates.
  - *Neonates* are more challenging to diagnose.
    - Little systemic inflammatory response is seen (CRP may be elevated but ESR is usually normal).
    - Bone scans are not helpful.
    - Diagnosis is typically made with MRI and bone aspiration.

TREATMENT

- Requires coordinated care among primary care physicians, orthopaedic surgeons, radiologists, and infectious disease specialists.
- Initial treatment includes the initiation of appropriate antibiotic therapy.
  - Treat for most likely pathogens.
  - Consider known antimicrobial resistance patterns.
  - Evaluate intrinsic host susceptibility (eg, neonate, immunocompromised host).
- Perform necessary procedures such as drainage of abscesses and debridement of necrotic tissue.
- Maintain close monitoring and follow-up.
- Adjust antibiotic regimens as needed based on culture results.
- Duration of antibiotic therapy is based on patient age, organism, and clinical course.
  - For *S aureus*, a minimum of 7 days intravenously followed by 21 to 35 days of oral antibiotics (4–6 weeks total course).
  - Six weeks of intravenous antibiotics are required for neonates.

EXPECTED OUTCOMES AND PROGNOSIS

- Prompt recognition and aggressive treatment are necessary for good long-term outcomes.
- Delayed diagnosis or inadequate treatment may lead to growth arrest, persistent joint stiffness and pain, avascular necrosis, pathologic fractures, and amputations.

WHEN TO REFER

- Refer the following to an infectious disease specialist:
  - — Cases of diagnostic uncertainty
  - — Children who are high risk because of associated diseases such as hemolytic anemias, diabetes mellitus, or immunocompromised status
  - — Invasive pathogens identified as causative agents that are associated with antimicrobial resistance
- Refer to an orthopaedic surgeon or interventional radiologist when diagnostic procedures are required such as bone biopsy or incision and drainage of an associated abscess.
- Children with significant systemic symptoms require critical supportive care.

RELEVANT *INTERNATIONAL CLASSIFICATION OF DISEASES, NINTH REVISION, CLINICAL MODIFICATION (ICD-9-CM)* CODE

- **730.0**   Osteomyelitis, acute or subacute

Subacute Osteomyelitis

INTRODUCTION/ETIOLOGY/EPIDEMIOLOGY

- Duration is longer than 3 weeks to several months.
- Patients are typically older than those with acute osteomyelitis.
- *S aureus* is the most common pathogen identified.

SIGNS AND SYMPTOMS

- Mild or intermittent pain over weeks
- Usually there are no or few signs of systemic illness.
- Thirty percent to 40% have had a trial of antibiotics and negative blood and tissue cultures.

DIFFERENTIAL DIAGNOSIS

- See Box 7-2.
- Rule out tumors such as chondroblastoma, which may have similar radiographic appearance.

MAKING THE DIAGNOSIS

- *Radiographs* usually show changes characteristic of osteomyelitis.

TREATMENT

- Promptly initiate antibiotic therapy.
- Surgical drainage and debridement have not been studied with randomized, prospective trials.

- Surgical intervention is indicated for
  — Frank pus found on needle aspiration of bone or an abscess
  — Penetrating injuries
  — Retained foreign bodies
  — Surgical drainage is essential for osteomyelitis of the femoral head or hip joint involvement.

EXPECTED OUTCOMES/PROGNOSIS

- Prompt initiation of appropriate antibiotic therapy results in rapid clinical improvement in pediatric patients.

WHEN TO REFER

- See Acute Hematogenous Osteomyelitis on page 78.

RELEVANT *ICD-9-CM* CODE

- **730.0**   Osteomyelitis, acute or subacute

Chronic Osteomyelitis

INTRODUCTION/ETIOLOGY/EPIDEMIOLOGY

- Sequela of undiagnosed, untreated, or inadequately treated acute osteomyelitis
- Develops in 19% of patients treated for less than 3 weeks, but only 2% of patients treated longer than 3 weeks.
- Usually affects the long bones.

SIGNS AND SYMPTOMS

- See Acute Hematogenous Osteomyelitis on page 78.
- Onset of symptoms is often subtle, resulting in a chronic condition.

DIFFERENTIAL DIAGNOSIS

- See Box 7-2.

MAKING THE DIAGNOSIS

- *Radiographs* reveal hallmark pathologic features of necrotic bone and involucrum formation (Figure 7-6).
- *Magnetic resonance imaging* may show variations in signal change within bone and chronic changes in surrounding soft tissues.
- Blood cultures are rarely positive.

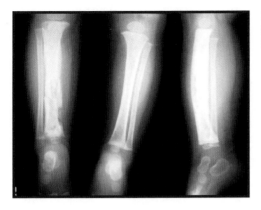

Figure 7-6. Three views of the tibia showing necrotic bone and involucrum formation in chronic osteomyelitis.

TREATMENT

- Requires surgical intervention and debridement, often repeated.
- Requires longer duration of antibiotic therapy than for acute osteomyelitis.

EXPECTED OUTCOMES/PROGNOSIS

- Compared with acute osteomyelitis,
  — Greater incidence of relapses and recurrent infections
  — Greater incidence of long-term complications such as growth arrest, abnormal limb function, or amputation
- Chronic drainage increases risk for squamous cell carcinoma of sinus tracts in adulthood.

WHEN TO REFER

- See Acute Hematogenous Osteomyelitis on page 78.

RELEVANT *ICD-9-CM* CODE

- **730.1**   Chronic osteomyelitis

Chronic Recurrent Multifocal Osteomyelitis (CRMO)

INTRODUCTION/ETIOLOGY/EPIDEMIOLOGY

- First described in 1972 as "an unusual from of multifocal bone lesions with subacute and chronic symmetrical osteomyelitis"
- Pathophysiology is poorly understood.
- Pathogens are rarely cultured from lesions, which have nonspecific histopathological findings.
- Lesions are frequently multifocal and do not form abscesses, fistulae, or sequestra.
- There are no characteristic laboratory findings, leading some to postulate that the disorder may be autoimmune, possibly a seronegative spondyloarthropathy.

- True incidence is unknown; a little more than 200 cases have been reported.
- Females seem to be affected more than males.

SIGNS AND SYMPTOMS

- Prolonged, fluctuating bone pain with recurrent episodes is typical.
- Often associated with skin diseases such as pustulosis palmoplantaris, acne vulgaris, psoriasis vulgaris, and pyoderma gangrenosum

DIFFERENTIAL DIAGNOSIS

- See Box 7-2.

MAKING THE DIAGNOSIS

- There are no characteristic laboratory findings.
- *Radiographs* demonstrate bony lesions similar in appearance to subacute or chronic osteomyelitis, but in unusual locations, predominantly on the clavicle and tubular bones, spine, and pelvis.

TREATMENT

- Typically does not respond to antibiotic treatment.
- Nonsteroidal anti-inflammatory drugs are the treatment of choice for pain control during the acute phase.
- Sulfasalazine and colchicine have also been effective.

EXPECTED OUTCOMES/PROGNOSIS

- Chronic recurrent multifocal osteomyelitis has an unpredictable clinical course but is usually self-limited without major sequelae when followed over 7 to 25 years.
- Limb-length inequality may occur because of growth arrest or impairment.

WHEN TO REFER

- May be best managed by pediatric rheumatologist because this is a chronic condition.

RELEVANT *ICD-9-CM* CODE

- **730.1**   Osteomyelitis, chronic

CHAPTER 8

Septic Arthritis

Introduction/Etiology/Epidemiology

- Also called *suppurative* arthritis (pus), septic arthritis (SA) results from bacterial invasion of a joint and subsequent inflammation (Figure 8-1), usually as a result of transient bacteremia, spread into the joint from a skin lesion, or extension from adjacent tissue.
- Rapid and progressive joint destruction occurs if urgent surgical drainage and irrigation is not undertaken.
- Viral, mycobacterial, and fungal invasions occur rarely.
- Common pathogens tend to be associated with specific populations (Table 8-1).
  — Since the era of *Haemophilus influenzae* type b (Hib) vaccination, *Kingella kingae* has supplanted Hib as a gram-negative cause of SA in children 2 months to 5 years of age (Hib infections are rare nowadays in immunized children).
  — The effect of the heptavalent pneumococcal vaccine on the incidence of *Streptococcal pneumoniae* in SA is still being investigated.
  — Reactive arthritis may occur as a complication of infection with *Salmonella, Shigella, Campylobacter, Yersinia, C trachomatis,* or *Neisseria meningitidis.*
- Fifty percent of SA cases occur in patients younger than 20 years.
- Children younger than 3 years are most commonly affected.
- Males are affected twice as often as females.
- Infection of the hip, knee, and ankle comprise 80% of cases.

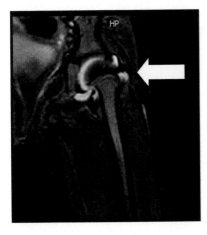

Figure 8-1. Arrow indicates hip effusion on T2-weighted magnetic resonance image in a 2-year-old child with fever and inability to bear weight consistent with a diagnosis of a septic hip.

Table 8-1. Microorganisms Causing Septic Arthritis and Commonly Affected Populations

Microorganism(s)	Commonly Affected Populations
Staphylococcus aureus	Most common (70%–90%) of all infections Methicillin-susceptible *S aureus* and methicillin-resistant *S aureus* (MRSA) (hospital-acquired MRSA and community-acquired MRSA—rapidly rising incidence)
Streptococcus (group A beta-hemolytic streptococci, *Streptococcus pneumoniae*), *Klebsiella kingae*	Non-neonates and older
Group B streptococcus, *Streptococcus agalactiae*, *Neisseria gonorrhoeae*, gram-negative enterics, and *Candida*	Neonates
N gonorrhoeae	Adolescents
Salmonella	Sickle cell disease
Borrelia burgdorferi	Deer tick exposure

- Children with sickle cell disease, diabetes mellitus, immunodeficiencies, preexisting joint damage, or compromised skin integrity from dermatologic conditions (eg, eczema, psoriasis) tend to be particularly susceptible.

Signs and Symptoms

- Focal erythema, edema, warmth, and effusion in the affected joint
- Limp or pseudoparalysis of the affected extremity
- Child typically holds the joint in a position that minimizes capsular stress (slightly flexed knee, flexed/abducted/externally rotated hip).
- Fever, anorexia, irritability, and malaise are common systemic symptoms.
- Multiple joint involvement is uncommon, but occurs in up to 50% of *N gonorrhoeae* infections.

Differential Diagnosis (Box 8-2)

Box 8-2. Differential Diagnosis for Septic Arthritis

Trauma
Accidental and non-accidental

Neoplasms
Primary bone tumors: Ewing sarcoma, osteosarcoma
Non-primary bone tumor involvement: leukemia, neuroblastoma

Idiopathic orthopaedic conditions
Slipped capital femoral epiphysis and Legg-Calve-Perthes disease

Noninfectious conditions
Synovitis, juvenile rheumatoid arthritis, hemarthrosis, inflammatory bowel disease, hyperostosis, osteitis syndrome, pustulosis, psoriasis, neutrophilic dermatosis, pyoderma gangrenosum, chronic recurrent multifocal osteomyelitis

Infectious conditions
Osteomyelitis, transient synovitis, post-infectious arthropathy, post-streptococcal arthritis, Lyme arthritis

Making the Diagnosis

- As with osteomyelitis, white blood cell (WBC) count, erythrocyte sedimentation rate (ESR), and C-reactive protein may be elevated.
- *Blood cultures* are positive one third of the time and may help identify an organism when synovial fluid cultures are negative.
- *Synovial fluid analysis* is the diagnostic gold standard.
  — Exudative appearing fluid
  — Leukocyte-predominant WBC count greater than 50,000 (seen also in some rheumatologic disease, so not pathognomonic for SA)
  — Up to one third of patients will have WBC count less than 50,000.
  — Gram stain is positive for organisms in 30% to 50%.
  — Protein level less than 40 mg/dL
  — Glucose level is usually less than serum glucose level.
  — Lactate is typically elevated except in gonococcal arthritis.
  — Culture of aspirated fluid is positive 50% to 80% of the time.
- *Neonates* may be more challenging to diagnose.
  — Predominant symptom is decreased limb movement.
  — Little systemic inflammatory response is seen.
  — Concomitant osteomyelitis is common (up to 76%).
- *Septic arthritis of the hip*
  — Difficult diagnosis requiring expertise and a high index of suspicion
  — All children presenting with hip, thigh, or knee pain or a limp should have a thorough examination of the hip joint.
  — Often pain is only elicited at the extreme range of motion with flexion, extension, and internal and external rotation.
  — Distinguish from *transient synovitis*, a post-viral, self-limited phenomenon. Children with transient synovitis typically have no or a low-grade fever, are well appearing, and may have more mild pain.
  — Kocher established 4 criteria for diagnosing SA of the hip—fever, inability to bear weight, ESR greater than 40 mm/hour, and peripheral WBC count greater than 12,000; when 3 or 4 of these criteria were met, kids had a better than 93% likelihood of having SA. In other prospective analyses of Kocher's criteria, the sensitivity has not been as high, and other clinical algorithms for diagnosing SA of the hip have been put forth.
  — Additional imaging or testing is often required to evaluate for other possible diagnoses such as osteomyelitis or pyomyositis.

Treatment

- *Surgical drainage and irrigation of the joint* is the cornerstone of treatment.
- *Antimicrobial therapy*
  - Instituted initially via an intravenous route
    - Empiric regimens should always include an anti-staphylococcal (anti–community-acquired methicillin-resistant *Staphylococcus aureus* [CA-MRSA]) agent.
    - Clindamycin or trimethoprim-sulfisoxazole is the antibiotic of choice for uncomplicated, suspected CA-MRSA infections.
      - D-testing should be performed.
    - For more severe, invasive, or systemic infections, vancomycin is the gold standard.
    - Broad-spectrum empiric regimens include nafcillin plus cefotaxime, cefuroxime, or ceftriaxone.
    - Most beta-lactams and second- or third-generation cephalosporins are effective against *K kingae*.
    - Anti-pseudomonal penicillin and an aminoglycoside are administered for *Pseudomonas aeruginosa*.
  - Transition to oral therapy depends on the clinical status of the patient (resolution of systemic symptoms and improving localized symptoms).
  - In general, antimicrobials are continued for 3 to 6 weeks because there is evidence that treatment for fewer than 3 weeks can lead to unacceptably high rates of relapse.
  - Intra-articular antibiotics do not seem to help and may cause chemical synovitis.

Expected Outcomes/Prognosis

- Varies, depending on site of infection and timing of diagnosis and intervention.

When to Refer

- Suspected septic arthritis is a surgical emergency and should be immediately referred to a pediatric orthopaedic surgeon for urgent evaluation and possible joint aspiration.
- Antimicrobial therapy for bone and joint infections in children should be undertaken in consultation with a local expert in infectious diseases.

Relevant *International Classification of Diseases, Ninth Revision, Clinical Modification* Code

- **711.0** Septic arthritis

CHAPTER 9

Miscellaneous Infections

Diskitis

INTRODUCTION/ETIOLOGY/EPIDEMIOLOGY

- Most commonly affects the lumbar spine in children younger than 5 years.
  — At this age discs derive rich blood supply from vertebral bodies.
- Starts in the vertebral end plates, then spreads to disc via vascular channels.

SIGNS AND SYMPTOMS

- Limp or refusal to walk; classic presentation is child with hands leaning on thighs to walk.
- Less commonly, patients have localized back pain (or referred abdominal pain).
- A low grade fever may be present.
- Physical findings are limited.

DIFFERENTIAL DIAGNOSIS

- Traumatic or non-traumatic orthopaedic conditions or neoplasms (see Chapter 14)

MAKING THE DIAGNOSIS

- Requires high index of suspicion.
- *Technetium 99m polyphosphate scan* will be positive.
- *Magnetic resonance imaging* is diagnostic test of choice.
  — Can identify diskitis, paravertebral abscess, and spinal cord involvement.
  — T1-weighted images demonstrate low signal intensity in disc while T2-weighted images show high signal intensity (Figure 9-1).
  — Infected area enhances with intravenous gadolinium contrast.
  — The whole spine should be imaged to look for multiple sites of infection.
- In chronic cases (2–3 weeks), hallmark findings of loss of disc space with associated degenerative changes can be seen on *plain radiographs*.
- Biopsy result is positive in 60% to 70% and may be helpful when there is a poor response to antibiotics.

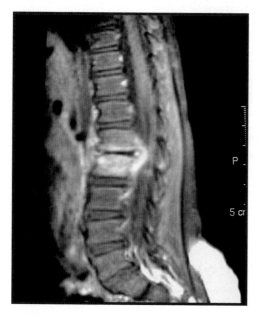

Figure 9-1. Magnetic resonance imaging of the lumbar spine revealing diskitis of the L1-L2 disc space, L1 and L2 osteomyelitis, and an epidural abscess.

TREATMENT

- Requires prolonged antimicrobial therapy (empiric coverage for *Staphylococcus aureus*) and a referral to a pediatric orthopaedic spine specialist.

EXPECTED OUTCOMES/PROGNOSIS

- Varies, depending on site of infection and timing of diagnosis and intervention.
- Rarely, complications include disc space narrowing, fusion of vertebral bodies, and persistent back pain.

WHEN TO REFER

- If imaging studies demonstrate the presence of vertebral disc infection, urgent referral to a pediatric orthopaedic spine specialist is warranted.
- Prolonged or unusual back pain, particularly when associated with systemic symptoms, should be referred to a pediatric orthopaedic surgeon.

RELEVANT *INTERNATIONAL CLASSIFICATION OF DISEASES, NINTH REVISION, CLINICAL MODIFICATION (ICD-9-CM)* CODE

- **722.90**   Diskitis

Vertebral Osteomyelitis

INTRODUCTION/ETIOLOGY/EPIDEMIOLOGY

- Can affect lumbar, cervical, or thoracic vertebrae.
- Usually occurs in children older than 5 years.
- *Staphylococcus aureus* is most common pathogen.

SIGNS AND SYMPTOMS

- Localized back pain and tenderness
- More significant systemic symptoms than in those with diskitis

DIFFERENTIAL DIAGNOSIS

- Traumatic or non-traumatic orthopaedic conditions or neoplasms (see Chapter 14)

MAKING THE DIAGNOSIS

- *White blood cell count* is normal or mildly elevated.
- *Elevated erythrocyte sedimentation rate (ESR)* is the most common laboratory finding.
- *Radiographs*
- Early: decrease in bone density
- Late: bone destruction
- *Technetium 99m polyphosphate scan* will be positive.
- *Magnetic resonance imaging* is diagnostic test of choice.
  — T1-weighted images demonstrate low bone marrow signal intensity, while T2-weighted images show high signal intensity (see Figure 9-1).
  — Infected area enhances with intravenous gadolinium contrast.
  — The whole spine should be imaged to look for multiple sites of infection.
- Biopsy result is positive in 60% to 70% and may be helpful when there is a poor response to antibiotics.

TREATMENT

- Requires prolonged antimicrobial therapy (empiric coverage for *S aureus*) and a referral to a pediatric orthopaedic spine specialist.

EXPECTED OUTCOMES/PROGNOSIS

- Varies depending on site of infection and timing of diagnosis and intervention.

WHEN TO REFER

- Prolonged or unusual back pain, particularly when associated with systemic symptoms, should be referred to a pediatric orthopaedic surgeon.

RELEVANT *ICD-9-CM* CODE

- **730.28**   Vertebral osteomyelitis

Pyomyositis

INTRODUCTION/ETIOLOGY/EPIDEMIOLOGY

- Purulent soft tissue infection of muscle
- Etiology is unclear; risk factors include direct trauma, viral infection, and malnutrition.
- Most commonly occurs in lower extremity muscles, especially quadriceps, gluteals, obturator internus, iliopsoas, and gastrocnemius.
- *S aureus* is the causative organism in the majority of cases.
- *Streptococcus* strains, gram negatives, *Mycobacterium*, anaerobes, yeast, and fungi can all be causative microorganisms.
- Children with HIV or other immunodeficiency are particularly prone.

SIGNS AND SYMPTOMS

- Muscle pain, swelling, tenderness, and induration
- Decreased joint function, but normal joint range of motion, of the affected limb (as opposed to intra-articular infections)
- Infections can spread hematogenously, resulting in severe systemic symptoms, such as fever and malaise.
- Pyomyositis of the psoas muscle may mimic appendicitis.

DIFFERENTIAL DIAGNOSIS

- Includes traumatic (eg, hematoma) and non-traumatic orthopaedic conditions or neoplasms, septic arthritis, osteomyelitis, cellulitis, polymyositis/dermatomyositis, and deep vein thrombosis.
- Distinguish pyomyositis from necrotizing fasciitis and clostridial myonecrosis, which tend to be much more aggressive and lethal processes.

MAKING THE DIAGNOSIS

- Requires high index of suspicion.
- White blood cell count and ESR are elevated.
- Serum creatine kinase and aldolase are usually normal.
- Blood cultures are rarely positive.
- Magnetic resonance imaging provides excellent visualization of soft tissue infections and can differentiate pyomyositis from osteomyelitis (see Figure 7-5).
- *Needle aspiration* can identify causative organism.

TREATMENT

- Requires prolonged antimicrobial therapy and a referral to an orthopaedic specialist.
- Prompt initiation of appropriate antibiotic therapy can obviate need for surgical drainage.
- Surgical drainage under ultrasonic or computed tomography guidance is often required, especially for large abscesses.

EXPECTED OUTCOMES/PROGNOSIS

- Varies depending on site of infection and timing of diagnosis and intervention.
- Underlying chronic disease, delays in diagnosis, and the presence of systemic symptoms increase the risk of morbidity and mortality, but little information is available in children to quantify to what degree.
- Life-threatening complications include sepsis and toxic shock syndrome.
- Recurrence rates are low in the absence of the previously mentioned risk factors.
- Patients treated rapidly while in the early stages of presentation tend to have excellent outcomes with intravenous antibiotic treatment alone.
- Intravenous antibiotics combined with surgical intervention for more severe cases are associated with excellent outcomes and low recurrence rates in patients without underlying chronic disease.

RELEVANT *ICD-9-CM* CODE

- **728.0**   Pyomyositis

Resources for Physicians and Families

- MedlinePlus definition of osteomyelitis (www.nlm.nih.gov/medlineplus/ency/article/000437.htm)
- eMedicine article on osteomyelitis (http://emedicine.medscape.com/article/967095-overview)
- eMedicine articles on septic arthritis (http://emedicine.medscape.com/article/236299-overview) (http://emedicine.medscape.com/article/1259337-overview)

Bibliography

Benjamin HJ, Nikore V, Takagishi J. Practical management: community-associated methicillin-resistant *Staphylococcus aureus* (CA-MRSA): the latest sports epidemic. *Clin J Sports Med.* 2007;17:393–397

Blyth MJ, Kincaid R, Craigen MA, Bennet GC. The changing epidemiology of acute and subacute haematogenous osteomyelitis in children. *J Bone Joint Surg Br.* 2001;83:99–102

Bocchini CE, Hulten KG, Mason EO Jr, Gonzalez BE, Hammerman WA, Kaplan SL. Panton-Valentine leukocidin genes are associated with enhanced inflammatory response and local disease in acute hematogenous *Staphylococcus aureus* osteomyelitis in children. *Pediatrics.* 2006;117:433–440

Butt WP. The radiology of infection. *Clin Orthop Relat Res.* 1973;96:20–30

Dahl LB, Høyland AL, Dramsdahl H, Kaaresen PI. Acute osteomyelitis in children: a population-based retrospective study 1965 to 1994. *Scand J Infect Dis.* 1998;30:573–577

Deysine M, Rafkin H, Russell R, Teicher I, Aufses AH Jr. The detection of acute experimental osteomyelitis with 67Ga citrate scannings. *Surg Gynecol Obstet.* 1975;141:40–42

Epps CH Jr, Bryant DD, Coles MJ, Castro O. Osteomyelitis in patients who have sickle-cell disease. Diagnosis and management. *J Bone Joint Surg Am.* 1991;73:1281–1294

Everett ED, Hirschmann JV. Transient bacteremia and endocarditis prophylaxis. A review. *Medicine (Baltimore).* 1977;56:61–77

Gafur OA, Copley LA, Hollmig ST, Browne RH, Thornton LA, Crawford SE. The impact of the current epidemiology of pediatric musculoskeletal infection on evaluation and treatment guidelines. *J Pediatr Orthop.* 2008;28:777–785

Gillespie WJ. Epidemiology in bone and joint infection. *Infect Dis Clin North Am.* 1990;4:361–376

Gutierrez K. Bone and joint infections in children. *Pediatr Clin North Am.* 2005;52:779–794

Jurik AG. Chronic recurrent multifocal osteomyelitis. *Semin Musculoskelet Radiol.* 2004;8:243–253

Kaplan SL. Osteomyelitis in children. *Infect Dis Clin North Am.* 2005;19:787–797

Kleinman PK. A regional approach to osteomyelitis of the lower extremities in children. *Radiol Clin North Am.* 2002;40:1033–1059

Lazzarini L, Mader JT, Calhoun JH. Osteomyelitis in long bones. *J Bone Joint Surg Am.* 2004;86-A:2305–2318

Ma LD, Frassica FJ, Bluemke DA, Fishman EK. CT and MRI evaluation of musculoskeletal infection. *Crit Rev Diagn Imaging.* 1997;38:535–568

McCarthy JJ, Dormans JP, Kozin SH, Pizzutillo PD. Musculoskeletal infections in children: basic treatment principles and recent advancements. *Instr Course Lect.* 2005;54:515–528

Modic MT, Pflanze W, Feiglin DH, Belhobek G. Magnetic resonance imaging of musculoskeletal infections. *Radiol Clin North Am.* 1986;24:247–258

Moutschen MP, Scheen AJ, Lefebvre PJ. Impaired immune responses in diabetes mellitus: analysis of the factors and mechanisms involved. Relevance to the increased susceptibility of diabetic patients to specific infections. *Diabete Metab.* 1992;18:187–201

Nair SP, Meghji S, Wilson M, Reddi K, White P, Henderson B. Bacterially induced bone destruction: mechanisms and misconceptions. *Infect Immun.* 1996;64:2371–2380

Offiah AC. Acute osteomyelitis, septic arthritis and discitis: differences between neonates and older children. *Eur J Radiol.* 2006;60:221–232

Paluska SA. Osteomyelitis. *Clin Fam Pract.* 2004;6:127–156

Saigal G, Azouz EM, Abdenour G. Imaging of osteomyelitis with special reference to children. *Semin Musculoskelet Radiol.* 2004;8:255–265

Small LN, Ross JJ. Tropical and temperate pyomyositis. *Infect Dis Clin North Am.* 2005;19:981–989

Sullivan DC, Rosenfield NS, Ogden J, Gottschalk A. Problems in the scintigraphic detection of osteomyelitis in children. *Radiology.* 1980;135:731–736

Treves S, Khettry J, Broker FH, Wilkinson RH, Watts H. Osteomyelitis: early scintigraphic detection in children. *Pediatrics.* 1976;57:173–186

Tröbs R, Möritz R, Bühligen U, et al. Changing pattern of osteomyelitis in infants and children. *Pediatr Surg Int.* 1999;15:363–372

Part 4: Evaluating the Limping Child

TOPICS COVERED

CHAPTER 10

General Approach and Differential Diagnosis

Introduction/Etiology/Epidemiology

- Limping—a common pediatric presenting complaint—may be secondary to pain, weakness, or musculoskeletal deformity (Table 10-1).
  — Growing pains usually *do not* cause limping.
- The hip is a common source of the pathology.
  — Toxic synovitis of the hip is a common cause of a limp in children younger than 5 years.
  — The overweight limping adolescent with knee, thigh, groin, or hip pain has a slipped capital femoral epiphysis until proven otherwise.
- Etiologies range from common to rare, and vary by age (Box 10-1).
- Narrow the differential diagnosis by classifying the limp according to
  — Gait pattern
  — Presence or absence of pain (figures 10-1 and 10-2)
  — Age of the child
  — Anatomic region involved

Abnormal Gait Patterns

ANTALGIC GAIT

- Limping because of pain
- Characterized by shortened stance phase duration on the affected limb
- Can be caused by pain in the lower extremity or back. When caused by back pain, the gait is not asymmetrical but slow and cautious with short steps.
- Commonly caused by trauma or infection
- Physical examination should focus on inspection, palpation, and range of motion to localize the pain source.

Table 10-1. Common Causes of a Limp

Cause	Common Age Range	Gait Pattern	Signs and Symptoms	Making the Diagnosis
Osteomyelitis	1–7 y	Antalgic	Localized pain, swelling, warmth, erythema, fever, malaise	Acute: Typical symptoms plus elevated WBC count, ESR, and CRP, and positive bone scan Subacute: Positive radiographs
Discitis	1–3 y	Antalgic; moves with back rigidly straight; or unwilling to walk	Infants and toddlers: Fever, irritability, refusal to walk In older children and adolescents: Back pain, worse with flexion	Early: Typical signs/symptoms plus elevated ESR or CRP and positive bone scan or MRI Late: Narrowed disc space on radiograph
Transient synovitis of the hip	1–8 y	Antalgic	Limited and painful hip range of motion, hip effusion, recent viral illness, nontoxic appearing	Typical clinical symptoms plus normal laboratory studies Imaging may show mild hip joint effusion.
Septic arthritis of the hip	1–8 y	Antalgic	Limited and painful hip range of motion, hip effusion, systemic symptoms (fever, malaise)	Suggested by elevated WBC, ESR, CRP, positive bone scan, or effusion on ultrasound. Confirmed by joint aspiration.
Toddler fracture	1–3 y	Antalgic	Tender at proximal tibia	Radiographs frequently negative, but may show periosteal reaction after 2 weeks (Figure 10-3).
Cerebral palsy	>1 y	Trendelenburg or steppage	Increased tone, spasticity, clonus, and flexion contracture in the affected limb(s)	Rule out neurodegenerative disorders; neurologist can confirm diagnosis.
Muscular dystrophy	Duchenne: Boys, 18 mo–4 y Becker: Boys, 2–21 y	Trendelenburg	Delayed motor milestones (not walking by 18 mo); weakness in proximal muscle groups, toe walking, calf pseudohypertrophy; Gower sign	Significantly elevated CPK, abnormal EMG, muscle biopsy

Table 10-1. Common Causes of a Limp, continued

Cause	Common Age Range	Gait Pattern	Signs and Symptoms	Making the Diagnosis
Developmental dysplasia of the hip	1–5 y; rarely mild dysplasia may present in adolescence.	Trendelenburg or equinus; when bilateral, exaggerated lumbar lordosis with waddling gait	In infants/toddlers: delayed walking (15–18 mo); in adolescents: activity-related pain, limb-length difference, limited hip range of motion, and mild hip flexion contracture	Radiographs (AP pelvis and frog lateral) (Figure 10-4)
Juvenile rheumatoid arthritis	Pauciarticular: 1–4 y Polyarticular: 1–3 y, adolescence	Antalgic	Joint pain with warmth, tenderness, swelling, and limited range of motion, possible iritis; 3–4 times more common in girls	Typical clinical symptoms plus may have elevated ESR, positive rheumatoid factor, or ANA
Ewing sarcoma	1–20 y	Antalgic	Pain, swelling of the overlying soft tissues; May cause systemic symptoms, low RBC count, low WBC, elevated ESR.	Radiographs reveal diaphyseal lesion with periosteal reaction; distinguished from osteomyelitis by biopsy.
Osteoid osteoma	10–20 y	Antalgic	Pain in tibia or spine, usually at night	Radiographs may reveal lucent nidus surrounded by sclerosis; bone scan is diagnostic.
Acute leukemia	Birth–adolescence; most common between 2 and 3 y	Antalgic	Joint pain or swelling, bruising, bleeding, hepatosplenomegaly, fever, and lethargy	Radiographs rarely show paraphyseal, lucent metaphyseal bands. Anemia, thrombocytopenia, elevated ESR, and high or low WBC. Bone marrow biopsy confirms diagnosis.
Neuroblastoma	Birth–10 y; Most present around 2 y	Antalgic	Bone pain, abdominal pain and swelling, fever, weight loss, subcutaneous nodules, orbital proptosis, and periorbital ecchymoses	Positive bone scan; increased levels of urine vanillylmandelic acid
Legg-Calve-Perthes disease	4–10 y	Trendelenburg or antalgic	Presents initially with a painless limp that becomes painful, then limits hip range of motion, especially adduction and rotation. If epiphysis collapses or fragments, there may be a leg length difference.	Radiographs may be normal early in the disease. Bone scan and MRI are diagnostic before radiographs (Figure 10-5).

Table 10-1. Common Causes of a Limp, continued

Cause	Common Age Range	Gait Pattern	Signs and Symptoms	Making the Diagnosis
Discoid lateral meniscus	3–12 y	Antalgic	Activity-related knee pain, clicking, and swelling; tenderness at the lateral knee joint; rare cause of limp	MRI
Leg-length discrepancy[a]	Any age; depends on etiology.	Circumduction and steppage gait most common; Trendelenburg for some etiologies	Can be painful or painless, depending on etiology. Patient's iliac crests not level when palpated from behind.	Measure leg length from the ASIS to the medial malleolus (accurate within 1 cm). Confirm and quantify on a standing plain radiograph with ruler (Figure 10-6). History and associated signs/symptoms usually suggest etiology.
Slipped capital femoral epiphysis	9–15 y	Trendelenburg or antalgic	Painful, limited hip range of motion	Radiographs (AP pelvis and frog lateral views [see Chapter 20])
Overuse syndromes (Osgood-Schlatter, Sever, patellofemoral pain)	Physically active children between 9 and 18 y	Antalgic	Activity-related pain, point tenderness, improves with rest	Clinical diagnosis. Imaging sometimes necessary to rule out other etiologies.
Osteochondritis dissecans of knee	9–18 y	Antalgic	Activity-related pain; may have swelling and reduced range of motion.	Radiographs (seen best on notch [tunnel] view); MRI to evaluate the stability of the lesion

WBC, white blood cell; ESR, erythrocyte sedimentation rate; CRP, C-reactive protein; MRI, magnetic resonance imaging; CPK, creatine phosphokinase; EMG, electromyogram; AP, anteroposterior; ANA, antinuclear antibody; RBC, red blood cell; ASIS, anterior superior iliac spine.

[a] Because of idiopathic hemihypertrophy, prior fracture with resulting overgrowth or undergrowth of bone, prior infection, neoplasm, metabolic disorders, or congenital anomalies.

Box 10-1. Causes of Limping in Children

Toddler (1–3 y)
Septic arthritis/osteomyelitis/myositis
Diskitis (spine)
Transient synovitis of the hip
Toddler fracture
Neuromuscular disease
Developmental dysplasia of the hip
Inflammatory disorders
Neoplasia (Ewing sarcoma, osteoid osteoma)
Metastatic disease (neuroblastoma, leukemia)

Child (4–10 y)
Transient synovitis of the hip
Perthes (Legg-Calve-Perthes disease)
Discoid meniscus
Leg-length discrepancy

Adolescent (11–16 y)
Slipped capital femoral epiphysis
Overuse syndromes
Developmental dysplasia of the hip
Osteochondritis dissecans

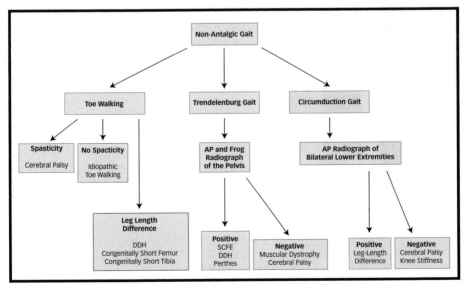

Figure 10-1. Algorithm for evaluating non-antalgic gait.

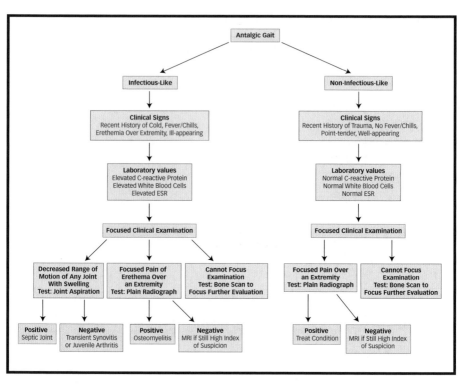

Figure 10-2. Algorithm for evaluating antalgic gait.

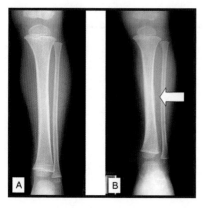

Figure 10-3. Anteroposterior radiographs of the tibia of a 2-year-old with a limp. A, Initial radiographs appear normal. B, Radiographs 4 weeks later demonstrate periosteal reaction (arrow).

TRENDELENBURG GAIT (ABDUCTOR LURCH)

- Results from weak hip abductors.
  - Hip abductors are responsible for maintaining a level pelvis during single limb stance.
  - Weakness causes the unsupported (contralateral) hip to drop during single limb stance (positive Trendelenburg sign [see Figure 4-24]).
  - To compensate, body weight is shifted over the weak hip during stance phase to lateralize the center of gravity.

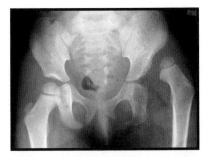

Figure 10-4. Anteroposterior radiograph of a 3-year-old's pelvis. The child was limping and the mothers complaint was a leg-length difference. Note the dislocated left hip.

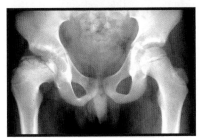

Figure 10-5. Anteroposterior radiograph of the pelvis of a 13-year-old boy. Right hip shows long-term changes seen in Legg-Calve-Perthes disease after remodeling with a loss of the round nature of the femoral head.

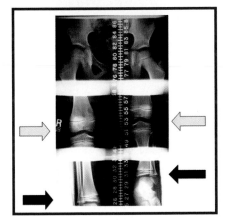

Figure 10-6. Anteroposterior standing scanogram radiograph of both lower extremities in an 8-year-old girl demonstrating left leg significantly shorter than right.

- Commonly seen in hip disorders or neuromuscular disease (eg, Legg-Calve-Perthes disease, developmental dysplasia of the hip, congenital coxa vara, slipped capital femoral epiphysis).

CIRCUMDUCTION

- Commonly results from a structural or functional limb-length inequality, but may also be seen as a pain avoidance pattern (ie, foot pain)
- During swing phase, the longer limb circumducts (swings around and to the side) to clear the ground and move forward.
- May be accompanied by vaulting of the short extremity, which involves early heel rise during stance phase to assist with clearance of the long side in swing phase.

STEPPAGE GAIT

- Increased hip and knee flexion during swing phase to help promote adequate clearance of the foot and ankle
- May be seen with limb-length inequality or weakness of the ankle dorsiflexors.

TOE WALKING (EQUINUS GAIT)

- Initial contact occurs at the forefoot instead of the heel.
- Caused by heel-cord contracture or muscle imbalance about the ankle
- Common causes include cerebral palsy, clubfoot deformity, idiopathic heel-cord contracture, or habitual toe walking.

Bibliography

Alexander JE, FitzRandolph RL, McConnell JR. The limping child. *Curr Probl Diagn Radiol.* 1987;16:229–270

Aronsson DD, Loder RT, Breur GJ, Weinstein SL. Slipped capital femoral epiphysis: current concepts. *J Am Acad Orthop Surg.* 2006;14:666–679

Barkin RM, Barkin SZ, Barkin AZ. The limping child. *J Emerg Med.* 2000;18:331–339

Beck RJ, Andriacchi TP, Kuo KN, Fermier RW, Galante JO. Changes in the gait patterns of growing children. *J Bone Joint Surg Am.* 1981;63:1452–1457

Bohne WH. Tarsal coalition. *Curr Opin Pediatr.* 2001;13:29–35

Cassas KJ, Cassettari-Wayhs A. Childhood and adolescent sports-related overuse injuries. *Am Fam Physician.* 2006;73:1014–1022

Crawford AH, Kucharzyk DW, Ruda R, Smitherman HC Jr. Diskitis in children. *Clin Orthop Relat Res.* 1991; 266:70–79

Dabney KW, Lipton G. Evaluation of limp in children. *Curr Opin Pediatr.* 1995;7:88–94

Davidson D, Letts M, Glasgow R. Discoid meniscus in children: treatment and outcome. *Can J Surg.* 2003;46:350–358

De Boeck H, Vorlat P. Limping in childhood. *Acta Orthop Belg.* 2003;69:301–310

Early SD, Kay RM, Tolo VT. Childhood diskitis. *J Am Acad Orthop Surg.* 2003;11:413–420

Flynn JM, Widmann RF. The limping child: evaluation and diagnosis. *J Am Acad Orthop Surg.* 2001;9:89–98

Grzegorzewski A, Synder M, Kozlowski P, Szymczak W, Bowen RJ. Leg length discrepancy in Legg-Calve-Perthes disease. *J Pediatr Orthop.* 2005;25:206–209

Guidera KJ, Helal AA, Zuern KA. Management of pediatric limb length inequality. *Adv Pediatr.* 1995;42:501–543

Habata T, Uematsu K, Kasanami R, et al. Long-term clinical and radiographic follow-up of total resection for discoid lateral meniscus. *Arthroscopy.* 2006;22:1339–1343

Hart JJ. Transient synovitis of the hip in children. *Am Fam Physician.* 1996;54:1587–1591, 1595–1596

Herring JA, Kim HT, Browne R. Legg-Calve-Perthes disease. Part I: classification of radiographs with use of the modified lateral pillar and Stulberg classifications. *J Bone Joint Surg Am.* 2004;86-A:2103–2120

Herring JA, Kim HT, Browne R. Legg-Calve-Perthes disease. Part II: prospective multicenter study of the effect of treatment on outcome. *J Bone Joint Surg Am.* 2004;86-A:2121–2134

Herring T, ed. *Tachdjian's Pediatric Orthopaedics.* Philadelphia, PA: Saunders; 2002:83–94

John SD, Moorthy CS, Swischuk LE. Expanding the concept of the toddler's fracture. *Radiographics.* 1997;17:367–376

Kalogrianitis S, Tan CK, Kemp GJ, Bass A, Bruce C. Does unstable slipped capital femoral epiphysis require urgent stabilization? *J Pediatr Orthop B.* 2007;16:6–9

Karabouta Z, Bisbinas I, Davidson A, Goldsworthy LL. Discitis in toddlers: a case series and review. *Acta Paediatr.* 2005;94:1516–1518

Karol LA. Surgical management of the lower extremity in ambulatory children with cerebral palsy. *J Am Acad Orthop Surg.* 2004;12:196–203

Kaufman KR, Miller LS, Sutherland DH. Gait asymmetry in patients with limb-length inequality. *J Pediatr Orthop.* 1996;16:144–150

Kaweblum M, Lehman WB, Bash J, Grant AD, Strongwater A. Diagnosis of osteoid osteoma in the child. *Orthop Rev.* 1993;22:1305–1313

Kocher MS, Klingele K, Rassman SO. Meniscal disorders: normal, discoid, and cysts. *Orthop Clin North Am.* 2003;34:329–340

Kocher MS, Zurakowski D, Kasser JR. Differentiating between septic arthritis and transient synovitis of the hip in children: an evidence-based clinical prediction algorithm. *J Bone Joint Surg Am.* 1999;81:1662–1670

Leet AI, Skaggs DL. Evaluation of the acutely limping child. *Am Fam Physician.* 2000;61:1011–1018

Lehmann CL, Arons RR, Loder RT, Vitale MG. The epidemiology of slipped capital femoral epiphysis: an update. *J Pediatr Orthop.* 2006;26:286–290

Leung AK, Lemay JF. The limping child. *J Pediatr Health Care.* 2004;18:219–223

MacEwen GD, Dehne R. The limping child. *Pediatr Rev.* 1991;12:268–274

Morresy R, Weinstein S. *Lovell and Winter's Pediatric Orthopaedics.* 5th ed. Philadelphia, PA: Lippincott, Williams, & Wilkins; 2001

Norlin R, Odenrick P, Sandlund B. Development of gait in the normal child. *J Pediatr Orthop.* 1981;1:261–266

Oudjhane K, Newman B, Oh KS, Young LW, Girdany BR. Occult fractures in preschool children. *J Trauma.* 1988;28:858–860

Perttunen JR, Anttila E, Sodergard J, Merikanto J, Komi PV. Gait asymmetry in patients with limb length discrepancy. *Scand J Med Sci Sports.* 2004;14:49–56

Phillips WA. The child with a limp. *Orthop Clin North Am.* 1987;18:489–501

Renshaw TS. The child who has a limp. *Pediatr Rev.* 1995;16:458–465

Richards BS. The limping child. In: Richards BS, ed. *Orthopaedic Knowledge Update Pediatrics.* Rosemont, IL: American Academy of Orthopaedic Surgeons; 1996:3–9

Ring D, Johnston CE II, Wenger DR. Pyogenic infectious spondylitis in children: the convergence of discitis and osteomyelitis. *J Pediatr Orthop.* 1995;15:652–660

Rogalsky RJ, Black GB, Reed MH. Orthopaedic manifestations of leukemia in children. *J Bone Joint Surg Am.* 1986;68:494–501

Romano CL, Frigo C, Randelli G, Pedotti A. Analysis of the gait of adults who had residua of congenital dysplasia of the hip. *J Bone Joint Surg Am.* 1996;78:1468–1479

Rouleau PA, Wenger DE. Radiologic evaluation of metastatic bone disease. In: Menendez LR, ed. *Orthopaedic Knowledge Update Musculoskeletal Tumors.* Rosemont, IL: American Academy of Orthopaedic Surgeons; 2002: 313–322

Sales de Gauzy J, Mansat C, Darodes PH, Cahuzac JP. Natural course of osteochondritis dissecans in children. *J Pediatr Orthop B.* 1999;8:26–28

Simon S, Whiffen J, Shapiro F. Leg-length discrepancies in monoarticular and pauciarticular juvenile rheumatoid arthritis. *J Bone Joint Surg Am.* 1981;63:209–215

Singer JI. The cause of gait disturbance in 425 pediatric patients. *Pediatr Emerg Care.* 1985;1:7–10

Song KM, Halliday S, Reilly C, Keezel W. Gait abnormalities following slipped capital femoral epiphysis. *J Pediatr Orthop.* 2004;24:148–155

Song KM, Halliday SE, Little DG. The effect of limb-length discrepancy on gait. *J Bone Joint Surg Am.* 1997;79:1690–1698

Storer SK, Skaggs DL. Developmental dysplasia of the hip. *Am Fam Physician.* 2006;74:1310–1316

Sutherland DH, Olshen R, Cooper L, Woo SL. The development of mature gait. *J Bone Joint Surg Am.* 1980;62:336–353

Thompson JD. Orthopedic aspects of cerebral palsy. *Curr Opin Pediatr.* 1994;6:94–98

Tosi L. Pediatric orthopaedic infections. In: Richards BS, ed. *Orthopaedic Knowledge Update Pediatrics.* Rosemont, IL: American Academy of Orthopaedic Surgeons; 1996:35–46

Wall E, Von Stein D. Juvenile osteochondritis dissecans. *Orthop Clin North Am.* 2003;34:341–353

Waters E. Toxic synovitis of the hip in children. *Nurse Pract.* 1995;20:44–46

Weinstein SL. Natural history and treatment outcomes of childhood hip disorders. *Clin Orthop Relat Res.* 1997;344:227–242

Westhoff B, Petermann A, Hirsch MA, Willers R, Krauspe R. Computerized gait analysis in Legg-Calve-Perthes disease—analysis of the frontal plane. *Gait Posture.* 2006;24:196–202

Youm T, Chen AL. Discoid lateral meniscus: evaluation and treatment. *Am J Orthop.* 2004;33:234–238

Part 5: Spinal Deformities

CHAPTER 11

Idiopathic Scoliosis

Overview

- Common in children and adolescents
- Prevalence is 2% to 3% in the general population.
- The etiology is unknown.
- Genetic factors increase the risk of developing idiopathic scoliosis.
  — Approximately 11.1% of patients have first-degree relatives with idiopathic scoliosis.
  — Frequency of idiopathic scoliosis in both monozygotic twins is 73% to 92%, compared with 36% to 63% in both dizygotic twins.
- Nongenetic factors may also contribute to development of idiopathic scoliosis.
  — Abnormalities of vertebral growth (as curve magnitude increases, vertebral wedging occurs), equilibrium, and vestibular function have been noted, but it is unclear whether these are primary or secondary.
  — Melatonin and the pineal gland may also play a role.
- Female-male prevalence
  — 1:1 for small curves of approximately 10 degrees
  — 5:1 for curves between 10 and 20 degrees
  — 10:1 for curves greater than 30 degrees

DIFFERENTIAL DIAGNOSIS

- The typical patient with *idiopathic scoliosis* is an adolescent female between 10 and 16 years of age with a thoracic curve having an apex to the right. Any deviation from this typical pattern warrants an investigation for an overt treatable underlying cause.
- When to suspect *non-idiopathic scoliosis*
  — Patients 10 years and younger have a higher incidence of non-idiopathic scoliosis than adolescent patients.
  — Atypical curve pattern (eg, thoracic curves with an apex to the left have a higher incidence of underlying neurologic cause)
  — Sacrum and pelvis included within the curve, resulting in pelvic obliquity
  — Associated kyphosis (May suggest a non-idiopathic cause such as neurofibromatosis.)
  — Significant pain (Idiopathic scoliosis is typically painless.)
  — Coexisting medical condition with a known association with scoliosis (eg, neurofibromatosis, connective tissue disorders, congenital heart disease)

- *Functional (nonstructural) scoliosis*
  - Most commonly caused by *limb-length discrepancy* or *muscle spasm* (eg, because of herniated intervertebral disc, spondylolysis/spondylolisthesis, discitis, tumor)
  - Functional curves are mild without any bony abnormalities.
  - Symptoms of underlying condition are present.
  - Curve corrects when the underlying problem is resolved.

MAKING THE DIAGNOSIS

- Diagnosis is based on history, physical examination, and radiographs.
- *Physical examination*
  - With the patient standing, inspect the shoulders, scapulae, ribs, and waist for asymmetry.
  - Palpate the top of the iliac crests, comparing height of right to left. If this reveals a limb-length discrepancy (which may cause nonstructural scoliosis), the hips and pelvis are made level by placing blocks (or office magazines) under the shorter limb. Once the pelvis is level, inspect the shoulders, scapulae, ribs, and waist for asymmetry (Figure 11-1).
- Perform the *Adams forward bend test* (Figure 11-2) by asking the patient to bend forward at the waist with knees straight and palms together. Scoliosis is associated with vertebral rotation. Vertebral rotation creates paraspinous asymmetry visible on the forward bend test.

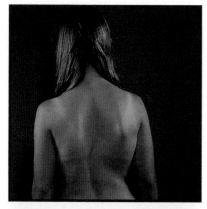

Figure 11-1. The first step in the physical examination of a patient with suspected scoliosis is inspection of the back. In this patient, the pelvis is level but the right hip appears elevated because of the waist asymmetry caused by scoliosis. The right scapula is more prominent than the left and the right shoulder is slightly elevated compared with the left.

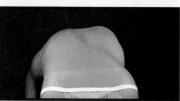

Figure 11-2. Next have the patient perform the Adams forward bend test. Vertebral rotation associated with scoliosis results in paraspinous rib prominence on the right.

- If asymmetry is present on Adams forward bend test, *full-length standing anteroposterior and lateral radiographs* should be obtained to evaluate and quantify the apparent scoliosis.
- The *Cobb technique* documents curve magnitude (Figure 11-3). Curves measuring 10 degrees or less are normal and should not be labeled as scoliosis.
- All patients with evidence of scoliosis should have a *simple neurologic examination* consisting of strength testing, deep tendon reflexes, and a check for upper motor neuron signs, including clonus at the ankles and the Babinski sign.
- *Magnetic resonance imaging (MRI) of the spinal cord* is indicated if there are any neurologic symptoms or physical examination findings.

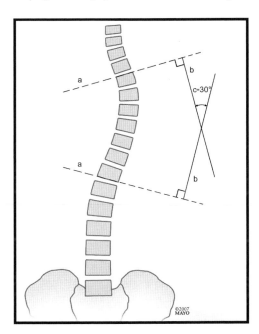

Figure 11-3. The standard method for measuring scoliosis curve magnitude is referred to as the Cobb technique. Lines are drawn along the endplates of the most tilted vertebrae (a). In a patient with a mild curvature, the endplate lines are almost parallel and do not intersect on the radiographic film, so a second pair of lines (b) are drawn perpendicular to the endplate lines. The angle created by the intersection of perpendicular lines (b) is the curve magnitude (c).

Adolescent Idiopathic Scoliosis

INTRODUCTION/ETIOLOGY/EPIDEMIOLOGY

- Onset from 11 years of age until skeletal maturity
- Most common type, representing approximately 89% of idiopathic scoliosis
- More common in females, especially curves greater than 30 degrees (10:1 female-male prevalence)
- Thoracic curves, apex to the right are most common.
- Curves with apex to the left are more likely to have an underlying neurologic cause.
- Primary risk factors for curve progression
  — Female sex
  — Skeletal immaturity
  — Large curve magnitude at presentation
  — Positive family history

- The relationship between patient age, curve magnitude, and the likelihood of curve progression has been nicely demonstrated (Table 11-1).

SIGNS AND SYMPTOMS

- Shoulder, waistline, or trunk asymmetry may be noted by patient or parent.
- Initial diagnosis is often made on annual physical examination (Box 11-1).
- Skeletally immature patients are asymptomatic, even when scoliosis is severe.

Table 11-1. Probability of Curve Progression: The Relationship Between Curve Magnitude and Age

Curve Magnitude (degrees)	Age in Years		
	10–12	13–15	>16
<19	25%	10%	0%
20–29	60%	40%	10%
30–59	90%	70%	30%
>59	100%	90%	70%

Scoliosis Research Society Prevalence and Natural History Committee Report

Box 11-1. Screening for Scoliosis

- Adolescent female patients 10 to 14 years of age should be evaluated for scoliosis as part of the general physical examination.
- School screening programs have been instituted in many areas but are no longer required in most states as recommended by the US Preventive Services Task Force.
  —School screening typically results in a referral rate of approximately 2 to 3 per 100 children screened, considerably higher than the 0.5% prevalence of scoliosis greater than 20 degrees that may benefit from active treatment.

TREATMENT

- There appears to be increasing intolerance of the cosmetic deformity associated with scoliosis.
- The goal of the treating physician is to identify those patients at risk of curve progression and in those patients *do as little as possible* but *as much as necessary* to alter the natural history and prevent the undesirable consequence of untreated disease.
- *Observation*
  — If spinal curvature measures less than 10 degrees, no scheduled follow-up is necessary.
  — Skeletally immature patients with mild curve magnitude between 10 and 25 degrees require monitoring with clinical evaluation and radiograph.
    ▪ In young patients with significant growth remaining and a curvature approaching 25 degrees, the follow-up interval is 4 months.
    ▪ In older patients and those with a curve closer to 10 degrees, the follow up interval is 6 to 12 months.

- *Bracing*
  — Skeletally immature patients with moderate curve magnitude between 25 and approximately 40 degrees require brace treatment (Figure 11-4 a, b).
  — Studies have demonstrated that brace treatment can change the natural history of idiopathic scoliosis, reducing the likelihood of progression when compared with no treatment.
  — The goal of brace treatment is to prevent progression; there is little evidence that bracing corrects the curvature.
  — Controversy exists regarding brace design, the optimal number of hours a brace should be worn each day, and how long the brace should be worn until it may be discontinued.
  — Compelling evidence suggests a dose-related brace effect. The more hours a brace is worn, the greater the beneficial effect.
  — Bracing is typically continued until skeletal maturity, which is confirmed by lack of growth documented on serial height measurements, or radiographic evidence.
  — A successful bracing program includes a skilled orthotist (Figure 11-5) and an empathetic health care professional to support patients and their families through the periodic brace adjustments necessitated by growth and the psychosocial aspects of brace treatment.

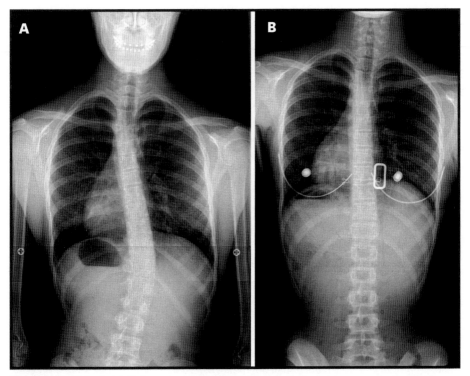

Figure 11-4. This skeletally immature patient has documented curve progression to 27 degrees (A). In the scoliosis brace, her flexible curvature corrects completely (B). Such an excellent initial response to brace treatment is associated with a favorable prognosis that curve progression and surgery can be prevented.

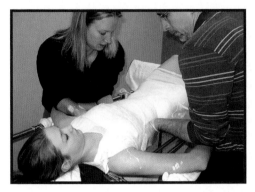

Figure 11-5. A skilled orthotist and assistant shape plaster around the torso of a scoliosis patient to create a mold for a custom brace. The brace applies corrective force to the spine through the ribs and paraspinous muscles. A seamless garment is worn beneath the brace, which is then worn beneath the patient's clothes.

— Flexibility of brace wear hours is important to allow participation in sports or other extracurricular activities, maintain good mental health, and improve patient compliance with the bracing program.

- *Other nonoperative treatments*
  — There is no high-level medical evidence that treatments such as physical therapy, electrical stimulation, or chiropractic manipulation change the natural history of scoliosis when compared with no treatment at all.
- *Surgical treatment*
  — Recommended for patients with severe curve magnitude (greater than 45–50 degrees). At 45 to 50 degrees, brace treatment is no longer effective, and the (untreated) natural history is associated with poor outcome as a result of cardiopulmonary problems, back pain, and dissatisfaction with appearance or self-image.
  — The rationale for surgery is to achieve a stable, well-balanced, painless spine while eliminating the risk of future progression and its associated consequences.
  — Surgery involves metal implants to correct the deformity as well as arthrodesis or fusion of the instrumented vertebrae to permanently preserve the correction. "Fusionless" surgical treatment methods are currently undergoing investigation.

EXPECTED OUTCOMES/PROGNOSIS

- In a 38-year follow-up study of 130 patients with untreated idiopathic scoliosis, the risk of mortality associated with idiopathic scoliosis approached that of the general population.
- Untreated patients with idiopathic scoliosis at the University of Iowa reported an increased incidence in back pain compared with a control group that did not have scoliosis (37% of patients complained of constant backache). They also reported an increase in psychological and cosmetic concerns.
- As curve magnitude increases, vital lung capacity and force expiratory volume decrease.
- A measurable decrease in pulmonary function occurs for thoracic curves in the 50- to 60-degree range, with a reduction of approximately 20% from normal as curve magnitude approaches 100 degrees.

WHEN TO REFER

- There are no uniform and simple referral guidelines that apply to all scoliosis patients of all ages.
- As a general rule, patients with curves less than 20 degrees may be observed by a primary care physician.
- Refer the following to a pediatric orthopaedic specialist with expertise in caring for spine deformities:
  — Patients with curves greater than 20 degrees
    - This recommendation is based on the fact that virtually all scoliosis patients who benefit from active treatment have a curve magnitude greater than 20 degrees.
  — Any patient with neurologic signs or symptoms
  — Patients who present with a *non-classic idiopathic scoliosis profile* (eg, adolescent female with a painless apex right thoracic curve).
- Consider the decision to refer in context of the physician's experience, clinical practice setting, and circumstances.
- Referral is also appropriate for patients with scoliosis presenting with findings that are outside a primary care physician's ability to comfortably evaluate and treat.

RELEVANT *INTERNATIONAL CLASSIFICATION OF DISEASES, NINTH REVISION, CLINICAL MODIFICATION (ICD-9-CM)* CODE

- **737.30**   Scoliosis, idiopathic

Infantile Idiopathic Scoliosis

INTRODUCTION/ETIOLOGY/EPIDEMIOLOGY

- Onset at 3 years or younger
- Represents only 1% of idiopathic scoliosis.
- Male predominance of 3:2
- Up to 90% of infantile curves resolve spontaneously, suggesting a fetal packing etiology.
- Occasionally, infantile scoliosis results from a spinal abnormality such as Chiari malformation or tumor.

SIGNS AND SYMPTOMS

- Painless deformity
- Curve apex is to the left in approximately 90% of patients.
- Often associated with plagiocephaly or hip dysplasia

TREATMENT

- *Observation*
  — For curves less than 20 degrees
- *Bracing*
  — For curves greater than 25 degrees
- *Surgical treatment*
  — Recommended for curves greater than 40 degrees

EXPECTED OUTCOMES/PROGNOSIS

- Up to 90% of infantile curves resolve spontaneously.
- Those who progress are a treatment challenge with the potential to sustain permanent deformity and pulmonary compromise. These patients tend to have an underlying spinal abnormality as the cause of the scoliosis.

WHEN TO REFER

- Refer all infants with curves greater than 20 degrees to an orthopaedic specialist.

RELEVANT *ICD-9-CM* CODES

- **737.31**   Scoliosis, idiopathic, infantile, progressing
- **737.32**   Scoliosis, idiopathic, infantile, resolving

Juvenile Idiopathic Scoliosis

INTRODUCTION/ETIOLOGY/EPIDEMIOLOGY

- Onset from 4 to 10 years of age
- Represents 10% of idiopathic scoliosis.
- Male predominance (1.6:1) in patients younger than 6 years
- Female predominance (2.7:1) in patients 6 to 10 years of age
- Twenty percent to 25% of curves greater than 20 degrees are associated with a spinal abnormality such as Chiari malformation or tumor.

SIGNS AND SYMPTOMS

- Painless deformity
- In patients younger than 6 years, left-sided curves predominate.
- In patients 6 to 10 years of age, right-sided curves predominate.

TREATMENT

- *Observation*
  — If the curve is mild (less than 20 degrees), typical, not progressive, and simple neurologic evaluation is unremarkable, observation is appropriate.
  — If the curve progresses beyond 20 degrees, MRI of the entire spine is indicated to evaluate for possible central neural axis abnormality.
- *Bracing*
  — Recommended for curves greater than 20 degrees
- *Surgical treatment*
  — Recommended for curves greater than 40 degrees

EXPECTED OUTCOMES/PROGNOSIS

- Juvenile scoliosis is *rarely self-limiting* and progresses at a rate of 1 to 3 degrees per year until age 10 years, when more rapid progression frequently occurs.

WHEN TO REFER

- Refer all patients with juvenile idiopathic scoliosis to an orthopaedic specialist.

RELEVANT *ICD-9-CM* CODE

- **737.30** Scoliosis, idiopathic

Congenital Scoliosis

INTRODUCTION/ETIOLOGY/EPIDEMIOLOGY

- Congenital scoliosis is a failure of vertebrae to develop normally during embryogenesis (Figure 11-7).
  — Failure of formation results in a hemivertebrae.
  — Failure of the column to fully segment leads to a bar or fusion between vertebrae, causing a tether on one side of the spine resulting in asymmetric growth.
- Congenital scoliosis occurs in many different patterns and combinations.

SIGNS AND SYMPTOMS

- Painless spinal asymmetry
- The patient with congenital scoliosis has a significant incidence of congenital cardiac (12%) and genitourinary (20%) abnormalities.
- There is a higher incidence of spinal cord abnormality with congenital scoliosis than with idiopathic scoliosis.

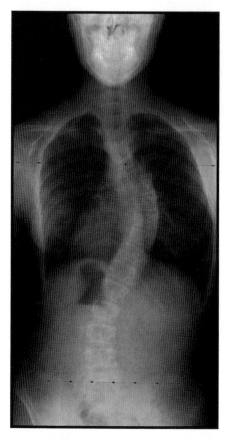

Figure 11-7. This patient has a thoracic congenital hemivertebrae (failure of formation) on the left. Fused ribs on the right opposite the hemivertebrae provide a clue to the presence of a contralateral bar between vertebrae (failure of segmentation). This patient also has failure of segmentation between several vertebrae in the lumbar spine.

MAKING THE DIAGNOSIS

- Diagnosis is based on history, physical examination, and radiographs (see "Making the Diagnosis" on page 114).
- *Radiographs* demonstrate hemivertebrae or fusions.
- *Magnetic resonance imaging of the spinal cord* is indicated if there are any neurologic signs or symptoms.
- *Renal ultrasound* should be preformed on diagnosis to evaluate for associated genitourinary abnormalities.
- *Echocardiogram* is necessary only for abnormalities on ausculatory examination.

TREATMENT

- Treatment consists of observation or surgery.
- Bracing is rarely effective for congenital scoliosis; however, a brace may be used to treat a compensatory curve in the adjacent normal spine.
- Treatment choice depends on the rate of progression, curve location, and curve pattern.
- Observation includes radiographs every 3 months during the first 3 years of life and during the pubertal growth spurt to evaluate rate of progression.

- Surgical indications
  — Curves due to unilateral bars
  — Curves approaching 40 degrees in a skeletally immature patient
  — Curves greater than 50 degrees in a skeletally mature patient

EXPECTED OUTCOMES/PROGNOSIS

- Like idiopathic scoliosis, congenital scoliosis is at greatest risk of progression during adolescent growth spurt.
- A hemivertebrae (extra growth) paired with a contralateral bar (reduced growth) is a pattern that always causes progressive scoliosis.
- Other patterns are not predictable and may never progress, requiring only periodic surveillance until skeletal maturity.

WHEN TO REFER

- Refer all patients with congenital scoliosis approaching 20 degrees to a pediatric orthopaedic surgeon.

RELEVANT ICD-9-CM CODE

- **754.2**   Scoliosis, congenital

Neuromuscular Scoliosis

INTRODUCTION/ETIOLOGY/EPIDEMIOLOGY

- Neuromuscular scoliosis is caused by a wide variety of neuromuscular disorders including cerebral palsy, myelodysplasia, muscular dystrophy, spinal muscle atrophy, and Friedreich ataxia, among others.

SIGNS AND SYMPTOMS

- Neuromuscular scoliosis appears as a long, sweeping, C-shaped curve.
- In contrast with idiopathic scoliosis, in which the sacrum and pelvis are not part of the curvature, *in neuromuscular scoliosis the sacrum and pelvis are frequently included within the curve,* resulting in pelvic obliquity (Figure 11-8).

TREATMENT

- *Nonoperative treatment*
  — Not effective at preventing scoliosis progression
  — Primary goal of nonoperative treatment is to preserve function.
  — Two main treatment options are wheelchair modification and bracing.
  — Brace treatment is a reasonable option if the physician and parent have shared, realistic expectations and are prepared for potential problems.

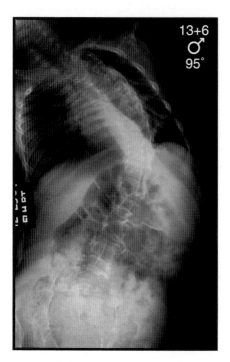

Figure 11-8. The long, sweeping C shape of neuromuscular scoliosis.

- *Surgical treatment*
  — Indications for surgical treatment vary depending on the underlying neuromuscular diagnosis, curve magnitude, coexisting medical conditions, and other factors.
  — Patients with Duchenne muscular dystrophy
    - Tend to develop a rapidly progressive curvature in early adolescence, which leads to restrictive lung disease, increasing the risk of pulmonary complications following surgery.
    - Indications for surgery include a progressive curvature above 30 degrees after patients become non-ambulatory.
  — Patients with cerebral palsy
    - Indications for surgery include curve progression above 40 degrees associated with pelvic obliquity, sitting difficulty, or truncal imbalance.

EXPECTED OUTCOMES/PROGNOSIS

- As in idiopathic and congenital scoliosis, the adolescent growth period is the time during which the risk of curve progression is greatest.
- Natural history of scoliosis is also influenced by the underlying neuromuscular disorder.
  - Scoliosis associated with progressive disorders such as muscular dystrophy follows a relentlessly progressive course.
- Across all diagnoses, neuromuscular scoliosis patients have notable functional problems.
  - Curve progression resulting in pelvic obliquity increases the difficulty of sitting. Comfortable, balanced sitting is important because the child may be non-ambulatory and may depend on comfortable sitting posture for mobility and function.
  - Progressive neuromuscular scoliosis causes significant trunk imbalance, which requires use of one or both upper extremities to support sitting, limiting the functional use of the arms.
- Medical problems associated with the underlying neuromuscular diagnosis may complicate scoliosis management—gastroesophageal reflux, malnutrition, restrictive lung disease, and cardiomyopathy.

WHEN TO REFER

- Refer all patients with neuromuscular scoliosis to an orthopaedic surgeon for management.

RELEVANT *ICD-9-CM* CODE

- **737.43**   Scoliosis associated with neuromuscular conditions

CHAPTER 12

Kyphosis

Introduction/Etiology/Epidemiology

- May be postural or structural.
- *Postural roundback* deformity of the thoracic or thoracolumbar spine is a common cause of kyphosis among teens and preteens.
  — Usually associated with a growth spurt
  — Considered a normal variant
- Structural kyphosis in otherwise healthy teens and preteens is most commonly caused by *Scheuermann disorder*. This classically involves the thoracic spine but may also occur in the thoracolumbar or lumbar spine.
- Unlike scoliosis, kyphosis is not associated with rotational abnormality.

Signs and Symptoms

- Postural roundback
  — May be associated with activity-related back pain or pain after prolonged sitting, but more frequently the complaint is purely cosmetic.
- Scheuermann kyphosis
  — More frequently causes pain.
  — There is often a family history of similar deformity.

Differential Diagnosis (Figure 12-1)

- Postural roundback
  — Kyphosis is flexible and can be consciously corrected.
  — Forward bending demonstrates a smooth hump.
- Scheuermann kyphosis
  — Kyphosis cannot be consciously corrected.
  — Forward bending demonstrates angular hump.

Making the Diagnosis

- Postural roundback
  — Diagnosis is based on physical examination.
  — Radiographs are normal.

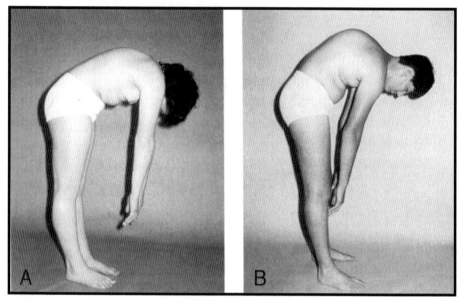

Figure 12-1. Adams forward bend test. Normal spine profiled (A). Angulated spine profile seen in a patient with Scheuermann disorder (B). Reproduced from Staheli L (ed): *Pediatric Orthopaedic Secrets*. Philadelphia, PA: Hanley & Belfus, Inc; 1998: 286, with permission from Elsevier.

- Scheuermann kyphosis
  — Diagnosis is based on a standing lateral radiograph of the entire spine.
  — Radiographic findings (Figure 12-2)
    ▪ Greater than 40 degrees of kyphosis as measured by Cobb technique
    ▪ Characteristic vertebral body wedging (greater than 5 degrees in at least 3 vertebrae)
    ▪ Endplate abnormalities
    ▪ Schmorl nodes may be present.

Treatment

- Postural roundback
  — Physical therapy to strengthen postural muscles
  — Occasionally, a brace may be used.
- Scheuermann kyphosis
  — Bracing and physical therapy are recommended for moderate deformities.
  — Nonsteroidal anti-inflammatory drugs may also be used to manage pain.
  — Surgery is rarely indicated for Scheuermann kyphosis, but when the kyphosis is *severe* (greater then 80 degrees) and symptomatic, surgery is appropriate.

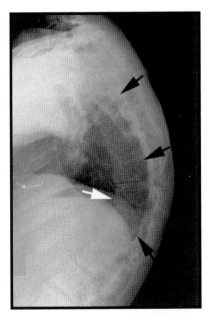

Figure 12-2. Lateral view of the thoracolumbar spine shows exaggerated thoracolumbar kyphosis (black arrows) associated with mild anterior wedging (white arrows) and end plate irregularity of the lower thoracic vertebral bodies. Reproduced with permission from Johnson TR, Steinbach LS (eds): *Essentials of Musculoskeletal Imaging.* Rosemont, IL: American Academy of Orthopaedic Surgeons; 2004.

Expected Outcomes/Prognosis

- Postural roundback
  - Pain responds to conservative treatment.
  - Does not lead to permanent deformity.
- Scheuermann kyphosis
  - Pain usually responds to conservative treatment.
  - Rarely, severe curves (greater than 100 degrees) can lead to cardiopulmonary compromise.

When to Refer

- Patients with kyphosis of more than 40 degrees should be referred to a pediatric orthopaedic specialist.

Relevant *International Classification of Diseases, Ninth Revision, Clinical Modification* Codes

- **737.10**   Kyphosis, postural
- **732.0**   Scheuermann kyphosis

CHAPTER 13

Spondylolysis and Spondylolisthesis

Introduction/Etiology/Epidemiology

- Spondylolysis and spondylolisthesis are common causes of low back pain in children and adolescents.
- *Spondylolysis* (common)
  - Acquired condition caused by repetitive hyperextension of the lumbar spine resulting in a stress reaction or fracture of the pars interarticularis
  - Rarely seen before age 5 years and then gradually increases to the adult prevalence of 4% to 6% by age 20 years.
  - More common in males than females (6:1)
  - More common in those participating in certain sports that require hyperextension and loading of the spine (eg, gymnastics, diving, football linemen, weight lifting, soccer, volleyball, softball pitching, wrestling)
- *Spondylolisthesis* (less common)
  - Forward translation (slip) of one vertebra on the adjacent caudal vertebra
  - Most frequently seen between L5 and S1, but can occur at more cranial levels.
  - Severity is graded by the amount of slip (Figure 13-1).
    - Grade 1: less than 25% of the vertebral body width
    - Grade 2: between 25% and 50%

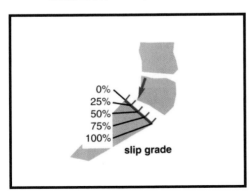

Figure 13-1. Severity is graded by the amount of vertebral slip. Reproduced with permission from Staheli LT. *Practice of Pediatric Orthopedics*. Philadelphia, PA: Lippincott Williams & Wilkins; 2001:165.

- Grade 3: between 50% and 75%
- Grade 4: more than 75%
- The term *spondyloptosis* is used when the posterior aspect of the cranial vertebral level "falls off" the anterior aspect of the inferior vertebral body.

Signs and Symptoms

- Activity-related back pain
  — Worse with extension; relieved with flexion
  — Occasional radiation to the buttock or posterior thigh
- Rarely, patients present with cauda equina syndrome (radicular symptoms, or sacral anesthesia and bowel and bladder dysfunction).
  — Usually associated with a high-grade slip (>50%) or dysplastic type (boxes 13-1 and 13-2)
- Paraspinal tenderness and spasms
- Limited lumbar mobility
  — Extension is limited by pain; as a result, patients often adopt a standing posture of slight lumbar flexion.
  — Forward flexion can be limited because of the extremely tight hamstrings but is not painful.
- Tight hamstrings
- Positive straight leg raise and weakness, particularly of the extensor hallucis longus and the peroneal muscles, may identify nerve root impingement, which can occur with spondylolysis but also may indicate disc herniation.

Differential Diagnosis

- Lumbar muscle strain
- Lumbar disc herniation

Box 13-1. Wilse-Newman Classification

I.	Dysplastic
II.	Isthmic
	IIA. Disruption of pars as a result of stress fracture
	IIB. Elongation of pars without disruption (repeated healed micro-fractures)
	IIC. Acute fracture through pars
III.	Degenerative
IV.	Traumatic
V.	Pathologic

Box 13-2. Marchetti-Bartolozzi Classification

Developmental

High dysplastic
    With lysis
    With elongation

Low dysplastic
    With lysis
    With elongation

Acquired

Traumatic
    Acute fracture
    Stress fracture

Post-surgery
    Direct surgery
    Indirect surgery

Pathologic
    Local pathology
    Systemic pathology

Degenerative
    Primary
    Secondary

Making the Diagnosis

- *Imaging is required for diagnosis.*
  - Radiographs
    - For a child or adolescent presenting with back pain, standing anteroposterior and lateral views of the lumbar spine and spot lateral radiograph of L5-S1
    - Additional images—standing right and left oblique views
    - In patients with spondylolysis, the pars defect has been described as having the appearance of a collar on a Scotty dog (Scotty dog sign) on the oblique view (Figure 13-2).
    - The spot lateral is the most sensitive view and is also important in quantifying the amount of forward displacement of L5 on S1 (Figure 13-3).
  - Single-photon emission computed tomography (SPECT) bone scan
    - Because radiographs often are normal, a SPECT scan of the lumbosacral spine is the best means of identifying a spondylolysis.
    - Shows increased activity at the level of the defect (Figure 13-4).
    - Contraindicated in the asymptomatic patient or in those with a long-standing radiographic pars defect.

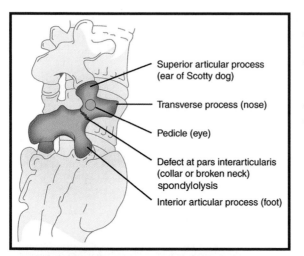

Superior articular process
(ear of Scotty dog)

Transverse process (nose)

Pedicle (eye)

Defect at pars interarticularis
(collar or broken neck)
spondylolysis

Interior articular process (foot)

Figure 13-2. Scotty dog with a collar. From Smith JA, Hu SS. Management of spondylolysis and spondylolisthesis in the pediatric and adolescent population. *Orthopedic Clinics of North America.* 1999;30(3): 487–499, ix. Copyright © 1999, Elsevier, with permission.

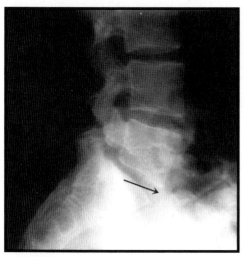

Figure 13-3. Spot lateral radiograph of a grade 2 to 3 spondylolisthesis at the lumbrosacral junction (arrow). Reproduced with permission from Griffin LY (ed): *Essentials of Musculoskeletal Care,* 3rd edition. Rosemont, IL: American Academy of Orthopaedic Surgeons; 2005.

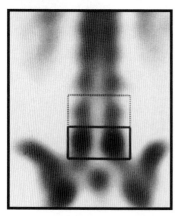

Figure 13-4. Pretreatment SPECT image of the lumbar spine demonstrating localization at L5 (solid rectangle). Courtesy of John F. Sarwark, MD.

—Thin-cut computed tomography (CT) scan of L5-S1
  ▪ More sensitive than radiographs
  ▪ Helpful in delineating bony morphology (Figure 13-5)
  ▪ Stress reactions of the pars identified by SPECT scans can be monitored with serial CT scans to assess healing of the lesions.
—Magnetic resonance imaging (MRI)
  ▪ Not as useful for imaging pars defects
  ▪ Helpful for evaluating nerve root compression, disc abnormalities, stenosis, or to rule out other sources of back pain such as tumor or infection in cases with higher grade slips
  ▪ *Do not order MRI for initial evaluation of spondylolysis.*

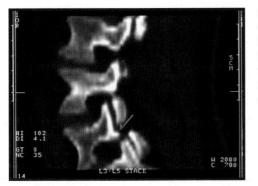

Figure 13-5. Sagittally reconstructed computed tomography scan of the lumbar spine shows a defect of the pars interarticularis on the left at L5. Reprinted with permission from eMedicine.com, 2008. Available at emedicine.medscape.com/article/95691-diagnosis.

Treatment

• The asymptomatic patient does not require treatment.
• Most children and adolescents presenting with symptomatic spondylolysis or spondylolisthesis can be managed nonoperatively.
• *Nonoperative treatment*
  —Acute spondylolysis (positive SPECT bone scan)
    ▪ The goal in cases of normal radiographs and a stress reaction of the pars diagnosed by SPECT or CT is to try to prevent progression to a fracture and fibrous union (spondylolysis).
    ▪ Activity modification is essential. Patients should avoid impact activities such as running and jumping and avoid lumbar hyperextension. This usually means complete rest from the sport.
    ▪ Full-time bracing (23 hours per day) with a lumbosacral orthosis (LSO) (Figure 13-6) in physiologic lordosis is recommended for a period of 6 to 12 weeks.
      ◆ Bracing with a rigid LSO leads to resolution of symptoms and may lead to healing of the defect.
      ◆ Early bracing has been shown to be superior to activity modification alone or bracing after a period of activity modification.
      ◆ The resolution of symptoms *or* repeat SPECT scan revealing diminution of uptake, can be used to monitor treatment and discontinue brace.

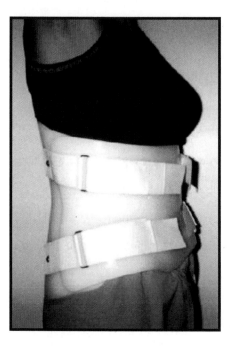

Figure 13-6. Custom-molded plastic lumbosacral orthosis. Reprinted with permission from eMedicine.com, 2008. Available at emedicine.medscape.com/article/95691-diagnosis.

- After bracing, patients undergo a supervised physical therapy program consisting of progressive abdominal, core, and back strengthening, and stretching of the lumbodorsal and hamstring muscles, followed by gradual resumption of sporting activities and close monitoring for symptom recurrence.
- Return to full participation in sports and activities is possible when pain is resolved, physical examination is normal, and core strength is adequate. This usually takes 2 to 4 months.

— Chronic spondylolysis (established nonunion of the pars interarticularis)
- Management focuses on pain reduction and return to function.
- Relative rest (avoiding only activities that cause pain), bracing as needed for symptom relief, and physical therapy to address any strength or flexibility deficits

— Spondylolisthesis (slip <50%)
- Management is the same as for symptomatic spondylolysis.

— Spondylolisthesis (slip >50%)
- Nonoperative management is rarely successful and referral of patients for surgical management is recommended.

- *Surgical treatment*
  — Reserved for
  - Slippage (listhesis) of greater than 50% on initial evaluation
  - The rare patient with uncontrolled pain after at least 6 months of nonoperative management
  — Direct surgical repair of the pars defect can be attempted using a variety of methods.

— The gold-standard surgery is a non-instrumented, in situ posterolateral fusion.
  ▪ For symptomatic spondylolysis or grade 1 or 2 slip, fusion is from L5 to S1.
  ▪ For higher grade slips, L4 is included.
— Reduction of the spondylolisthesis at surgery is controversial.
  ▪ The goal of reduction is to restore spinal pelvic balance, but there is a significant neurologic risk.
  ▪ Surgeons advocate a partial reduction, which mitigates the neurologic risk while allowing significant improvement in the patient's posture.
— Surgery results in high levels of patient satisfaction.
— Return to full participation in sports and activities after surgery usually takes 6 to 8 months.

Expected Outcomes/Prognosis

- The natural history of spondylolysis and low-grade spondylolisthesis is a benign course with infrequent episodes of low back pain and discomfort.
- After proper treatment, almost all patients are able to return to their previous level of sports and activities.
- There is no evidence that participation in sports increases the risk for slip progression.
- Less than 5% may have persistent low back pain or sports-related back pain.
- Early diagnosis and treatment may improve outcomes.

Prevention

- Maintaining adequate core strength and hamstring flexibility may reduce the risk for recurrent pain after treatment for spondylolysis or spondylolisthesis.
- During the preparticipation physical evaluation, the need for core strengthening or hamstring flexibility exercises can be assessed.

When to Refer

- Refer to a sports medicine physician.
  — Persistent low back pain
  — Sports-related back pain
  — Pain with hyperextension on physical exertion
  — Evidence of spondylolysis or listhesis on radiographs or SPECT scan
    ▪ Athletes with spondylolysis or low-grade spondylolisthesis can benefit from consultation with a sports medicine physician who can provide guidance on sports-specific activity modifications during the acute period, prescribe and monitor response to physical therapy, and provide clearance for full return to sport.
- Refer to an orthopaedic surgeon.
  — High-grade slips (>50%)
  — Persistent pain after 6 months of nonoperative management

Resources for Physicians and Families

- www.aaos.org
- MedLinePlus.gov

Relevant *International Classification of Diseases, Ninth Revision, Clinical Modification* Codes

- **756.11**   Spondylolysis, congenital
- **756.12**   Spondylolisthesis, congenital
- **738.4**   Spondylolysis, spondylolisthesis, acquired

Bibliography

Adams W. *Lectures on Pathology and Treatment of Lateral and Other Forms of Curvature of the Spine.* London, England: Churchill Livingston; 1865

Albanese M, Pizzutillo PD. Family study of spondylolysis and spondylolisthesis. *J Pediatr Orthop.* 1982;2:496–499

Anderson K, Sarwark JF, Conway JJ, Logue ES, Schafer MF. Quantitative assessment with SPECT imaging of stress injuries of the pars interarticularis and response to bracing. *J Pediatr Orthop.* 2000;20:28–33

Bellah RD, Summerville DA, Treves ST, Micheli LJ. Low-back pain in adolescent athletes: detection of stress injury to the pars interarticularis with SPECT. *Radiology.* 1991;180:509–512

Beutler WJ, Fredrickson BE, Murtland A, Sweeney CA, Grant WD, Baker D. The natural history of spondylolysis and spondylolisthesis: 45-year follow-up evaluation. *Spine (Phila Pa 1976).* 2003;28:1027–1035

Blanda J, Bethem D, Moats W, Lew M. Defects of pars interarticularis in athletes: a protocol for nonoperative treatment. *J Spinal Disord.* 1993;6:406–411

Boxall D, Bradford DS, Winter RB, Moe JH. Management of severe spondylolisthesis in children and adolescents. *J Bone Joint Surg Am.* 1979;61:479–495

Brooks HL, Azen SP, Gerberg E, Brooks R, Chan L. Scoliosis: a prospective epidemiological study. *J Bone Joint Surg Am.* 1975;57:968–972

Cobb J. Outline for the study of scoliosis. *Instr Course Lect.* 1948;5:261

Congeni J, McCulloch J, Swanson K. Lumbar spondylolysis. A study of natural progression in athletes. *Am J Sports Med.* 1997;25:248–253

El Rassi G, Takemitsu M, Woratanarat P, Shah SA. Lumbar spondylolysis in pediatric and adolescent soccer players. *Am J Sports Med.* 2005;33:1688–1693

Fernandez-Feliberti R, Flynn J, Ramirez N, Trautmann M, Algeria M. Effectiveness of TLSO bracing in the conservative treatment of idiopathic scoliosis. *J Pediatr Orthop.* 1995;15:176–181

Fredrickson BE, Baker D, McHolick WJ, Yuan HA, Lubicky JP. The natural history of spondylolysis and spondylolisthesis. *J Bone Joint Surg Am.* 1984;66:699–707

Harris IE, Weinstein SL. Long-term follow-up of patients with grade-III and IV spondylolisthesis. Treatment with and without posterior fusion. *J Bone Joint Surg Am.* 1987;69:960–969

Kesling KL, Reinker KA, Scoliosis in twins. A meta-analysis of the literature and report of six cases. *Spine (Phila Pa 1976).* 1997;22:2009–2015

Lamberg T, Remes V, Helenius I, Schlenzka D, Seitsalo S, Poussa M. Uninstrumented in situ fusion for high-grade childhood and adolescent isthmic spondylolisthesis: long-term outcome. *J Bone Joint Surg Am.* 2007;89: 512–518

Lonstein JE, Winter RB. The Milwaukee brace for the treatment of adolescent idiopathic scoliosis. A review of one thousand and twenty patients. *J Bone Joint Surg Am.* 1994;76:1207–1221

Machida M, Dubousset J, Imamura Y, Iwaya T, Yamada T, Kimura J. An experimental study in chickens for the pathogenesis of idiopathic scoliosis. *Spine (Phila Pa 1976).* 1993;18:1609–1615

Marchetti PG, Bartolozzi P. Classification of spondylolisthesis as a guideline for treatment. In: Bridwell KH, DeWald RL, eds. *The Textbook of Spinal Surgery.* 2nd ed. Philadelphia, PA: Lippincott-Raven; 1997:1211–1254

Meyerding HW. Spondylolisthesis. *Surg Gynecol Obstet.* 1932;54:371–377

Micheli LJ. Back injuries in dancers. *Clin Sports Med.* 1983;2:473–484

Micheli LJ. Back injuries in gymnastics. *Clin Sports Med.* 1985;4:85–93

Nachemson A. A long term follow-up study of non-treated scoliosis. *Acta Ortho Scand.* 1968;39:446–476

Nachemson A, Lonstein J, Weinstein S. Report of the SRS Prevalence and Natural History Committee 1982. Presented at the SRS Meeting, Denver, CO; 1982

Nachemson AL, Peterson LE. Effectiveness of treatment with a brace in girls who have adolescent idiopathic scoliosis. A prospective, controlled study based on data from the Brace Study of the Scoliosis Research Society. *J Bone Joint Surg Am.* 1995;77:815–822

O'Sullivan PB, Phyty GD, Twomey LT, Allison GT. Evaluation of specific stabilizing exercise in the treatment of chronic low back pain with radiologic diagnosis of spondylolysis or spondylolisthesis. *Spine (Phila Pa 1976).* 1997;22:2959–2967

Poussa M, Schlenzka D, Seitsalo S, Ylikoski M, Hurri H, Osterman K. Surgical treatment of severe isthmic spondylolisthesis in adolescents. Reduction or fusion in situ. *Spine (Phila Pa 1976).* 1993;18:894–901

Riseborough EJ, Wynne-Davies R. A genetic survey of idiopathic scoliosis in Boston, Massachusetts. *J Bone Joint Surg Am.* 1973;55:974–982

Rosenberg NJ, Bargar WL, Friedman B. The incidence of spondylolysis and spondylolisthesis in nonambulatory patients. *Spine (Phila Pa 1976).* 1981;6:35–38

Rowe GG, Roche MB. The etiology of separate neural arch. *J Bone Joint Surg Am.* 1953;35-A:102–110

Stewart TD. [The age incidence of neural-arch defects in Alaskan natives, considered from the standpoint of etiology.]. *J Bone Joint Surg Am.* 1953;35-A:937–950

Sys J, Michielsen J, Bracke P, Martens M, Verstreken J. Nonoperative treatment of active spondylolysis in elite athletes with normal X-ray findings: literature review and results of conservative treatment. *Eur Spine J.* 2001;10:498–504

Ward CV, Latimer B. Human evolution and the development of spondylolysis. *Spine (Phila Pa 1976).* 2005;30:1808–1814

Weinstein SL. Idiopathic scoliosis. Natural history. *Spine (Phila Pa 1976).* 1986;11:780–783

Weinstein SL, Zavala DC, Ponseti IV. Idiopathic scoliosis: long-term follow-up and prognosis in untreated patients. *J Bone Joint Surg Am.* 1981;63:702–712

Wiltse LL, Newman PH, Macnab I. Classification of spondylolisis and spondylolisthesis. *Clin Orthop Relat Res.* 1976;117:23–29

Wynne-Davies R, Scott JH. Inheritance and spondylolisthesis: a radiographic family survey. *J Bone Joint Surg Br.* 1979;61-B:301–305

Part 6: Back Pain

TOPICS COVERED

CHAPTER 14

General Approach and Differential Diagnosis

Back pain is an uncommon presenting complaint in young children but increases in presentation during adolescence.

- Fifty percent of individuals will have one episode of back pain by age 20 years and evidence suggests that back pain in children, especially idiopathic, correlates directly with continued back pain as adults.
- Retrospective review of children with back pain demonstrated no specific diagnosis was made in 78% of cases. Even so, children and adolescents are more likely than adults to have a specific diagnosis assigned to their back pain.
- Causes range from relatively benign, with little concern for long-term consequences; to somewhat concerning, such as infections, with the potential for lasting repercussions; to malignancies, which have potential for immediate harm (Table 14-1).
- Patient age can help narrow the differential diagnosis (Table 14-2).

Table 14-1. Distinguishing Features of Common Causes of Back Pain in Children and Adolescents

Causes of Back Pain	Distinguishing Signs/Symptoms	Evaluation/Treatment
Diskitis	Inflammatory condition in disc space commonly seen in ages 4 years and younger Presents with back/abdominal pain. May refuse to walk. Likely infectious, although pathogen often difficult to identify Most commonly identified pathogen is *Staphylococcus aureus*.	CBC, CRP, ESR, and blood cultures Radiographs are negative for 10–14 d, then show disc space narrowing and vertebral end plate changes. Bone scan helpful for diagnosis MRI also good for diagnosis and for identifying abscess or neural compression (see Figure 9-1). Treated with 5–7 d IV antibiotics then transition to oral antibiotics
Osteomyelitis	May have fever and chills, generalized malaise, anorexia, and weight loss.	CBC, CRP, ESR typically elevated Blood cultures positive in 50% Radiographs are negative for 10–14 d, then show periosteal thickening or elevation, and focal osteopenia. Bone scan or MRI helpful for diagnosis Treated with 5–7 d IV antibiotics then transition to oral antibiotics
Benign tumors **Osteoid osteoma**	Small, benign lesion causing a dull, well-localized pain, worse at night Pain often relieved by NSAIDs May lead to scoliosis	Involvement of the pedicle may lead to characteristic obliteration of the pedicle on AP radiograph known as the "winking owl sign" (Figure 14-1). Typically resolves over the course of several years; some may benefit from surgery. Requires referral to orthopaedic specialist.
Bone cyst (unicameral or aneurysmal)	Benign cystic lesions that usually affect posterior elements of the spine Usually chronic, dull pain, or may present with pathologic fracture. PE often normal, but aneurysmal cysts may have neurologic symptoms secondary to cord or nerve root impingement.	Usually identified on plain radiographs MRI features are diagnostic. Require referral to orthopaedic specialist.

Table 14-1. Distinguishing Features of Common Causes of Back Pain in Children and Adolescents, continued

Causes of Back Pain	Distinguishing Signs/Symptoms	Evaluation/Treatment
Eosinophilic granuloma	Benign tumor of anterior portion of spine Can be isolated or part of Letterer-Siwe or Hand-Schüller-Christian disease. Rarely, presents with fever and leukocytosis.	Radiographs show flattened lesion of vertebra, "vertebra plana" (Figure 14-2). Biopsy necessary to confirm diagnosis Skeletal survey helpful to look for other lesions Requires referral to orthopaedic specialist.
Malignant tumors	Unrelenting, deep, and progressively more severe pain, especially at night May have fever and chills, generalized malaise, anorexia, and weight loss. Most common in children <4 y Osteosarcoma and Ewing sarcoma most common primary bone tumors affecting spine May also be caused by leukemia or metastatic disease. Metastatic disease in children frequently involves the spine.	Back pain caused by leukemia has no characteristic radiographic features but may demonstrate compression fractures. Bone scan is the best study to evaluate for skeletal metastases. Intraspinal tumors that present with neurologic signs and symptoms require urgent referral to a neurosurgeon.
Herniated intervertebral disc	Usually seen in adults, but can also occur in adolescents. Can occur at any level; lower lumbar most common. Usually sudden onset of severe "burning" or "shooting" back pain, with or without radicular leg pain True radicular pain will radiate to the foot in a dermatomal pattern. Exacerbated by straining as with coughing or sneezing. May have positive straight leg raise test, and weakness or sensory changes on examination.	MRI will confirm diagnosis. High rate of resolution with nonoperative care including anti-inflammatory medications and physical therapy Pediatric sports medicine physician can assist with management. Large disc herniations associated with bowel or bladder dysfunction and saddle anesthesia (cauda equina syndrome) require emergent MRI and surgical decompression.
Slipped vertebral ring apophysis	May present similar to herniated disc. Injury unique to growing children Typically occurs with a flexion injury such as with extreme straining during weight lifting. Pain is usually of intense, sudden onset.	Avulsed bony fragment may be small and difficult to visualize on radiographs; if seen, will be within the spinal canal. MRI helpful to diagnose and differentiate from disc herniation Requires urgent referral to orthopaedic specialist. Often requires surgical treatment.

Table 14-1. Distinguishing Features of Common Causes of Back Pain in Children and Adolescents, continued

Causes of Back Pain	Distinguishing Signs/Symptoms	Evaluation/Treatment
Spondylolysis and spondylolisthesis	Activity-related pain, worse with hyperextension, relieved with flexion Common in sports requiring repetitive back extension (eg, gymnastics, football lineman, volleyball, weight lifting, soccer)	Oblique radiographs may reveal classic Scotty dog (see Figure 13-2) of spondylolysis. Lateral view can identify spondylolisthesis (see Figure 13-3). Bone scan for suspicious cases with normal radiographs Majority respond to nonoperative treatment of rest, bracing, and physical therapy. Refer to pediatric sports medicine specialist or orthopaedist if no response to 6 months of nonoperative treatment.
Postural roundback	Pain may be activity related or after prolonged sitting. Roundback can be consciously corrected. Forward bend test reveals smooth hump (Figure 12-1).	Radiographs are normal. Treatment includes strengthening and postural training.
Scheuermann kyphosis	Activity-related pain Roundback cannot be consciously corrected. Forward bending demonstrates angular hump (Figure 12-1).	Radiographs show >40–45 degrees kyphosis, characteristic vertebral body wedging, endplate abnormalities, and Schmorl nodes. Refer to orthopaedic specialist. Most respond to bracing and physical therapy.
Mechanical back pain	Usually chronic and intermittent Often related to overuse or poor mechanics May have paraspinal muscle tenderness and tight hamstrings, but usually no specific findings on examination.	Diagnosis of exclusion Treated with activity modification, physical therapy, and NSAIDs Avoid bed rest because it leads to deconditioning. When other diagnoses have been excluded and patient fails to respond to these modalities, referral to a pain management specialist is appropriate.

CBC, complete blood count; CRP, C-reactive protein; ESR, erythrocyte sedimentation rate; MRI, magnetic resonance imaging; IV, intravenous; NSAID, nonsteroidal anti-inflammatory drug; AP, anteroposterior; PE, physical examination.

Table 14-2. Common Causes of Back Pain

Birth–4 y	5–11 y	12 y–maturity
Diskitis	Benign tumors	Mechanical back pain
Osteomyelitis	• Osteoid osteoma	Spondylolysis
Malignant tumors	• Unicameral bone cyst	Spondylolisthesis
	• Aneurysmal bone cyst	Kyphosis
	• Eosinophilic granuloma	• Postural
	Diskitis	• Scheuermann disorder
	Osteomyelitis	Slipped vertebral ring apophysis

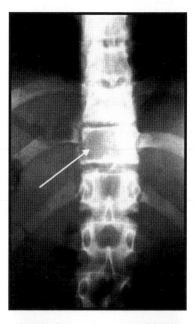

Figure 14-1. "Winking owl" sign in osteoid osteoma. Reproduced with permission from Griffin LY (ed): *Essentials of Musculoskeletal Care,* 3rd edition. Rosemont, IL: American Academy of Orthopaedic Surgeons; 2005.

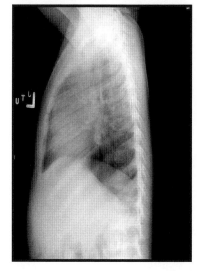

Figure 14-2. Lateral radiograph of thoracic spine showing characteristic vertebra plana caused by eosinophilic granuloma.

Approach to the Evaluation

- History
  - Duration, location, timing, character, and intensity of pain, as well as aggravating and alleviating factors
  - Constitutional symptoms such as fever, weight loss, and fatigue
  - Change in bowel or bladder function is a red flag requiring urgent evaluation.
  - Dysuria, gait changes, and lower extremity numbness indicate a neurologic disorder.
- Physical examination
  - Inspect for sacral dimple or hair patch that may indicate spinal dysraphism, and skin changes that may indicate neurofibromatosis.
  - Assess for leg-length inequalities.
  - Evaluate spine range of motion in flexion, extension, lateral bending, and rotation.
    - Pain with hyperextension is commonly seen with spondylolysis and spondylolisthesis.
    - Pain with flexion, but relief in extension, is commonly seen with herniated disc.
  - Perform a single-leg extension test (Stork test) for spondylolysis and spondylolisthesis (see Figure 4-10).
  - Measure the popliteal angle to assess hamstring flexibility (see Figure 4-5).
    - Hamstring tightness has been correlated with mechanical back pain.
  - Examine extremities for muscle strength, sensation, deep tendon reflexes, and long tract findings.
  - Check umbilical reflex.
    - Stroke the 4 quadrants of the abdomen to ensure that the umbilicus moves to the lateral half of the body each time.
    - May be abnormal with intraspinal pathology.
  - Observe gait.
    - Stiff gait seen with muscular strains
    - Slap-foot or drop-foot gait seen with tibialis anterior weakness resulting from nerve impingement
    - Crouched gait at the knees may be seen with hamstring spasticity related to spondylolysis or spondylolisthesis.

Making the Diagnosis

- In some cases, the diagnosis can be made by history and physical examination.
- Radiographs
  - When to order
    - 4 years or younger
    - Presence of any red flags (Box 14-1)
    - Duration of symptoms longer than 6 weeks

Box 14-1. Red Flags Pertaining to the History

Fevers, chills, malaise, anorexia
Weight loss
Decreased appetite
Unrelenting pain
Night pain
Associated radicular pain
Dysuria
Loss of bowel or bladder control

Clinical Pearl

When possible, order the lumbar radiograph in the standing position to assess alignment.

- — What to order
  - ▪ Obtain radiographs prior to any advanced imaging (eg, magnetic resonance imaging [MRI], computed tomography).
  - ▪ Views—thoracic (anteroposterior [AP] and lateral), lumbar (standing AP and lateral)
  - ▪ Additional oblique lumbar films may help visualize spondylolysis.
- Bone scan
  - — Extremely sensitive and relatively inexpensive test
  - — Helpful when diagnosis cannot be made by history, physical examination, and radiographs
  - — Order single-photon emission computed tomography scan to evaluate for spondylolysis.
  - — Study may require sedation in younger children.
- Magnetic resonance imaging
  - — Not the initial imaging choice
  - — May show abnormalities in asymptomatic patients, so must correlate history and physical examination with MRI findings.
  - — Good at evaluating intraspinal abnormalities, tumors, and infection
  - — Obtain with and without contrast to evaluate for tumor or infection.
- Computed tomography
  - — Limited role in workup of back pain in children
  - — Helpful for evaluating bony anatomy
  - — Helpful to localize a small tumor such as an osteoid osteoma
- Laboratory studies
  - — If concern for infection, malignancy, or inflammatory arthropathy, complete blood count with differential, erythrocyte sedimentation rate, and C-reactive protein should be obtained.
  - — Urinalysis should be ordered for flank pain or tenderness, dysuria, or abdominal pain.
  - — HLA-B27 testing can be ordered if concern for ankylosing spondylitis or Reiter syndrome (see Chapter 8).

Treatment

- Additional information about treatment of specific diagnoses can be found in other chapters.
  — Osteomyelitis (Chapter 7), diskitis (Chapter 9), kyphosis (Chapter 12), spondylolysis and spondylolisthesis (Chapter 13), benign and malignant tumors (chapters 50 and 51).

Backpack-Induced Back Pain

- Back pain is common in adolescents and proving casual relationship between backpacks and back pain has been inconclusive.
- Some studies have demonstrated a correlation between weight of the backpack and back pain.
- Other studies have failed to demonstrate this effect and found that psychosomatic factors had more influence on back pain.
- Suggestions to manage backpack-related pain include limiting pack weight to no more than 15% of body weight, obtaining a second set of books for home and school, or using a rolling bag instead of a backpack.

Resources for Physicians and Families

- http://orthoinfo.aaos.org/topic.cfm?topic=A00036
- http://orthoinfo.aaos.org/menus/spine.cfm

Relevant *International Classification of Diseases, Ninth Revision, Clinical Modification* Code

- **724.2**   Low back pain

Bibliography

American Academy of Pediatrics. Back to school tips. Available at: http://www.aap.org/advocacy/releases/augschool.cfm. Accessed February 10, 2010

Clifford SN, Fritz JM. Children and adolescents with low back pain: a descriptive study of physical examination and outcome measurement. *J Orthop Sports Phys Ther.* 2003;33:513–522

Dai LY, Ye H, Qian QR. The natural history of cervical disc calcification in children. *J Bone Joint Surg Am.* 2004;86-A:1467–1472

Feldman DS, Hedden DM, Wright JG. The use of bone scan to investigate back pain in children and adolescents. *J Pediatr Orthop.* 2000;20:790–795

Grubb MR, Currier BL, Pritchard DJ, Ebersold MJ. Primary Ewing's sarcoma of the spine. *Spine (Phila Pa 1976).* 1994;19:309–313

Heinrich SD, Gallagher D, Warrior R, Phelan K, George VT, MacEwen GD. The prognostic significance of the skeletal manifestations of acute lymphoblastic leukemia of childhood. *J Pediatr Orthop.* 1994;14:105–111

Leboeuf-Yde C, Kyvik KO. At what age does low back pain become a common problem? A study of 29,424 individuals aged 12–41 years. *Spine (Phila Pa 1976)*. 1998;23:228–234

Leeson MC, Makley JT, Carter JR. Metastatic skeletal disease in the pediatric population. *J Pediatr Orthop*. 1985;5:261–267

Lonstein JE. Spondylolisthesis in children. Cause, natural history, and management. *Spine (Phila Pa 1976)*. 1999;24:2640–2648

Mirovsky Y, Jakim I, Halperin N, Lev L. Non-specific back pain in children and adolescents: a prospective study until maturity. *J Pediatr Orthop B*. 2002;11:275–278

Negrini S, Carabalona R, Sibilla P. Backpack as a daily load for schoolchildren. *Lancet*. 1999;354:1974

Ogilvie JW, Sherman J. Spondylolysis in Scheuermann's disease. *Spine (Phila Pa 1976)*. 1987;12:251–253

Ovadia D, Metser U, Lievshitz G, Yaniv M, Wientroub S, Even-Sapir E. Back pain in adolescents: assessment with integrated 18F-fluoride positron-emission tomography-computed tomography. *J Pediatr Orthop*. 2007;27:90–93

Pediatric Orthopaedic Society of North America. Backpack safety. American Academy of Orthopaedic Surgeons Web site. Available at: http://orthoinfo.aaos.org/fact/thr_report.cfm?Thread_ID=105&topcategory=Children. Accessed February 10, 2010

Sheir-Neiss GI, Kruse RW, Rahman T, Jacobson LP, Pelli JA. The association of backpack use and back pain in adolescents. *Spine (Phila Pa 1976)*. 2003;28:922–930

Shives TC, Dahlin DC, Sim FH, Pritchard DJ, Earle JD. Osteosarcoma of the spine. *J Bone Joint Surg Am*. 1986;68:660–668

Siambanes D, Martinez JW, Butler EW, Haider T. Influence of school backpacks on adolescent back pain. *J Pediatr Orthop*. 2004;24:211–217

Sward L, Hellstrom M, Jacobsson B, Nyman R, Peterson L. Acute injury of the vertebral ring apophysis and intervertebral disc in adolescent gymnasts. *Spine (Phila Pa 1976)*. 1990;15:144–148

Tertti MO, Salminen JJ, Paajanen HE, Terho PH, Kormano MJ. Low-back pain and disk degeneration in children: a case-control MR imaging study. *Radiology*. 1991;180:503–507

van Gent C, Dols JJ, de Rover CM, Hira Sing RA, de Vet HC. The weight of schoolbags and the occurrence of neck, shoulder, and back pain in young adolescents. *Spine (Phila Pa 1976)*. 2003;28:916–921

Wall EJ, Foad SL, Spears J. Backpacks and back pain: where's the epidemic? *J Pediatr Orthop*. 2003;23:437–439

Weinstein SL. Natural history. *Spine (Phila Pa 1976)*. 1999;24:2592–2600

Young AI, Haig AJ, Yamakawa KS. The association between backpack weight and low back pain in children. *J Back Musculoskel Rehabil*. 2006;19:25–33

Part 7: Pediatric Cervical Spine

CHAPTER 15

Basic Radiographic Interpretation

General Considerations

- The pediatric cervical spine has unique anatomic features.
- The pediatric cervical spine reaches adult proportions between 8 and 10 years of age, at which point the spectrum of diagnoses and treatment are the same as in adults.
- The younger the child, the higher the risk for an upper cervical spine injury because of hypermobility secondary to ligamentous laxity, shallow and angled facet joints, anterior vertebral body wedging, variation of the fulcrum of movement (C2-C3 in children vs C5-C6 in adults), and a large head relative to the body.
- Initial radiographic evaluation for a cervical spine injury should include anteroposterior and lateral views.
  — Flexion and extension views may be added to look for signs of instability.
  — Open-mouth odontoid views are routinely ordered in cases of trauma.
- Computed tomography with multiplanar reformatting is used to evaluate bony detail.
- Magnetic resonance imaging is useful to discern soft tissue injury and to evaluate for instability or spinal cord injury without radiologic abnormality.

Normal Anatomic Variants

- Normal variations in apophyses, synchondroses, and ossification (Table 15-1) should be distinguished from fractures. Fractures have irregular edges whereas normal apophyses (secondary centers of growth) appear smooth and regular and can have sclerotic margins.
- Children younger than 16 years may show an absence of cervical lordosis (Figure 15-1) as a normal variant on lateral films.
- Lateral radiographs may show a large prevertebral soft tissue space that may be mistaken for injury. Up to 6 mm of prevertebral space (Figure 15-2) at C3 is normal in children. This normal widening compared with adults may be because of expiration, so repeat radiographs on inspiration may be useful in discerning true injury from artifact. True widening of the prevertebral space is suggestive of a cervical spine injury.

Table 15-1. Normal Cervical Spine Ossification Centers in Children

Level	Ossification Centers	Appearance	Fusion
C1	Three: Anterior arch and 2 neural arches	Neural arches are present at birth. Anterior arch—20% are present at birth, visible ossification at age 1 y.	Neural arches fuse posteriorly by age 3 y. Anterior arch fuses with neural arches at age 7 y.
C2	Four: 2 neural arches, vertebral body, odontoid process	All 4 are present at birth. Os terminale (a secondary ossification center at apex of odontoid process) appears by 3–6 y.	Posterior neural arches fuse at 2–3 y. Posterior neural arches fuse with odontoid process at 3–6 y. Body of C2 fuses with odontoid process at 3–6 y; fusion line (subdental synchondrosis) visible until 11 y. Os terminale fuses by 12 y.
C3-C7	Three: Vertebral body, 2 neural arches	Present at birth	Posterior neural arches fuse at 2–3 y. Vertebral body fuses with neural arches at 3–6 y. Fusion of secondary ossification centers at tips of transverse and spinous processes, superior and inferior aspects of vertebral bodies are varied—can persist until third decade.

Information from Jagannathan J, Sansur CA, Shaffrey CI. Iatrogenic spinal deformity. *Neurosurgery*. 2008;63:104–116

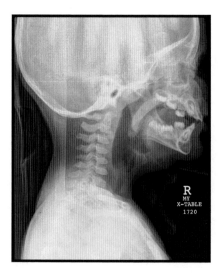

Figure 15-1. Lateral view of the cervical spine in a 17-month-old child demonstrates absence of normal cervical lordosis and pseudosubluxation of C2 on C3.

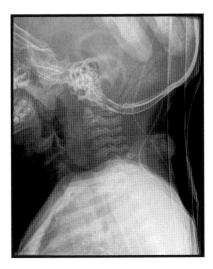

Figure 15-2. Lateral view of the cervical spine in a 1-year-old child demonstrates normal prominence of prevertebral soft tissues.

Pseudosubluxation (Figure 15-3)

- Anterior subluxation of C2-C3 or C3-C4 up to 2 mm caused by physiologic hypermobility of the pediatric upper cervical spine facet joints
- Seen on lateral neutral and flexion radiographs
- May be mistaken for injury in children up to 14 years of age.
- On lateral radiographs, the line drawn along the anterior aspects of the C1 and C3 spinous processes and the posterior cervical line should be within 1 mm of each other on flexion and extension films. Lines that do not overlap the anterior aspect of C2 by 2 mm or more suggest injury and possibly a hangman fracture (spondylolysis) of C2.
- Pseudosubluxation may correct on extension films and may be accentuated with muscle spasm.
- Magnetic resonance imaging is useful if radiographs or history create uncertainty.

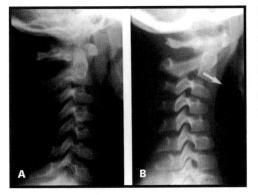

Figure 15-3. The normal alignment of the cervical spine (A). Pseudosubluxation with C2 displaced forward on C3 is indicated by the yellow arrow (B). From Staheli LT. *Practice of Pediatric Orthopedics.* Philadelphia, PA: Lippincott Williams & Wilkins; 2001:178. Reprinted by permission.

Pseudo-Jefferson Fracture

- Odontoid views can show widening of the lateral masses relative to the dens, which can be mistaken for a fracture.
- This pseudo-spread of the atlas on the axis can show up to 6 mm of displacement of the lateral masses in children up to 7 years of age.
- True displacement can result from an axial load to the head causing a burst fracture of atlas.

CHAPTER 16

Torticollis

Overview

- Torticollis (wry neck) is a condition in which the head is tilted toward one side and the chin is turned toward the other.
- Derived from Latin—torqueo, "to twist," and collum, or "neck."
- A spectrum of conditions may precipitate torticollis in a child. An appropriate history and physical examination (Box 16-1) will narrow the differential diagnosis. Congenital muscular torticollis, by far, is the most common.

> ### Clinical Pearls
> **All patients with torticollis should have screening anteroposterior and lateral cervical radiographs.**

Congenital Muscular Torticollis

INTRODUCTION/ETIOLOGY/EPIDEMIOLOGY

- Most common form of torticollis
- Incidence is 1% to 2% of live births.
- More common in boys and in breech presentation births
- Involves the right side more than the left.
- Etiology is unknown.
  - Ultrasound studies suggest that intrauterine malpositioning may play a role by causing injury to the sternocleidomastoid muscle (SCM). This may cause compartment-like syndrome leading to subsequent fibrosis.
  - Heredity may also be a factor.
  - Other potential etiologies include trauma (muscle stretch with intracompartmental hemorrhage), infection, and venous occlusion.
- *Developmental dysplasia of the hip* may coexist with congenital muscular torticollis at a rate of about 2% to 29%.
  - Boys are more likely than girls to develop both conditions regardless of which diagnosis was made.
  - Both seem to occur in association with breech presentation, but a causal relationship has not been firmly established.

Box 16-1. History and Physical Examination for Various Causes of Torticollis

History or Physical Examination Finding	Diagnoses to Consider
Present since birth	Congenital muscular torticollis Klippel-Feil/congenital cervical abnormality Neurogenic causes
First appears in late infancy	Ocular torticollis if flexible and painless
Sudden onset	Atlantoaxial rotatory subluxation
Worsened over *weeks or months*	Neurogenic causes
Worsened over *years*	Klippel-Feil/congenital cervical abnormality
Intermittent	Neurogenic causes Sandifer syndrome Paroxysmal torticollis of infancy
History of trauma	Atlantoaxial rotatory subluxation Other subluxation Fracture
Recent fever	Vertebral osteomyelitis or diskitis Grisel syndrome (inflammatory atlantoaxial rotatory subluxation)
Painful	Traumatic 　　Atlantoaxial rotatory subluxation 　　Other subluxation 　　Fracture Inflammatory 　　Grisel syndrome (inflammatory atlantoaxial rotatory subluxation) 　　Diskitis/osteomyelitis 　　Juvenile rheumatoid arthritis Neoplastic 　　Eosinophilic granuloma 　　Osteoid osteoma/osteoblastoma
Flexible (no SCM contracture or range of motion deficit)	Ocular torticollis Sandifer syndrome
Neurologic signs or symptoms	CNS tumors (cervical cord, brainstem, or posterior fossa) Chiari malformation[a] Syringomyelia[a] Basilar invagination[a]

SCM, sternocleidomastoid muscle; CNS, central nervous system.
[a]Especially suspect in the presence of other known skeletal abnormalities.

SIGNS AND SYMPTOMS

- Typically present at 2 to 4 weeks of age .
- The head is tilted toward the involved SCM and the chin is tilted away (chin left and occiput right, or chin right and occiput left).

- A palpable, firm mass usually at the distal third of the SCM
- Range of motion is decreased.
- When the defect is long-standing, plagiocephaly, facial asymmetry, and a unilateral epicanthal fold may be noted.

DIFFERENTIAL DIAGNOSIS

- Ocular torticollis
- Klippel-Feil/congenital cervical abnormality

MAKING THE DIAGNOSIS

- Diagnosis is based on the history and physical examination described previously *and* normal radiographs.
- *Anteroposterior (AP) and lateral cervical spine radiographs*
  — Will rule out bony malformation or C1-C2 subluxation, and are necessary to confirm diagnosis prior to starting physical therapy.
- Ultrasound
  — Can help differentiate congenital muscular torticollis from other pathologies in the neck such as tumors or cysts, and may help evaluate for resolution of the mass, but is not typically necessary for diagnosis or follow-up.

TREATMENT

- *Nonoperative*
  — Manual stretching is the treatment of choice and is 90% effective, particularly if the child is younger than 1 year.
    - Also includes home program of active stretching (after instruction by an occupational or physical therapist).
- *Operative*
  — Surgery may be indicated if satisfactory improvement is not achieved after 6 months of stretching exercises and after 1 year of age. This is rare.
  — The goal of surgery is cosmetic and functional improvement in those patients who fail conservative measures or who present late.
  — While many consider the optimal time for surgery to be between 1 and 4 years of age, surgical treatment beyond 10 years of age may be of benefit.
  — The preferred surgical technique varies.
  — Factors associated with less satisfactory outcomes of surgery include older age at operation, longer duration of disease, and more severe deformity before surgery.

EXPECTED OUTCOMES/PROGNOSIS

- The mass may slowly increase in size over 2 to 3 months and then gradually will regress or disappear, in most cases by 4 to 6 months. The mass is a pseudotumor and must not be misdiagnosed as a pediatric tumor or malignancy.

- If congenital muscular torticollis persists beyond 1 year of age, it is less likely to resolve spontaneously.

> **Clinical Pearls**
>
> **Congenital muscular torticollis is the most common form of congenital torticollis and responds to a stretching program. Patients with the diagnosis should be evaluated for hip dysplasia.**

WHEN TO REFER

- Refer to an orthopaedic surgeon
  - — If satisfactory improvement is not achieved after 6 months of stretching exercises
  - — Those who present after 1 year of age

RELEVANT *INTERNATIONAL CLASSIFICATION OF DISEASES, NINTH REVISION, CLINICAL MODIFICATION (ICD-9-CM)* CODE

- **723.5** Congenital muscular torticollis

Ocular Torticollis (Congenital Superior Oblique or Lateral Rectus Palsy)

INTRODUCTION/ETIOLOGY/EPIDEMIOLOGY

- Ocular torticollis is a compensatory mechanism that children with strabismus, ptosis, or nystagmus adopt to obtain the best vision.
- Presents most commonly in children older than 2 years, although may present as young as 6 months.
- Signs or symptoms may be present for years by the time of presentation.
- The diagnosis is frequently made as an incidental finding on examination for another condition.

SIGNS AND SYMPTOMS

- Torticollis with *no sternocleidomastoid contracture* is the most common presentation.
- Head tilting is not present at sleep.
- Patients are able to demonstrate full active, pain-free neck range of motion when eyes are closed.
- Not associated with pain or other neurologic symptoms
- Strabismus, nystagmus, ptosis, and rarely, diplopia, may be present.

MAKING THE DIAGNOSIS

- Diagnosis is based on the history and physical examination described previously *and* normal cervical radiographs.

DIFFERENTIAL DIAGNOSIS

- Congenital muscular torticollis (SCM contracture)
- Paroxysmal torticollis of infancy (intermittent)
- Congenital cervical spine deformities (abnormal radiographs)

TREATMENT AND EXPECTED OUTCOMES AND PROGNOSIS

- Surgical treatment of the ocular abnormality can correct the torticollis.

WHEN TO REFER

- Refer to an ophthalmologist for formal assessment.

RELEVANT *ICD-9-CM* CODE

- **781.93**   Ocular torticollis

Paroxysmal Torticollis of Infancy

INTRODUCTION/ETIOLOGY/EPIDEMIOLOGY

- This uncommon condition is usually first noted in infancy, almost always prior to 9 months of age.
- Typically occurs in otherwise healthy infants.

SIGNS AND SYMPTOMS

- The child will have a recurrent head tilt, usually to one side, but may alternate sides.
- The symptoms present periodically, usually every several days or weeks.
- The trunk may bend in the same direction as the head, and the posterior neck muscles may contract.
- Accompanying symptoms may include drowsiness, irritability, vomiting, and ataxia, but usually there are no accompanying symptoms.
- The torticollis is usually the only notable physical finding.

DIFFERENTIAL DIAGNOSIS

- *Sandifer syndrome*
  — Characterized by intermittent, abnormal head and neck posturing associated with gastroesophageal reflux and esophagitis, sometimes from hiatal hernia
  — The torticollis may be the child's attempt to decrease the pain of the esophagitis.
  — Medical management for the gastrointestinal symptoms, and sometimes fundoplication, resolve the condition.

MAKING THE DIAGNOSIS

- Any child with a torticollis should have *AP and lateral radiographs of the cervical spine*; these should be negative in benign paroxysmal torticollis.
- No other imaging is typically indicated.

TREATMENT AND EXPECTED OUTCOMES AND PROGNOSIS

- Benign paroxysmal torticollis typically resolves spontaneously between 1 and 3 years of age, after which the child remains symptom free.
- May herald the onset of migraine later in childhood.

WHEN TO REFER

- Refer to a pediatric orthopaedic specialist if no resolution by 3 years of age.

RELEVANT *ICD-9-CM* CODE

- **723.5**   Paroxysmal torticollis

Congenital Cervical Abnormalities/ Klippel-Feil Syndrome

INTRODUCTION/ETIOLOGY/EPIDEMIOLOGY

- Congenital abnormalities of the cervical spine are a common cause of fixed torticollis in the young patient.
- Defects in segmentation or formation (Figure 16-1) of the cervical spine lead to fixed, sometimes progressive deformity, as well as pain and neurologic symptoms.
- *Klippel-Feil syndrome*
  - — Represents 50% of all congenital cervical abnormalities.
  - — Patients have abnormal number of cervical vertebrae or fusion of hemivertebrae into one osseous mass, leading to the clinical triad of short neck, low posterior hairline, and limitation of neck range of motion.
- Incidence has been estimated at 1 per 40,000 live births.
- Usually appears sporadically, but may be familial (6%–16% of cases in one series).

SIGNS AND SYMPTOMS

- The presentation of congenital cervical abnormality is heterogeneous.
- Some patients are asymptomatic and the condition is discovered only incidentally.
- Eighteen percent of patients present with a fixed torticollis.
  - — Occasionally appreciated in the infant or toddler, but commonly does not receive attention until later in life.
  - — The deformity may be gradually progressive, typically over years.
- Limitation of neck range of motion in lateral bending or rotation
- Webbed neck may be present.

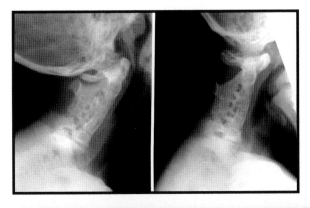

Figure 16-1. Defects in segmentation or formation of cervical spine. Reprinted with permission from eMedicine.com, 2008. Available at emedicine.medscape.com/article/1260442-overview.

> ### Clinical Pearls
>
> **All patients with congenital cervical anomalies should have a renal ultrasound, a hearing evaluation, radiographs of the thoracolumbar spine, and cardiac assessment.**

- Patients with Klippel-Feil syndrome have the triad of short neck, low posterior hairline, and limitation of neck range of motion.
- Neck pain or neurologic complaints (radiculopathy or myelopathy) may rarely be a presenting complaint, typically at adolescence or older.
- Neurologic findings may include cranial nerve abnormalities (swallowing or speaking difficulties, mirror image movements), myelopathy (spasticity or hyperreflexia), or radiculopathy.
- Blurred vision or headaches may indicate an associated basilar invagination.
- Several conditions are associated with congenital cervical spine abnormalities.
  - Congenital scoliosis of the thoracic or lumbar spine (50%)
  - Sprengel deformity (maldescent of the shoulder girdle) (20%–30%)
  - Hearing abnormalities (30%)
  - Congenital cardiac disease (4%–29%)
  - Renal abnormalities (30%): agenesis is the most common, but malrotation, horseshoe kidney, or ectopic kidney may be present.
  - Cleft palate has also been associated.

MAKING THE DIAGNOSIS

- In most cases, the diagnosis can be made on *radiographs of the cervical spine (AP and lateral)*.
- In some cases, *computed tomography or magnetic resonance imaging of the cervical spine* is necessary for diagnosis.
  - When upper cervical anomalies are suspected but radiographs are inconclusive
  - In the infant, the cervical vertebrae are largely cartilaginous, and abnormalities may be difficult to distinguish.

— For congenital abnormalities of the upper cervical spine, usually C1, which may also be difficult to distinguish on plain radiographs

— Magnetic resonance imaging of the cervical spine is indicated if the patient has neurologic findings, to assess for stenosis, myelopathy, or nerve root compromise.

- To evaluate for associated conditions, all patients diagnosed with congenital cervical anomalies should have
  — Radiographs of the thoracolumbar spine
  — Renal ultrasound
  — Hearing evaluation
  — Cardiac assessment

DIFFERENTIAL DIAGNOSIS

- Congenital muscular torticollis (normal radiographs)
- Ocular torticollis (flexible torticollis and normal radiographs)

TREATMENT

- The patient is followed for progression of deformity or symptoms.
- For those with neck pain, activity restriction and occasionally orthoses or traction can be helpful.
- Surgery is indicated for progression of deformity, progressive instability, or neurologic compromise, fusion of the hypermobile segments.
- Prophylactic surgical intervention is not typically recommended.
- Individuals with high-risk anomalies (see the following) should be cautioned to avoid contact sports and situations highly risky for a blow to the head.

EXPECTED OUTCOMES/PROGNOSIS

- The natural history is highly variable.
- The condition may present and remain asymptomatic or minimally symptomatic.
- Because of the cervical spine fusion(s) present, however, hypermobility of the adjacent open segments can lead to stenosis and osteoarthritis over time.
- Of those who become symptomatic, 1 out of 5 do so before 5 years of age.
- More frequently, symptoms are not apparent until the teenage years and twenties, with 65% symptomatic by age 30 years.
- Three patterns of congenital cervical anomalies carry a particularly high risk for neurologic injury or sequelae.
  — Fusion of the occiput to C1; C1 to C2; or C2 to C3
  — A long cervical fusion with an abnormal occipitocervical junction
  — Two fused segments with a single open intervening interspace

WHEN TO REFER

- Refer all patients with congenital cervical spine abnormality to an orthopaedic surgeon. The referral can be routine unless there are neurologic signs or symptoms.

RELEVANT *ICD-9-CM* CODES

- **756.16**   Klippel-Feil syndrome
- **756.10**   Anomaly of spine
- **756.14**   Hemivertebra
- **756.15**   Congenital fusion of spine

CHAPTER 17

Atlantoaxial Rotatory Subluxation or Fixation

Introduction/Etiology/Epidemiology

- Common causes of torticollis in older children (acquired torticollis)
- Regional inflammation or trauma can precipitate rotatory subluxation of the C1 facet joints relative to C2, which may become fixed, with an associated torticollis.
  — Grisel syndrome, also referred to as viral torticollis, may follow an upper respiratory infection such as otitis media or pharyngitis.
- Atlantoaxial rotatory subluxation should be suspected in any case of new-onset, painful torticollis.
- Can present at any time during childhood, with a peak incidence between 6 and 8 years of age.

Signs and Symptoms

- New-onset, fixed torticollis
- History of recent upper respiratory infection or recent trauma
- Pain may be associated, sometimes at rest, but especially while attempting to rotate the head toward the midline.
- A spasm of the sternocleidomastoid muscle may be noted on the side *contralateral* to the head tilt.

Differential Diagnosis

- Less common causes of painful, new-onset torticollis include
  — Traumatic injuries
  — Diskitis or osteomyelitis (see Chapter 7)
  — Osteoid osteoma or osteoblastoma (see Chapter 50)
- Eosinophilic granuloma
  — Painful torticollis that occasionally presents with neurologic compromise
  — Flattened vertebrae (vertebra plana) with bone lysis may be seen on cervical spine radiographs.
  — Biopsy confirms the diagnosis.

— Without neurologic involvement, symptoms typically resolve completely without intervention.

— Surgery or radiation therapy may be indicated when neurologic compromise is present.

• Cervical and posterior fossa tumors

— The torticollis seen may be fixed or with rhythmic twisting.

— Photophobia, headache, weakness, and other neurologic signs may be associated.

• Juvenile idiopathic arthritis (JIA)

— Neck pain because of cervical spine involvement occurs in about half of patients with polyarticular JIA and frequently in those with systemic onset disease.

— Torticollis is a less common presentation (about 1% of patients with JIA).

— Juvenile rheumatoid arthritis patients may be more prone to developing atlantoaxial rotatory subluxation.

— Other radiographic findings can include erosions of the odontoid, ankylosis of vertebrae, and subluxations in the lower cervical spine.

Making the Diagnosis

• *Anteroposterior and lateral radiographs of the cervical spine* should be ordered first if atlantoaxial rotatory subluxation is suspected.

— Oblique view of C1 and C2 may be produced and therefore, a lateral view of the skull may be helpful to determine the relationship of C1 and C2.

— Radiographs may help differentiate between an atlantoaxial rotatory subluxation and the other conditions noted previously.

• Computed tomography (CT) scan of C1 and C2 is the definitive imaging study for diagnosis of atlantoaxial rotatory subluxation.

— Will demonstrate a fixed relationship (no reducibility) between the facets of C1 and C2 despite rotation in each direction (Figure 17-1).

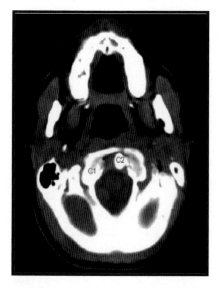

Figure 17-1. Computed tomography demonstrates a fixed subluxation between the facets of C1 and C2. © 2006 Al Kaissi et al; licensee BioMed Central Ltd. Available at: www.scoliosisjournal.com/content/1/1/15.

Treatment

- Symptoms present for less than 1 week
  - The child may be treated with a soft collar, analgesics, rest, and heat.
  - Frequently spontaneous reduction may occur; however, appropriate follow-up *must be facilitated and should not be assumed.* Delay in treatment can greatly decrease the likelihood of reduction with conservative measures.
- Symptoms present for more than 1 week
  - Spontaneous reduction is unlikely to occur.
  - Inpatient management with cervical halter traction, muscle relaxants, greater analgesia, and close clinical follow-up.
  - Reduction is heralded by improved rotational range of motion in the previously restricted direction, and may be confirmed with a follow-up CT scan.
  - If halter traction fails to yield a reduction, a halo is applied to allow greater traction weight to be applied to facilitate reduction. After reduction, this is followed by halo vest immobilization for 6 to 12 weeks.
  - Finally, if use of halo traction does not facilitate reduction, or if reduction cannot be maintained, atlantoaxial arthrodesis may be performed.

Expected Outcomes/Prognosis

- When reduced promptly, the likelihood of recurrence is low.
- The greater the delay to reduction, the greater the likelihood of requiring more aggressive means to achieve reduction.

When to Refer

- Refer to a pediatric orthopaedic specialist *promptly* on diagnosis or suspicion of atlantoaxial rotatory subluxation.

Relevant *International Classification of Diseases, Ninth Revision, Clinical Modification* Code

- **723.5** Atlantoaxial rotatory subluxation

Clinical Pearls

Any child with new-onset torticollis, particularly after recent infection, surgery, or trauma, must be suspected to have atlantoaxial rotatory subluxation. Prompt referral and initiation of treatment are essential to optimize likelihood of a good outcome. Two-view radiographs of the cervical spine are imperative prior to the initiation of physical therapy.

When torticollis is painful and plain films are non-diagnostic, further imaging should be pursued until a diagnosis is made.

Magnetic resonance imaging should be ordered when torticollis is associated with neurologic signs or symptoms.

Bibliography

Ain MC, Chaichana KL, Schkrohowsky JG. Retrospective study of cervical arthrodesis in patients with various types of skeletal dysplasia. *Spine (Phila Pa 1976)*. 2006;31:E169–E174

Amacher AL, Eltomey A. Spinal osteoblastoma in children and adolescents. *Childs Nerv Syst*. 1985;1:29–32

Bethem D, Winter RB, Lutter L. Disorders of the spine in diastrophic dwarfism. *J Bone Joint Surg Am*. 1980;62:529–536

Binder H, Eng GD, Gaiser JF, Koch B. Congenital muscular torticollis: results of conservative management with long-term follow-up in 85 cases. *Arch Phys Med Rehabil*. 1987;68:222–225

Bixenman WW. Diagnosis of superior oblique palsy. *J Clin Neuroophthalmol*. 1981;1:199–208

Bratt HD, Menelaus MB. Benign paroxysmal torticollis of infancy. *J Bone Joint Surg Br*. 1992;74:449–451

Brown CW, Jarvis JG, Letts M, Carpenter B. Treatment and outcome of vertebral Langerhans cell histiocytosis at the Children's Hospital of Eastern Ontario. *Can J Surg*. 2005;48:230–236

Canale ST, Griffin DW, Hubbard CN. Congenital muscular torticollis. A long-term follow-up. *J Bone Joint Surg Am*. 1982;64:810–816

Chan YL, Cheng JC, Metreweli C. Ultrasonography of congenital muscular torticollis. *Pediat Radiol*. 1992;22:356–360

Chandler FA. Congenital muscular torticollis. *Bull Hosp Joint Dis*. 1953;14:158–171

Cheng JC, Au AW. Infantile torticollis: a review of 624 cases. *J Pediatr Orthop*. 1994;14:802–808

Cheng JC, Tang SP. Outcome of surgical treatment of congenital muscular torticollis. *Clin Orthop Relat Res*. 1999;362:190–200

Cheng JC, Wong MW, Tang SP, Chen TM, Shum SL, Wong EM. Clinical determinants of the outcome of manual stretching in the treatment of congenital muscular torticollis in infants. A prospective study of eight hundred and twenty-one cases. *J Bone Joint Surg Am*. 2001;83-A:679–687

Coventry MB, Harris LE. Congenital muscular torticollis in infancy; some observations regarding treatment. *J Bone Joint Surg Am*. Jul 1959;41-A:815–822

Davids JR, Wenger DR, Mubarak SJ. Congenital muscular torticollis: sequela of intrauterine or perinatal compartment syndrome. *J Pediatr Orthop*. 1993;13:141–147

Davidson RI, Shillito J Jr. Eosinophilic granuloma of the cervical spine in children. *Pediatrics*. 1970;45:746–752

Demirbilek S, Atayurt HF. Congenital muscular torticollis and sternomastoid tumor: results of nonoperative treatment. *J Pediatr Surg.* 1999;34:549–551

Drigo P, Carli G, Laverda AM. Benign paroxysmal torticollis of infancy. *Brain Dev.* 2000;22:169–172

Dudkiewicz I, Ganel A, Blankstein A. Congenital muscular torticollis in infants: ultrasound-assisted diagnosis and evaluation. *J Pediatr Orthop.* 2005;25:812–814

Engin C, Yavuz SS, Sahin FI. Congenital muscular torticollis: is heredity a possible factor in a family with five torticollis patients in three generations? *Plast Reconstr Surg.* 1997;99:1147–1150

Fried JA, Athreya B, Gregg JR, Das M, Doughty R. The cervical spine in juvenile rheumatoid arthritis. *Clin Orthop Relat Res.* 1983;179:102–106

Girodias JB, Azouz EM, Marton D. Intervertebral disk space calcification. A report of 51 children with a review of the literature. *Pediatr Radiol.* 1991;21:541–546

Gray SW, Romaine CB, Skandalakis JE. Congenital fusion of the cervical vertebrae. *Surg Gynecol Obstet.* 1964;118:373–385

Healey D, Letts M, Jarvis JG. Cervical spine instability in children with Goldenhar's syndrome. *Can J Surg.* 2002;45:341–344

Helmi C, Pruzansky S. Craniofacial and extracranial malformations in the Klippel-Feil syndrome. *Cleft Palate J.* 1980;17:65–88

Hensinger RN. Spondylolysis and spondylolisthesis in children. *Instr Course Lect.* 1983;32:132–151

Hensinger RN, DeVito PD, Ragsdale CG. Changes in the cervical spine in juvenile rheumatoid arthritis. *J Bone Joint Surg Am.* 1986;68:189–198

Hensinger RN, Lang JE, MacEwen GD. Klippel-Feil syndrome; a constellation of associated anomalies. *J Bone Joint Surg Am.* 1974;56:1246–1253

Herman MJ. Torticollis in infants and children: common and unusual causes. *Instr Course Lect.* 2006;55:647–653

Herring JA. *Tachdjian's Pediatric Orthopaedics.* 3rd ed. Philadelphia, PA: WB Saunders; 2002

Herring JA, Hensinger RN. Cervical disc calcification. *J Pediatr Orthop.* 1988;8:613–616

Hobbs WR, Sponseller PD, Weiss AP, Pyeritz RE. The cervical spine in Marfan syndrome. *Spine (Phila Pa 1976).* 1997;22:983–989

Hsu TC, Wang CL, Wong MK, Hsu KH, Tang FT, Chen HT. Correlation of clinical and ultrasonographic features in congenital muscular torticollis. *Arch Phys Med Rehabil.* 1999;80:637–641

Hummer CD, MacEwen GD. The coexistence of torticollis and congenital dysplasia of the hip. *J Bone Joint Surg Am.* 1972;54:1255–1256

Inglefinger FJ. *Dorland's Medical Dictionary.* Philadelphia, PA: Saunders Press; 1980

Ippolito E, Tudisco C, Massobrio M. Long-term results of open sternocleidomastoid tenotomy for idiopathic muscular torticollis. *J Bone Joint Surg Am.* 1985;67:30–38

Johnston CE 2nd, Birch JG, Daniels JL. Cervical kyphosis in patients who have Larsen syndrome. *J Bone Joint Surg Am.* 1996;78:538–545

Jones MC. Unilateral epicanthal fold: diagnostic significance. *J Pediatr.* 1986;108:702–704

Keuter EJ. Non-traumatic atlanto-axial dislocation associated with nasopharyngeal infections (Grisel's disease). *Acta Neurochir (Wien).* 1969;21:11–22

Kumandas S, Per H, Gumus H, et al. Torticollis secondary to posterior fossa and cervical spinal cord tumors: report of five cases and literature review. *Neurosurg Rev.* 2006;29:333–338

Lin JN, Chou ML. Ultrasonographic study of the sternocleidomastoid muscle in the management of congenital muscular torticollis *J Pediatr Surg.* 1997;32:1648–1651

Ling CM. The influence of age on the results of open sternomastoid tenotomy in muscular torticollis. *Clin Orthop Relat Res.* 1976;116:142–148

MacEwen D. Proceedings: the Klippel-Feil syndrome. *J Bone Joint Surg Br.* 1975;57:261

Morrison DL, MacEwen GD. Congenital muscular torticollis: observations regarding clinical findings, associated conditions, and results of treatment. *J Pediatr Orthop.* 1982;2:500–505

Murphy WJ, Gellis SS. Torticollis with hiatus hernia in infancy. Sandifer syndrome. *Am J Dis Child.* 1977;131:564–565

Nucci P, Kushner BJ, Serafino M, Orzalesi N. A multi-disciplinary study of the ocular, orthopedic, and neurologic causes of abnormal head postures in children. *Am J Ophthalmol.* 2005;140:65–68

Ozaki T, Liljenqvist U, Hillmann A, et al. Osteoid osteoma and osteoblastoma of the spine: experiences with 22 patients. *Clin Orthop Relat Res.* 2002;397:394–402

Panjabi MM, White AA 3rd, Keller D, Southwick WO, Friedlaender G. Stability of the cervical spine under tension. *J Biomech.* 1978;11:189–197

Phillips WA, Hensinger RN. The management of rotatory atlanto-axial subluxation in children. *J Bone Joint Surg Am.* 1989;71:664–668

Pizzutillo PD, Woods M, Nicholson L, MacEwen GD. Risk factors in Klippel-Feil syndrome. *Spine (Phila Pa 1976).* 1994;19:2110–2116

Porter SB, Blount BW. Pseudotumor of infancy and congenital muscular torticollis. *Am Fam Physician.* 1995;52:1731–1736

Ramenofsky ML, Buyse M, Goldberg MJ, Leape LL. Gastroesophageal reflux and torticollis. *J Bone Joint Surg Am.* 1978;60:1140–1141

Raskas DS, Graziano GP, Herzenberg JE, Heidelberger KP, Hensinger RN. Osteoid osteoma and osteoblastoma of the spine. *J Spinal Disord.* 1992;5:204–211

Rouvreau P, Glorion C, Langlais J, Noury H, Pouliquen JC. Assessment and neurologic involvement of patients with cervical spine congenital synostosis as in Klippel-Feil syndrome: study of 19 cases. *J Pediatr Orthop B.* 1998;7:179–185

Sarnat HB, Morrissy RT. Idiopathic torticollis: sternocleidomastoid myopathy and accessory neuropathy. *Muscle Nerve.* 1981;4:374–380

Sonnabend DH, Taylor TK, Chapman GK. Intervertebral disc calcification syndromes in children. *J Bone Joint Surg Br.* 1982;64:25–31

Svensson O, Aaro S. Cervical instability in skeletal dysplasia. Report of 6 surgically fused cases. *Acta Orthop Scand.* 1988;59:66–70

Theiss SM, Smith MD, Winter RB. The long-term follow-up of patients with Klippel-Feil syndrome and congenital scoliosis. *Spine (Phila Pa 1976).* 1997;22:1219–1222

Thomsen MN, Schneider U, Weber M, Johannisson R, Niethard FU. Scoliosis and congenital anomalies associated with Klippel-Feil syndrome types I-III. *Spine (Phila Pa 1976).* 1997;22:396–401

Tracy MR, Dormans JP, Kusumi K. Klippel-Feil syndrome: clinical features and current understanding of etiology. *Clin Orthop Relat Res.* 2004;424:183–190

Ventura N, Huguet R, Salvador A, Terricabras L, Cabrera AM. Intervertebral disc calcification in childhood. *Int Orthop.* 1995;19:291–294

von Heideken J, Green DW, Burke SW, et al. The relationship between developmental dysplasia of the hip and congenital muscular torticollis. *J Pediatr Orthop.* 2006;26:805–808

Walsh JJ, Morrissy RT. Torticollis and hip dislocation. *J Pediatr Orthop.* 1998;18:219–221

Weiner DS. Congenital dislocation of the hip associated with congenital muscular torticollis. *Clin Orthop Relat Res.* 1976;121:163–165

Wetzel FT, La Rocca H. Grisel's syndrome. *Clin Orthop Relat Res.* 1989;240:141–152

Wong CC, Pereira B, Pho RW. Cervical disc calcification in children. A long-term review. *Spine (Phila Pa 1976).* 1992;17:139–144

Yong-Hing K, Kalamchi A, MacEwen GD. Cervical spine abnormalities in neurofibromatosis. *J Bone Joint Surg Am.* 1979;61:695–699

Part 8: Hip Disorders

TOPICS COVERED

CHAPTER 18

Developmental Dysplasia of the Hip

Introduction/Etiology/Epidemiology

- Broad diagnosis that includes a spectrum of hip disorders representing varying degrees of distortion in the relationship between the femoral head and acetabulum
- Ranges from radiologic diagnosis with normal examination to clinically dislocated hip.
- Most children are diagnosed as infants, but initial detection may occur at almost any age.
- Incidence of unstable hip is 1 to 1.5 per 1,000 births; incidence is higher if defined by ultrasound changes and not gross dislocation.
- May also be seen in association with neuromuscular disorders (eg, cerebral palsy, arthrogryposis, spina bifida).
- Etiology multifactorial with mechanical and biologic causes
- Risk factors include breech positioning, ligamentous laxity, female sex, first born, family history, oligohydramnios, postnatal positioning (eg, hips held in adduction in papoose), and race (most common in whites and Native American groups).

Signs and Symptoms

- Symptoms depend on age of child.
  - Typically asymptomatic in infants and toddlers. May be associated with other intrauterine molding disorders such as metatarsus adductus and torticollis.
  - School-aged children may have some vague activity-related discomfort caused by leg-length discrepancy.
  - Teenagers and young adults are usually asymptomatic but may have activity-related groin or buttock pain.
- Dislocated hip may demonstrate decreased abduction.

Differential Diagnosis

- In infants or walking child the leg shortening or hip instability may be related to congenital coxa vara, congenital short femur, or proximal femoral focal deficiency. Post-septic hip dislocation can also occur and result in limp and hip instability.
- In the older child, other etiologies of hip or knee pain should be considered including slipped capital femoral epiphysis and Perthes disease.

Making the Diagnosis

- Infants younger than 6 months
  - In newborns, the proximal femoral epiphysis is not ossified, limiting the usefulness of plain radiographs.
  - *Ultrasound*
    - Useful for assessing anatomy and following treatment in this age group
    - Ultrasound allows for a static and dynamic examination.
    - Ultrasound screening before 6 weeks of age may be overly sensitive and result in overtreatment.
  - *Ortolani sign:* Considered positive when a hip that is dislocated can be reduced and felt as a clunk. Occurs by bringing the involved hip into a flexed and abducted position (Figure 18-1a).
  - *Barlow sign:* Positive when a reduced hip can be dislocated by clunk associated with flexion and adduction of the hip (Figure 18-1b).
  - *Galeazzi sign:* Adduct both hips so that the thighs are vertical and assess the knee heights. Asymmetry indicates a unilaterally shortened thigh segment and is a positive Galeazzi sign (see Figure 4-23).
  - *Klisic sign:* Helpful with bilateral dislocated hips.
    - Line drawn on the child from tip of the greater trochanter to the ipsilateral anterior superior iliac spine should pass above the umbilicus.
    - If line passes below the umbilicus, the hip is likely dislocated.
- Children older than 6 months
  - Once a child is older than 6 months, developmental dysplasia of the hip (DDH) can be assessed with radiographs (Figure 18-2 a,b).
  - An anteroposterior view of the pelvis is typically obtained with the legs in neutral position and in a frog lateral position.
  - Arthrography is a dynamic study typically done in the operating room that involves injecting contrast dye into the joint to see the outline of the cartilage and soft tissue structures of the joint.

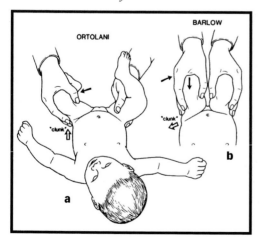

Figure 18-1. Technique for performing the Ortolani (a) and Barlow (b) maneuvers. The Ortolani sign is obtained by gently abducting the leg and a palpable "clunk" is felt as the femoral head slides over the posterior rim of the acetabulum into the socket. This is called the sign of entry. The Barlow provocative test is obtained by adducting the hip and pushing gently on the knee and a palpable "clunk" is felt as the femoral head slides over the posterior rim of the acetabulum and out of the socket. This is called the sign of exit. From Aronsson DD, Goldberg MJ, Kling TF Jr, Roy DR. Developmental dysplasia of the hip. *Pediatrics.* 1994;94:201–208.

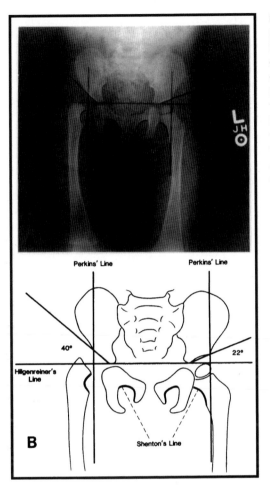

Figure 18-2. A, An anteroposterior pelvis radiograph of an 8-month-old infant with developmental dysplasia of the hip (DDH) on the right. B, The drawing of the radiograph shows Hilgenreiner line connecting the top of the triradiate cartilages. Perkins line is perpendicular to Hilgenreiner line through the lateral ossified margin of the acetabulum. Shenton line forms a continuous contour between the obturator foramen and the medial border of the femoral neck. There is DDH on the right with a delay in the appearance of the ossific nucleus, lateral displacement of the proximal femoral metaphysis, an elevated acetabular index (40°), and a "break" in Shenton line. From Aronsson DD. Goldberg MJ, Kling TF Jr, Roy DR. Developmental dysplasia of the hip. *Pediatrics.* 1994;94:201–208.

— Computed tomography can be useful to assess reduction in a spica cast or for planning reconstructive osteotomies.

— Magnetic resonance imagery arthrography is useful for confirming reduction of the hip in a spica cast, and in an older child, may identify other causes of pain such as labral or chondral injuries.

Treatment

- Goals are to maintain a concentrically reduced hip joint and avoid complications.
- Based on the principle that placing the immature femoral head and acetabulum together positively influence the development of both
- Remodeling potential is related to age, so early diagnosis usually results in less need for invasive procedures.
- High rate of resolution of hip instability seen in the immediate perinatal period

- Infants with clinical instability (positive Barlow/Ortolani) are treated with abduction splinting, typically in a Pavlik harness.
  — Pavlik harness holds legs flexed and abducted to hold concentric hip reduction.
  — Harness treatment typically for 6 to 12 weeks
  — Avoid extremes of leg positioning, which may result in femoral nerve injury or avascular necrosis.
- Children aged 6 to 18 months typically require closed reduction and arthrograms in the operating room with placement of a hip spica cast.
  — Cast is changed every 4 to 6 weeks.
  — Cast treatment typically lasts 2 to 4 months, followed by bracing for several months.
  — If hip remains irreducible or unstable, open reduction is performed.
- Open reduction is performed in those patients with hips that cannot safely be reduced by closed methods.
  — These children are usually walking but not yet in primary school.
  — Other procedures such as adductor tenotomy and femoral shortening osteotomy may be required in addition to open reduction to avoid excessive pressure on the hip following reduction.
- Following reduction of the hip, acetabular remodeling should occur to give the hip a more normal shape. Incomplete remodeling with growth may require additional procedures such as pelvic osteotomy to reorient the acetabulum. Pelvic osteotomies are usually performed from age 18 months to adulthood.

Expected Outcomes/Prognosis

- Developmental dysplasia of the hip is a spectrum of conditions, so outcomes also follow a spectrum from normal hip to early arthritis.
- Long-term sequelae are dependent on degree of deformity.
- Unilateral dislocation typically reduces in a child up to 8 years of age; bilateral dislocations up to 6 years of age.
- Unilateral dislocation
  — Typically results in leg-length discrepancy and can lead to altered gait mechanics, scoliosis, and lower back symptoms.
  — Hip pain and arthritis typically develop in the fourth decade.
- Bilateral dislocations
  — Lead to lordosis of the lumbar spine and a waddling gait.
  — May function well into the sixth decade.
- A persistently subluxated hip leads to increased force concentration on the lateral edge of the acetabulum, predisposing to early arthritis in the fourth decade of life.

Prevention

- Universal screening at birth is effective but not 100% sensitive. No countries have been successful in identifying all children with DDH despite universal screening programs.

When to Refer

- Infants and children with DDH should be referred to a pediatric orthopaedic surgeon at time of diagnosis or when instability is detected on clinical examination.

Resource for Physicians and Families

- http://orthoinfo.aaos.org/topic.cfm?topic=A00347

Relevant *International Classification of Diseases, Ninth Revision, Clinical Modification* Code

- **754.30**   Developmental dysplasia of the hip

CHAPTER 19

Perthes Disease

Introduction/Etiology/Epidemiology

- Develops secondary to a vascular event of the proximal femoral epiphysis.
- Generally affects children between 4 and 12 years of age.
- More common in males than females (4–5:1)
- Typically unilateral
- Often seen in very active children
- Etiology is unknown; proposed mechanisms include trauma, hypercoagulability, environment, and hereditary.

Signs and Symptoms

- Typically present with a limp and activity-related thigh or knee pain. *Always consider hip etiology in a limping child with knee pain.*
- Some complain of hip discomfort.
- Physical examination shows guarding at the extremes of hip range of motion, limited hip abduction and internal rotation, and antalgic gait.
- Some may have a hip flexion contracture.

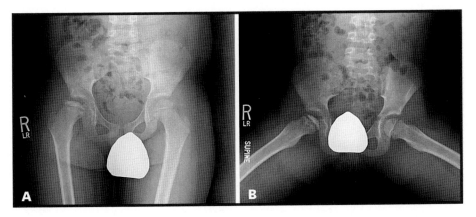

Figure 19-1. Anteroposterior (AP) (A) and frog lateral (B) of radiograph of a patient with Perthes disease. Note the difference in the proximal femur with comparing B, with Legg-Perthes disease, and A, which is normal. There is collapse and increased density of the proximal epiphysis on the AP pelvic radiograph, as well as the frog lateral.

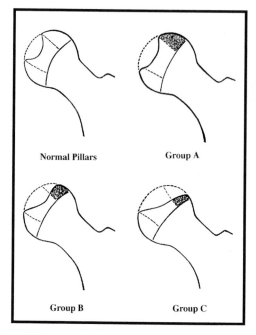

Figure 19-2. The lateral pillar (Herring) classification of Legg-Perthes disease. The epiphysis is divided into 3 segments. The most lateral aspect is analyzed with respect to height. Normal pillar is depicted. Group A is a normal height. In group B, more than 50% of the lateral pillar is maintained; in group C, less than 50% of the high to lateral pillar is maintained. The lateral pillar B-C border is between B and C (not pictured).

Differential Diagnosis

- Slipped capital femoral epiphysis
- Transient synovitis of the hip
- Septic arthritis
- Developmental hip dysplasia
- Multiple epiphyseal dysplasia
- Muscle strain or pelvic avulsion fracture should be considered in cases with acute onset during activity, especially in adolescents.
- Femoral stress fracture should be considered in cases preceded by repetitive overuse, such as running, also more common in adolescents.

Making the Diagnosis

- Diagnosis is made on radiographs.
  — Obtain anteroposterior (AP) and frog lateral views of both hips.
  — Early in the disease, radiographs will demonstrate increased density of the involved epiphysis.
  — Later stage involves fragmentation of the epiphysis, which may demonstrate a subchondral lucency on the epiphysis (crescent sign), or the epiphysis may look as though it is breaking up or collapsing (Figure 19-1 a, b).

— Severity is based on degree of femoral head involvement as indicated by lateral pillar classification on AP view. The height of the lateral third of the epiphysis is compared with the uninvolved side (Figure 19-2).
  ▪ Group A: no loss of height
  ▪ Group B: less than 50% loss of height
  ▪ Group C: more than 50% loss of height
- *Magnetic resonance imaging or bone scan* is not necessary for diagnosis but may be used in specific indications such as assessing the severity or morphology.

Treatment

- Somewhat controversial
- Treatment varies based on age, symptoms, range of motion, and amount of femoral head involvement.
- Goal of treatment is containment, or keeping the involved or remodeling portion of the epiphysis in the acetabulum. This helps the head remodel as spherically as possible.
- Nonsteroidal anti-inflammatory drugs and limited weight bearing can help when the hip is symptomatic.
- Nonsurgical treatment includes physical therapy for abduction stretching, bracing, or casting.
- Surgical treatment includes a varus osteotomy of the proximal femur or an acetabular surgery to reorient the acetabulum.

Expected Outcomes/Prognosis

- Outcomes for children younger than 6 years are generally favorable.
- Long-term prognosis is dependent on the overall shape of the femoral head at the time of healing (Stulberg classification 1–5).
  — Stulberg 1, 2, and 3 have a round femoral head and a generally good prognosis.
  — Stulberg 4 and 5 generally have early osteoarthritis and may require hip arthroplasty at a younger age.

When to Refer

- All patients with a new diagnosis of Perthes disease should be referred to an orthopaedist at the time of diagnosis.

Resource for Physicians and Families

- http://orthoinfo.aaos.org/topic.cfm?topic=A00070

Relevant *International Classification of Diseases, Ninth Revision, Clinical Modification* Code

- **732.1** Perthes disease

CHAPTER 20

Slipped Capital Femoral Epiphysis

Introduction/Etiology/Epidemiology

- Slipped capital femoral epiphysis (SCFE) is an orthopaedic hip condition in which the proximal femoral metaphysis shifts and displaces anterior and superior relative to the capital femoral epiphysis (not acetabulum).
- The incidence is approximately 2 per 100,000.
- Average age of presentation is 13.5 years for boys and 12 years for girls.
- Boys are slightly more often affected, comprising 60% of patients.
- Obesity is a risk factor.
  - More than half of all patients with SCFE are at or above the 95th percentile for weight for their age.
  - Obesity is associated with a deeper acetabulum, increased femoral retroversion, and increased physeal obliquity. The combination of these factors increases the shear stress across the physis and contributes to failure.
- Endocrine etiologies account for 5% to 8% of SCFE and are more likely in those outside the typical age range (younger than 10 or older than 15 years).
  - Testosterone decreases, while estrogen increases physeal strength.
  - Proper development of the physis requires thyroid hormone, vitamin D, and calcium. Thus, hypothyroidism and renal osteodystrophy have been associated with SCFE.

Signs and Symptoms

- Patients typically present in early adolescence.
- Groin pain, medial knee pain, or both are present.
- There may be a limp.
- There may be a history of acute trauma, but most present insidiously.
- Knee pain may be the only presenting symptom. *It is important to evaluate the hip of every patient who presents with knee pain.*
- Patients will hold the hip in external rotation and have limited internal rotation and limited hip flexion.

Differential Diagnosis

- Muscle strain or pelvic avulsion fracture should be considered in cases with acute onset during activity, especially in adolescents.
- Femoral stress fracture should be considered in cases preceded by repetitive overuse, such as running, especially in adolescents.
- Legg-Calve-Perthes disease
- Septic arthritis
- Transient synovitis of the hip
- Developmental dysplasia of the hip

Making the Diagnosis

- Diagnosis is made with *radiographs* (anteroposterior [AP] and frog lateral of the pelvis).
  — Slipped capital femoral epiphysis is most easily identified on a frog lateral view of the pelvis (Figure 20-1).
  — On the AP view, *Klein line* is used to diagnose SCFE. This is a line drawn along the superior femoral neck that should intersect the capital femoral epiphysis (Figure 20-2).
  — *Findings should be reviewed prior to discharging the patient.*
- *Magnetic resonance imaging* of the hips and pelvis
  — Indicated if radiographs are normal but strong clinical suspicion for SCFE.
  — Reveals increased signal along both sides of the physis.
- *Classification*
  — Slip severity is defined by the amount of displacement of the proximal femoral relative to the capital femoral epiphysis (Figure 20-3).
    - Mild: less than 33% slip
    - Moderate: 33% to 50% slip
    - Severe: greater than 50% slip
  — Slipped capital femoral epiphysis may also be categorized into *stable* and *unstable*, a classification that helps guide treatment.
    - Stable SCFE: the patient is able to bear weight on the affected extremity.
    - Unstable SCFE: the patient is unable to bear weight because of pain.
- Consider endocrine etiologies in patients younger than 10 or older than 15 years.
- Consider growth hormone deficiency in patients with short stature. (No clear relationship between growth hormone deficiency and SCFE has been demonstrated.)

Treatment

- Patients diagnosed with SCFE are *immediately* made non-weight bearing on the affected extremity (eg, crutches, walker, bed rest) and referred to an orthopaedic surgeon for urgent treatment.
- Untreated slips may progress, with risk for development of later complications including osteonecrosis and degenerative joint disease.

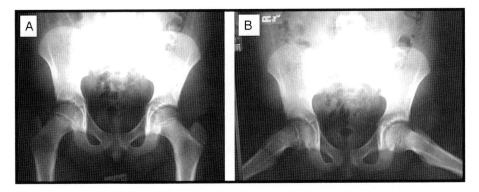

Figure 20-1. Pelvis radiographs of a 13-year-old with right-sided groin and knee pain. A, Anteroposterior radiographs showing a normal relationship between the epiphysis and metaphysis of the right femur. B, Frog leg pelvis radiographs showing the posterior slip of the epiphysis of the right proxmial femur. Please note that this abnormality was not seen until a frog leg pelvis radiograph was ordered.

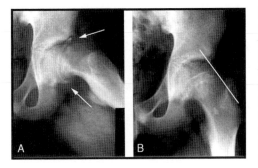

Figure 20-2. Radiographs of the pelvis showing mild slipped capital femoral epiphysis (SCFE) of the right hip. A, Posterior displacement of the femoral head (arrows) is indicated on the frog lateral radiographs. B, On the anteroposterior view mild degrees of medial displacement can be identified by drawing a line along the lateral aspect of the femoral neck. SCFE is present if the line misses the femoral head or transects it less than on the uninvolved hip. Reproduced with permission from Griffin LY (ed): *Essentials of Musculoskeletal Care,* 3rd edition. Rosemont, IL: American Academy of Orthopaedic Surgeons; 2005.

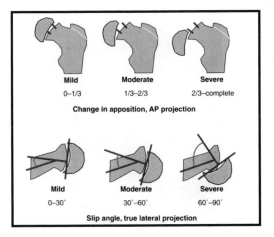

Figure 20-3. Severity of slipped capital femoral epiphysis can be expressed as a grade based on the displacement scan in the anteroposterior projection. A more accurate measurement is the slip angle measured from a true lateral radiograph. From Staheli LT. *Practice of Pediatric Orthopedics.* Philadelphia, PA: Lippincott Williams & Wilkins; 2001:153. Reprinted by permission.

- Stable slips
  — Surgical method of treatment is percutaneous in situ fixation with a single screw under general anesthesia.
  — Postoperatively, patients are non-weight bearing on the affected extremity for 4 to 6 weeks (author preference) followed by weight bearing as tolerated.
  — Other treatment options include bone graft epiphysiodesis, multiple pin fixation, and SPICA casting.
- Unstable slips
  — Fixation is similar; however, consensus is that *urgency for treatment is greater* (stemming from compromise of the blood supply to the femoral head occurring in unstable slips) with increased risk for late osteonecrosis.
  — Surgeons may atraumatically reduce the slip degree when examining the hip under anesthesia, thus performing an incidental reduction.
  — Following surgery, patients are non-weight bearing on the affected extremity for 6 to 8 weeks (crutches or walker).
  — Some patients will have bilateral involvement. For this reason, some surgeons prophylactically pin the contralateral hip.

Expected Outcomes/Prognosis

- Long-term outcomes are generally favorable in the uncomplicated case.
- Severity of slip at the time of diagnosis affects outcome, with moderate to severe slips having increased risk for late osteonecrosis, degenerative joint changes, and chondrolysis.
- Patients may demonstrate limited internal rotation and hip flexion after in situ fixation; however, this limitation may remodel with time. If disabling, a number of corrective orthopaedic surgical procedures may be undertaken.

When to Refer

- Patients diagnosed with SCFE should be *immediately* made non-weight bearing on the affected extremity (eg, crutches, walker, bed rest) and referred to an orthopaedic surgeon for urgent treatment.

Relevant *International Classification of Diseases, Ninth Revision, Clinical Modification* Code

- **732.2**   SCFE

CHAPTER 21

Snapping Hip

Introduction/Etiology/Epidemiology

- Audible, sometimes painful, snapping sensation caused by 1 of 2 etiologies.
  - *External snapping hip*: a tight or inflamed iliotibial band snaps across the greater trochante.
  - *Internal snapping hip*: a tight or inflamed iliopsoas tendon subluxes over the iliopectineal eminence (figures 21-1 and 21-2a, b).
- The snapping can be painful or painless, or cause a sensation of relief.
- It can be unilateral or bilateral.
- It usually presents during the adolescent growth spurt and is more common in girls.
- Incidence is highest in athletes who perform repetitive hip flexion such as gymnasts and dancers. One study of adolescent dancers reported snapping hip in approximately 50%.

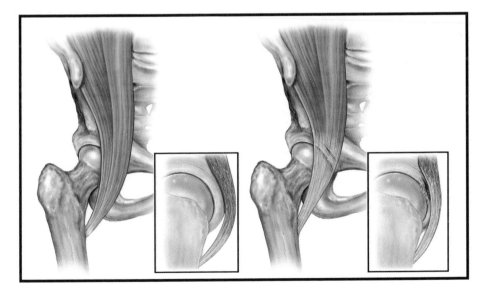

Figure 21-1. A portion of the psoas, running outside the joint (in most cases), becomes symptomatic, in that it tightens causing it to snap (internal snapping hip) across the rim of the acetabulum or the femoral head. The psoas itself can become painful from this repetitive motion. In other cases, the psoas compresses the labrum resulting in crushing and sometimes tearing of the labral tissue due to the close proximity of the 2 structures.
Copyright Randal S. McKenzie. Used with permission.

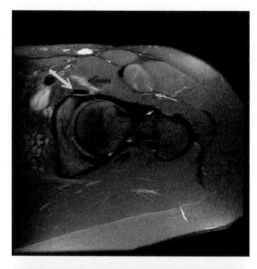

Figure 21-2a. Fifteen-year-old female with snapping left hip, referred for magnetic resonance imaging to see if snapping is intra-articular (usually due to a labral tear) or extra-articular in origin. Oblique axial T2-weighted image reveals local soft tissue edema associated with the iliopsoas tendon.
Courtesy Vic David, MD.

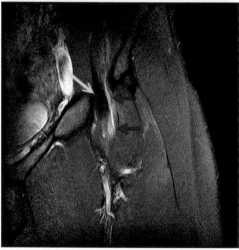

Figure 21-2b. Oblique coronal T2-weighted image confirms the edema tracking along the iliopsoas tendon. Courtesy Vic David, MD.

External Snapping Hip

SIGNS AND SYMPTOMS

- Patients report pain or audible snapping on the lateral aspect of the hip with flexion and external rotation.
- Onset is usually insidious, but may also be triggered by direct trauma to the lateral hip.
- On physical examination, pain and snapping can be reproduced when the patient actively flexes and rotates the hip but not when the examiner passively moves the hip.
- Most patients will be able to voluntarily reproduce the snapping.
- There is usually tenderness over the greater trochanter and proximal iliotibial band.

DIFFERENTIAL DIAGNOSIS

- Hip abductor muscle strain, trochanteric bursitis, greater trochanter apophysitis, or avulsion

MAKING THE DIAGNOSIS

- External snapping hip is a clinical diagnosis. Imaging is not required.
- Radiographs (anteroposterior [AP] view of the pelvis and frog lateral of both hips) are indicated only to evaluate for other causes of hip pain in a patient with atypical signs and symptoms.

TREATMENT

- Rest from irritating activities
- Nonsteroidal anti-inflammatory drugs
- A comprehensive physical therapy program for hip muscle strengthening, stretching, and soft tissue massage to the tight iliotibial band

EXPECTED OUTCOMES/PROGNOSIS

- The pain associated with external snapping hip usually resolves with physical therapy, but this may take 6 months or longer.
- Full return to prior level of activity is expected.
- Many adolescents will also outgrow this on reaching full skeletal maturity.
- The snapping often persists even when pain is resolved.

WHEN TO REFER

- Persistent symptoms despite several months of physical therapy

PREVENTION

- Maintain good hip muscle strength and flexibility.
- Avoid repetitive hip flexion activities.

RELEVANT *INTERNATIONAL CLASSIFICATION OF DISEASES, NINTH REVISION, CLINICAL MODIFICATION (ICD-9-CM)* CODE

- **719.65** Snapping hip

Internal Snapping Hip

SIGNS AND SYMPTOMS

- Patients report anterior (groin) hip pain and snapping with hip flexion or external rotation.
- There may be tenderness in the groin over the iliopsoas tendon.
- Snapping can usually be voluntarily reproduced with active hip flexion.
- Range of motion is usually normal, although flexion and external rotation may be limited because of pain.

DIFFERENTIAL DIAGNOSIS

- Labral tear: The labrum is a layer of cartilage that forms a cup around the acetabulum. It can be injured by direct trauma or overuse. On examination, a labral tear will usually cause pain with passive, rather than active, hip flexion.
- Slipped capital femoral epiphysis (SCFE)
- Perthes disease
- Anterior inferior iliac spineapophysitis or avulsion
- Hip adductor muscle strain (groin pull)

MAKING THE DIAGNOSIS

- While the diagnosis can be made clinically, radiographs (AP view of the pelvis and frog lateral of both hips) should be performed to rule out other causes of anterior hip pain (eg, SCFE, Perthes, apophysitis, avulsion). Radiographs are normal in internal snapping hip syndrome.
- Ultrasound may demonstrate the subluxing iliopsoas tendon.
- Magnetic resonance imaging of the hip with interarticular contrast (arthrogram) can distinguish iliopsoas tendonitis from a labral tear. (See Figure 21-2a,b.)

TREATMENT

- A rehabilitation program for hip muscle strengthening and stretching usually alleviates the pain, although the snapping may persist.
- A corticosteroid injection of the iliopsoas tendon sheath may help patients with persistent pain after physical therapy.

EXPECTED OUTCOMES/PROGNOSIS

- The pain usually resolves with physical therapy but may take 6 months or longer.
- The snapping often persists even when pain is resolved.
- Full return to prior level of activity is expected.

WHEN TO REFER

- Persistent symptoms despite several months of physical therapy

PREVENTION

* Same as for external snapping hip syndrome

RELEVANT *ICD-9-CM* CODES

* **719.65**   Snapping hip

Bibliography

Aronsson DD, Loder RT, Breur GJ, Weinstein SL. Slipped capital femoral epiphysis: current concepts. *J Am Acad Orthop Surg.* 2006;14:666–679

Barlow TG. Early diagnosis and treatment of congenital dislocation of the hip. *J Bone Joint Surg Br.* 1962;44-B:292–301.

Carney BT, Weinstein SL, Noble J. Long-term follow-up of slipped capital femoral epiphysis. *J Bone Joint Surg Am.* 1991;73:667–674

Eldridge JC. Slipped capital femoral epiphysis. In: Sponseller PD, ed. *Orthopaedic Knowledge Update Pediatrics* Rosemont, IL: American Academy of Orthopaedic Surgeons; 2002:143–152

Harding MG, Harcke HT, Bowen JR, Guille JT, Glutting J. Management of dislocated hips with Pavlik harness treatment and ultrasound monitoring. *J Pediatr Orthop.* 1997;17:189–198

Herring JA, Kim HT, Browne R. Legg-Calve-Perthes disease. Part I: classification of radiographs with use of the modified lateral pillar and Stulberg classifications. *J Bone Joint Surg Am.* 2004;86-A:2103–2120

Herring JA, Kim HT, Browne R. Legg-Calve-Perthes disease. Part II: prospective multicenter study of the effect of treatment on outcome. *J Bone Joint Surg Am.* 2004;86-A:2121–2134

Jones GT, Schoenecker PL, Dias LS. Developmental hip dysplasia potentiated by inappropriate use of the Pavlik harness. *J Pediatr Orthop.* 1992;12:722–726

Kay RM. Slipped capital femoral epiphysis. In: Morrissy RT, Weinstein SL. *Lovell & Winter's Pediatric Orthopaedics.* 6th ed. Philadelphia, PA: Lippincott Williams & Wilkins; 2006

Kitadai HK, Milani C, Nery CA, Filho JL. Wiberg's center-edge angle in patients with slipped capital femoral epiphysis. *J Pediatr Orthop.* 1999;19:97–105

Leunig M, Werlen S, Ungersbock A, Ito K, Ganz R. Evaluation of the acetabular labrum by MR arthrography. *J Bone Joint Surg Br.* 1997;79:230–234

Lindstrom JR, Ponseti IV, Wenger DR. Acetabular development after reduction in congenital dislocation of the hip. *J Bone Joint Surg Am.* 1979;61:112–118

Loder RT. The demographics of slipped capital femoral epiphysis. An international multicenter study. *Clin Orthop Relat Res.* 1996;322:8–27

Loder RT, Aronsson DD, Dobbs MB, Weinstein SL. Slipped capital femoral epiphysis. *Instr Course Lect.* 2001;50:555–570

Loder RT, Richards BS, Shapiro PS, Reznick LR, Aronson DD. Acute slipped capital femoral epiphysis: the importance of physeal stability. *J Bone Joint Surg Am.* 1993;75:1134–1140

Loder RT, Starnes T, Dikos G, Aronsson DD. Demographic predictors of severity of stable slipped capital femoral epiphyses. *J Bone Joint Surg Am.* 2006;88:97–105

Luhmann SJ, Schoenecker PL, Anderson AM, Bassett GS. The prognostic importance of the ossific nucleus in the treatment of congenital dysplasia of the hip. *J Bone Joint Surg Am.* 1998;80:1719–1727

Ponseti IV. Growth and development of the acetabulum in the normal child. Anatomical, histological, and roentgenographic studies. *J Bone Joint Surg Am.* 1978;60:575–585

Ramsey PL, Lasser S, MacEwen GD. Congenital dislocation of the hip. Use of the Pavlik harness in the child during the first six months of life. *J Bone Joint Surg Am.* 1976;58:1000–1004

Schoenecker PL, Anderson DJ, Capelli AM. The acetabular response to proximal femoral varus rotational osteotomy. Results after failure of post-reduction abduction splinting in patients who had congenital dislocation of the hip. *J Bone Joint Surg Am.* 1995;77:990–997

Segal LS, Boal DK, Borthwick L, Clark MW, Localio AR, Schwentker EP. Avascular necrosis after treatment of DDH: the protective influence of the ossific nucleus. *J Pediatr Orthop.* 1999;19:177–184

Sucato DJ, Johnston CE 2nd, Birch JG, Herring JA, Mack P. Outcome of ultrasonographic hip abnormalities in clinically stable hips. *J Pediatr Orthop.* 1999;19:754–759

Wedge JH, Wasylenko MJ. The natural history of congenital dislocation of the hip: a critical review. *Clin Orthop Relat Res.* 1978;137:154–162

Weinstein SL. Natural history of congenital hip dislocation (CDH) and hip dysplasia. *Clin Orthop Relat Res.* 1987;225:62–76

Part 9: Rotational and Angular Deformities

TOPICS COVERED

CHAPTER 22

General Treatment Guidelines

- Angular and rotational lower limb variations in children are common presenting complaints to pediatricians and primary care practitioners, most often with *no* treatment interventions required.
- Usually described with reference to the position of the foot (in-toeing and out-toeing) or the knee (bowlegs and knock-knees) in relationship to the midline axis of the body
- Adult patterns of lower limb rotation and angulation develop in a predictable fashion during the first decade of life and are not present at birth.
  — Wide variations of normal have been documented.
    - Rotational variation within normal limits for age is termed *version*.
    - Rotation that exceeds 2 standard deviations from the mean is termed *torsion*.
- Knowledge of normal development of limb alignment during growth is the cornerstone of diagnosis in these patients.
  — The femur and tibia rotate laterally with growth, so internal tibial torsion and medial femoral torsion decrease with age, while lateral femoral torsion and external tibial torsion increase with age.
- Parents and other family members are often concerned about the long-term functional, degenerative, and cosmetic implications of these conditions and most often the treatment intervention is *reassurance* of normal development.
- Families may attribute a child's clumsiness, disinterest in sports, or frequent falls to an observed rotational or angular pattern.
- Parental reaction may be colored by personal experience, and it is common to discover that a family member has received treatment for a similar disorder in the past.

Rotational Deformities

- The use of braces and other devices has waned over the past 30 years because research studies have demonstrated that the natural history in most of these conditions is spontaneous resolution.
- It is important to provide appropriate *education* and *reassurance* to families.
- Persistent alignment abnormalities associated with significant functional or cosmetic concern may be corrected surgically; however, this is rarely required.

In-toeing

INTRODUCTION/ETIOLOGY/EPIDEMIOLOGY

- In-toeing is a general term for deviation of the feet toward the midline. In lay terminology this may be referred as pigeon-toed.
- In-toeing may be unilateral or bilateral; it is often more visually striking when there is asymmetry.
- In-toeing may be explained by one of the following anatomic variants: *medial femoral torsion, internal tibial torsion,* or *metatarsus adductus.*
  — Metatarsus adductus presents in the first year of life.
  — Internal tibial torsion presents in toddlers.
  — Medial femoral torsion presents in children older than 3 years.
- More than one rotational variant may coexist, accentuating or compensating for the index deformity (eg, a patient with coexistent medial femoral torsion and external tibial torsion will exhibit a neutral gait pattern).

EVALUATION

- *History*
  — Young children are generally asymptomatic and present to the physician's office because of an adult's concern.
  — Older children are usually aware of the condition and may describe functional problems such as tripping or may be self-conscious.
- *Physical examination*
  — Assess lower limb alignment in standing position with particular attention to the angle produced by the intersection of the long axes of the femur and tibia.
  — Evaluate the foot progression angle (FPA) during gait.
    - Foot progression angle is the angle produced by the long axis of the foot and the line of forward travel of the body.
    - When the foot points towards the midline, the FPA is defined as negative.
    - When the foot points away from the midline, FPA is positive.
    - Normal FPA ranges from -5 to +20 degrees.
  — Determine the rotational profile of the femur, tibia, and feet in the prone position.
    - Femur: Measure hip internal and external rotation in prone position with the knees in flexion (Figure 22-1 a, b).
    - Tibia: Measure the thigh-foot angle (TFA) in the prone position. With the hips extended and the knees flexed to 90 degrees, measure the angle between the long axis of the foot and the long axis of the thigh (Figure 22-2).
      + In infants, normal TFA ranges from -17 to +5 degrees.
      + In children and adults, normal TFA ranges from -5 to +30 degrees with a mean of 10 to 15 degrees.
    - Feet: The lateral border of the foot should be straight.

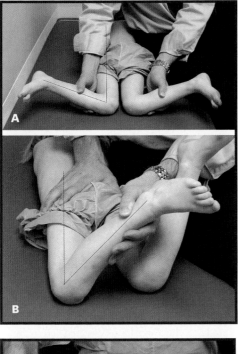

Figure 22-1. Measurement of hip internal (A) and external rotation (B) with patient prone, knees together. Normal ranges vary by age and sex. Excessive internal rotation may signal joint laxity, femoral anteversion, or spasticity. Femoral anteversion is likely present when internal rotation is significantly greater than external rotation.

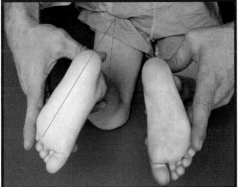

Figure 22-2. Thigh-foot angle (TFA) is assessed by having the patient lie prone with the knees flexed to 90 degrees and the feet in a relaxed position. TFA is formed by the axis of the foot and the axis of the thigh. Note any asymmetry.

— Very young children (2 years and younger) may be unwilling to lie prone and therefore may be examined sitting on the parent's lap to lessen anxiety and encourage cooperation. In this position, hip range of motion is examined supine and tibial rotation can be quantified by comparing the position of the second toe to that of the tibial tubercle.

DIFFERENTIAL DIAGNOSIS

- Clarify the exact presenting complaint because other musculoskeletal conditions such as pes planus may be misidentified by laypeople as in-toeing.
- Differentiate rotational profile variants from underlying neurologic disorders (eg, cerebral palsy) by looking for clues such as delayed motor development or a regression of motor skills.

MEDIAL FEMORAL TORSION

Introduction/Etiology/Epidemiology

- Usually symmetrical and commonly noted between 3 and 6 years of age (see Box 22-1)
- The ratio of affected girls to boys is 2:1.

Box 22-1. Femoral Torsion

The angular difference between the axes of the femoral neck and the transcondylar axis of the knee

Has been measured to be as high as 40 degrees in normal infants, decreasing to between 10 and 15 degrees by adulthood.

While femoral rotation can be measured radiographically (methods using biplanar radiographs, ultrasound, computed tomography scans, and magnetic resonance imaging have all been described), it is more commonly estimated by quantifying the internal and external rotation of a patient's hips in the prone position.

Signs and Symptoms

- There is often a family history of similar deformity.
- Children with medial femoral torsion often avoid sitting cross-legged, preferring to sit on their knees with their hips internally rotated and the lower limbs directed externally (often called the W position).
- Parents or patients may report clumsiness and frequent tripping.
- Physical examination—negative FPA and hip internal rotation greater than 70 degrees
  - Mild: internal rotation 70 to 80 degrees; external rotation 10 to 20 degrees
  - Moderate: internal rotation 80 to 90 degrees; external rotation 0 to 10 degrees
  - Severe: internal rotation greater than 90 degrees; external rotation less than 0 degrees
- With running, the legs rotate laterally at the knee during swing phase—described as an *eggbeater* pattern.

Making the Diagnosis

- Diagnosis is made by history and physical examination.
- Imaging studies are not necessary for making the diagnosis and are only recommended if motion is markedly asymmetrical or as part of preoperative planning.

Treatment

- The initial intervention is *reassurance* and *education* for the child and family that the natural history of medial femoral torsion is one of resolution in more than 80% of children.
- Nonoperative treatment including shoe wedges, twister cables, and night splints have been shown to be ineffective in altering the natural history of femoral version.
- There is no evidence that discouraging W-sitting has a positive effect.
- In rare instances, surgical correction involves proximal femoral derotational osteotomy. This is indicated only for severe deformity (more than 80 degrees of medial hip rotation and more than 50 degrees of measured medial femoral torsion) and functional problems.

Expected Outcomes/Prognosis

- Medial femoral torsion decreases by 1.5 degrees per year during normal skeletal growth.
- Most children have achieved a normal adult rotational profile in the upper femur by 8 to 10 years of age.
- Researchers have demonstrated that the physical performance of adults and adolescents with medial femoral torsion is not impaired.
- Medial femoral torsion has been implicated by some in the development of hip osteoarthritis; however, comparison of arthritic and control hips has revealed no difference in medial femoral torsion between the 2 groups. Therefore, prophylactic surgical correction of the rotational alignment is not recommended on this basis.
- There is ongoing debate about the effect of medial femoral torsion on the knee joint. The "miserable malalignment syndrome" has been described, where medial femoral torsion combines with external tibial torsion to create patellofemoral dysfunction and pain. Isolated medial femoral torsion, however, seems to be more benign.

When to Refer

- If a child has persistent, symptomatic medial femoral torsion beyond 8 years of age, refer to an orthopaedic specialist.

Relevant **International Classification of Diseases, Ninth Revision, Clinical Modification (ICD-9-CM)** *Code*

- **755.60**   Medial femoral torsion (congenital)

INTERNAL TIBIAL TORSION

Introduction/Etiology/Epidemiology

- Common in infants and toddlers
- Caused by intrauterine factors. Not found in preterm infants.
- Bilateral in two thirds of cases
- Unlike medial femoral torsion, there is no gender-related difference.

Signs and Symptoms

- In-toeing because of internal tibial torsion is noted in the second year of life. At this early stage of gross motor development, *frequent falls are not unusual* and parents may attribute falls to observed rotational malalignment.
- In-toeing may be more pronounced when the child is running, fatigued, or wearing bulky footwear because the necessary compensatory hip external rotation may be more challenging. This may cause parents to think that the deformity waxes and wanes over time.

Making the Diagnosis

- Physical examination reveals a negative TFA and negative FPA, with the patella pointing anteriorly and the foot pointing medially.
- It is important to evaluate for genu varum or foot deformity because internal tibial torsion may be associated with other lower limb abnormalities such as clubfoot or tibia vara (Blount disease).

Treatment

- Because *spontaneous resolution is expected in almost all cases of internal tibial torsion,* education and reassurance play a major role in managing internal tibial torsion.
- Although most isolated cases of internal tibial torsion do not require treatment or intervention, a night splint was formerly recommended. It has not been shown to alter the natural history of resolution of internal tibial torsion.
- Surgical treatment (rare) includes a rotational osteotomy, most commonly performed in the distal region of the tibia. This is generally indicated in patients with a TFA of -10 degrees or less who are at least 8 to 20 years of age.

Expected Outcomes/Prognosis

- *Spontaneous resolution is expected in almost all cases of internal tibial torsion.*
  — Correction is generally complete by 8 years of age.
- While persistent internal tibial torsion may be of cosmetic concern, it rarely causes a functional problem.
- Some authors have postulated that this rotational variation may actually improve performance in certain sports such as sprinting.

When to Refer

- Refer internal tibial torsion to an orthopaedic specialist
  — When associated with foot deformity or significant amount of genu varum
  — If it fails to correct spontaneously by age 8 years

Relevant ICD-9-CM Code

- **755.60**   Internal tibial torsion (congenital)

METATARSUS ADDUCTUS

Introduction/Etiology/Epidemiology

- A congenital molded foot that causes medial deviation of the foot at the tarsometatarsal joint (Figure 22-3)
- Unilateral or bilateral
- Secondary to intrauterine positioning. As with internal tibial torsion, it is not found in preterm newborns.
- Prone sleeping may perpetuate the condition.

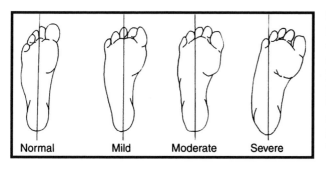

Figure 22-3. Heel bisector line to evaluate medial deviation of the foot at the tarsometatarsal joint. Reprinted with permission from Bleck WW. Developmental orthopaedics. III: Toddlers. *Develop Med Child Neurol.* 1982;24:533–534.

Signs and Symptoms

- Identified at or shortly after birth by the characteristic kidney bean shape of the foot, where the lateral border of the foot is convex.
- Flexibility of the deformity is variable; more rigid feet may have a medial or plantar crease.

Making the Diagnosis

- Diagnosis is made based on physical examination, by estimating the position of the heel bisector line (a line drawn along the plantar surface that bisects the U shape of the heel).
  — In a normal foot, the heel bisector line falls between the second and third toes.
  — In metatarsus adductus, the heel bisector line falls lateral to the third toe.

Differential Diagnosis

- Dynamic hallux varus: the foot appears adducted in stance because of an overactive abductor hallucis muscle, but unlike metatarsus adductus, the foot shape is normal at rest.
- Clubfoot: the forefoot deformity is accompanied by varus of the hindfoot and equinus of the ankle (see Chapter 42).
- Skew foot: Combination of metatarsus adductus and excessive hindfoot valgus

Treatment

- Mild, flexible deformities require observation only.
- Moderate deformities may benefit from parental stretching that involves gentle lateral pressure applied to the medial aspect of the foot for several minutes with every diaper change.
- For severe or persistent deformities, serial casts are applied.
  — This is most effective if initiated before 8 months of age.
  — Correction is usually achieved in 4 to 6 weeks.
  — Some advocate the use of reverse last shoes to maintain the correction following casting.
- If the deformity is identified late, surgical correction may be indicated to improve cosmesis and shoe fitting.
  — Tarsometatarsal capsulotomies are no longer recommended for this condition because of poor long-term results; a variety of other procedures ranging from soft tissue releases to midfoot osteotomies have been described for this condition.

Expected Outcomes/Prognosis

- Most cases of metatarsus adductus diagnosed before walking age correct spontaneously.
- Persistent deformity causes difficulty with footwear and cosmesis.
- Metatarsus adductus has not been associated with foot pain or degenerative disease in adulthood.

When to Refer

- If the deformity persists beyond 3 months of age, refer to an orthopaedic specialist.

Relevant ICD-9-CM Code

- **754.53**   Metatarsus adductus

Out-toeing

INTRODUCTION/ETIOLOGY/EPIDEMIOLOGY

- Out-toeing is defined as an FPA greater than the upper limit of normal (20 degrees in infancy and 15 degrees at skeletal maturity).
- Out-toeing may come from the hip, femur, or tibia.
- Pes plano valgus and pronation may also contribute to out-toeing.

DIAGNOSIS AND TREATMENT

- *Infantile lateral rotation contractures of the hips*
  - Common finding in normal infants; produces an externally rotated posture of the lower limb. May be present at onset of walking.
  - Feet turn out when the infant is placed in an upright position.
  - Reassurance is usually all that is required because these contractures resolve over the first year of life.
- *Slipped capital femoral epiphysis (SCFE)*
  - It is important to evaluate for SCFE in the obese teenager with a new onset of unilateral or bilateral externally rotated gait (see Chapter 20).
  - Physical examination usually reveals obligate hip external rotation with flexion, and pain with passive hip rotation.
  - *Anteroposterior (AP) and lateral radiographs of the hips must be obtained* if this diagnosis is suspected.
- *Lateral femoral torsion*
  - Rare deformity that may be developmental or result from SCFE
  - Associated with obesity; postulated to be caused by excessive femoral remodeling secondary to mechanical forces.
  - On physical examination, hip internal rotation is less than 25 degrees.
  - Does not improve with growth.
  - Can lead to hip pain and a degenerative hip joint.

- *External tibial torsion*
  - — Thigh-foot angle greater than 30 degrees
  - — Less common than internal tibial torsion
  - — Excessive tibial torsion (>40 degrees) may cause disability including medial foot pain, patellofemoral pain, patellofemoral instability, and osteochondritis dissecans of the knee.
  - — Tight iliotibial band or Achilles tendon contribute to the out-toeing; in these cases, routine stretching can reduce the apparent deformity.
  - — Tibial osteotomy (rare) is recommended only for severe, symptomatic deformity that persists beyond 8 to 10 years of age.

WHEN TO REFER

- Any symptomatic deformity that persists beyond 8 to 10 years of age should be referred to an orthopaedic specialist.
- Slipped capital femoral epiphysis requires immediate referral to an orthopaedic surgeon.

RELEVANT *ICD-9-CM* CODES

- **755.63**　　Infantile hip contracture
- **736.89**　　Lateral femoral torsion (acquired)
- **755.60**　　Lateral femoral torsion (congenital)
- **732.2**　　SCFE
- **755.60**　　External tibial torsion (congenital)

Angular Deformities

GENU VARUM (BOWLEGS) AND GENU VALGUM (KNOCK-KNEES)

Introduction/Etiology/Epidemiology

- *Physiologic*
  - — Angular variations at the knee (bowlegs or knock-knees) that fall within 2 standard deviations of the mean
  - — Angular orientation of the lower limbs follows a predictable pattern of normal development during childhood (Figure 22-4).
    - ▪ Before 2 years of age, most children demonstrate physiologic genu varum, in some cases as much as 15 degrees.
    - ▪ By 2 years of age, neutral alignment is the norm.
    - ▪ Children then proceed to develop exaggerated valgus, which peaks by about 3 years of age and then corrects towards the normal adult value of 5 to 7 degrees of valgus.
    - ▪ Physiologic genu varum and valgum are typically symmetrical.

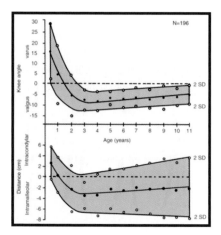

Figure 22-4. Normal values for the knee angle are shown in degrees and intracondylar in intramalleolar distance. Reprinted from Heath CH, Staheli LT. Normal limits of knee angle in white children—genu varum and genu valgum. *J Pediatr Orthop* 1993;13:259–262, with permission form Wolters Kluwer Health.

- *Idiopathic*
  - Angular variations at the knee (bowlegs or knock-knees) that fall outside 2 standard deviations of the mean.
  - May be familial.
  - Idiopathic genu valgum is most commonly seen in obese girls.
    - In supine position with the knees fully extended, the distance between the medial malleoli is greater than 8 to 10 cm.
  - Idiopathic genu varum is most commonly seen in Asians.
- *Pathologic*
  - *Rickets* may cause genu varum or valgum (see Chapter 61).
    - Usually associated with short stature
    - Radiographs show characteristic widening of the physes and help to establish the diagnosis along with serum calcium studies.
  - *Blount disease* is a pathologic cause of varus deformity at the knee.
    - Focal growth disturbance of medial proximal tibial epiphysis produces tibia vara.
    - Occurs commonly in children who walk at an early age and in those who are obese or of African descent.
    - Often associated with significant internal tibial torsion
    - Radiographs demonstrate metaphyseal-diaphyseal angle in the proximal tibia (Drennan angle) greater than 15 degrees; more advanced cases are identified by deformity of the medial tibial physis.
  - *Skeletal dysplasias* can be associated with genu varum (see Chapter 60).
    - Identified by positive family history, short stature, abnormal body proportions, or characteristic radiologic findings.
  - *Post-traumatic genu valgum*
    - Typically unilateral
    - Occurs after a seemingly benign undisplaced upper tibial metaphyseal fracture in young children.

Treatment

- Physiologic genu varum and valgum require no treatment other than *reassurance* and *education.*
- For equivocal cases at the upper limit of normal, evaluate the deformity with a standing photograph taken in the AP plane and repeat within 6 months to identify whether there has been resolution or progression.
- Shoe wedges and bracing are not effective
- If angular malalignment is severe or persists beyond the expected age of correction, surgical treatment (rare) may be indicated to prevent degenerative arthritis of the knee.
  — Prior to physeal closure, correction may be achieved by physeal stapling or hemi-epiphysiodesis.
  — After skeletal maturity, osteotomy is required to correct angular deformity.

Expected Outcomes/Prognosis

- Severe or pathologic deformities can lead to a degenerative knee joint.
  — Excessive valgus wears out the lateral knee joint while excessive varus wears out the medial joint.

When to Refer

- Deformities that are severe, pathologic, or persist beyond the expected age of correction should be referred to an orthopaedic specialist.

Relevant ICD-9-CM Codes

- **736.41**   Genu valgum (acquired)
- **736.42**   Genu varum (acquired)
- **755.64**   Genu valgum or varum (congenital)
- **732.4**   Tibia vara (Blount disease)

Bibliography

Asirvatham R, Stevens PM. Idiopathic forefoot-adduction deformity: medial capsulotomy and abductor hallucis lengthening for resistant and severe deformities. *J Pediatr Orthop.* 1997;17:496–500

Bleck EE. Metatarsus adductus: classification and relationship to outcomes of treatment. *J Pediatr Orthop.* 1983;3:2–9

Bramer JAM, Mass M, Dallinga RJ, te Slaa RL, Vergroesen DA. Increased external tibial torsion and osteochondritis dissecans of the knee. *Clin Orthop Relat Res.* 2004;422:175–179

Bruce WD, Stevens PM. Surgical correction of miserable malalignment syndrome. *J Pediatr Orthop.* 2004; 24:392–396

Engel GM, Staheli LT. The natural history of torsion and other factors influencing gait in childhood. *Clin Orthop.* 1974;99:12–17

Fuchs R, Staheli LT. Sprinting and intoeing. *J Pediatr Orthop.* 1996;16:489–491

Heinrich SD, Sharps CH. Lower extremity torsional deformities in children: a prospective comparison of two treatment modalities. *Orthopedics.* 1991;14:655–659

Hubbard DD, Staheli LT, Chew DE, Mosca VS. Medial femoral torsion and osteoarthritis. *J Pediatr Orthop.* 1988;8:540–542

Hudson D, Royer T, Richards J. Ultrasound measurements of torsions in the tibia and femur. *J Bone Joint Surg Am.* 2006;88:138–143

Hunziker UA, Largo RH, Due G. Neonatal metatarsus adductus, joint mobility, axis and rotation of the lower extremity in preterm and term children 0-5 years of age. *Eur J Pediatr.* 1988;148:19–23

Kingsley PC, Olmstead KL. A study to determine the angle of anteversion of the neck of the femur. *J Bone Joint Surg Am.* 1948;30A:745–751

Kling TF, Hensinger RN. Angular and torsional deformities of the lower limbs in children. *Clin Orthop Relat Res.* 1983;176:136–147

Krengel WF, Staheli LT. Tibial rotation osteotomy for idiopathic torsion. A comparison of the proximal and distal osteotomy levels. *Clin Orthop Relat Res.* 1992;283:285–289

Lichtblau S. Section of the abductor hallucis tendon for correction of metatarsus varus deformity. *Clin Orthop Relat Res.* 1975;110:227–232

Ponseti IV, Becke JR. Congenital metatarsus adductus: the results of treatment. *J Bone and Joint Surg Am.*1966;48:702–711

Salenius P, Vankka E. The development of the tibiofemoral angle in children. *J Bone Joint Surg Am.* 1975; 57:259–261

Savva N, Ramesh R, Richards RH. Supramalleolar osteotomy for unilateral tibial torsion. *J Pediatr Orthop B.* 2006;15:190–193

Schneider B, Laubenberger J, Jemlich S, Groene K, Weber HM, Langer M. Measurement of femoral antetorsion and tibial torsion by magnetic resonance imaging. *Br J Radiol.* 1997;70:575–579

Schwarze DJ, Denton JR. Normal values of neonatal lower limbs: an evaluation of 1,000 neonates. *J Pediatr Orthop.* 1993;13:758–760

Staheli LT. Rotational problems in children. *J Bone and Joint Surg.* 1993;75-A:939–949.

Staheli LT, Corbett M, Wyss C, King H. Lower-extremity rotational problems in children. Normal values to guide management. *J Bone Joint Surg Am.* 1985;67:39–47

Staheli LT, Lippert F, Denotter P. Femoral anteversion and physical performance in adolescent and adult life. *Clin Orthop Relat Res.* 1977;129:213–216

Svenningsen S, Apalset K, Terjesen T, Anda S. Regression of femoral anteversion. A prospective study of intoeing children. *Acta Ortho Scand.* 1989;60:170–173

Wedge JH, Munkacsi I, Loback D. Anteversion of the femur and idiopathic osteoarthrosis of the hip. *J Bone Joint Surg Am.* 1989;71:1040–1043

Part 10: Upper Extremity Problems

TOPICS COVERED

CHAPTER 23

Brachial Plexus Injuries

Newborn Brachial Plexus Injuries

INTRODUCTION/ETIOLOGY/EPIDEMIOLOGY

- Frequency is 0.1% to 0.2% of live births.
- Most are traction injuries to the brachial plexus (tables 23-1 and 23-2) caused by excessive lateral flexion or hyperextension of the neck during delivery, resulting in varying degrees of arm muscle weakness, which can lead to progressive glenohumeral joint deformity and dislocation.
- Shoulder dystocia is documented in about 50% of cases.
- Risk factors are listed in Table 23-3.
- Plexus injuries most commonly occur in macrosomic newborns without macrocephaly.
  — This body shape allows the head to be delivered easily but traps the shoulders against the pubic bone.
  — Downward pressure on the head is commonly used to deliver the body of the newborn, which places traction on the plexus.
- Plexus injuries can occur without shoulder dystocia.
  — Because of abnormal abdominal and uterine expulsive forces or an abnormal sacral promontory
  — These injuries are more severe, take longer to resolve, and are more frequently associated with clavicular fracture.
- Cesarean delivery does not preclude the possibility of plexus injury.
- Comorbidities
  — *One percent to 5% have diaphragmatic paralysis.* C3, C4, and C5 nerve roots contribute to the phrenic nerve, which innervates the ipsilateral hemidiaphragm. Suspect this in any newborn with a brachial plexus injury and respiratory distress, including mild tachypnea.
  — Five percent to 30% have Horner syndrome. Disruption of sympathetic nerves that arise from the nerve roots in the upper thoracic spinal cord results in miosis, ptosis, enophthalmos, and anhidrosis on the ipsilateral face.

Table 23-1. Brachial Plexus Injuries and Associated Deficits

Injury	Sensory Deficit	Motor Deficit
C5 root	Lateral shoulder	Shoulder external rotation and abduction
C6 root	Cubital fossa Tip of thumb	Elbow flexion Extensor carpi radialis longus
C7 root	Thumb, index, and middle fingers Dorsal radial hand	Flexor carpi radialis Brachioradialis Pronator teres
C8 root	Fourth and fifth fingers Dorsal ulnar hand	Wrist and finger flexion
T1 root	None or minimal	Intrinsic muscles of the hand
Upper trunk	Lateral shoulder Thumb, index, and middle fingers	Shoulder external rotation and abduction Pronator teres Flexor carpi radialis
Middle trunk	Thumb, index, and middle fingers Radial forearm Radial dorsal hand	Elbow extension Brachioradialis Wrist and finger extension
Lower trunk	Fourth and fifth fingers Medial arm and forearm	Most of wrist and finger flexors Median and ulnar intrinsics
Posterior cord	Lateral shoulder	Shoulder abduction
Lateral cord	Thumb, index, and middle fingers Cubital fossa Radial forearm	Pronator teres Flexor carpi radialis Elbow flexion
Medial cord	Fourth and fifth fingers Medial arm and forearm	Most of wrist and finger flexors Median and ulnar intrinsics

- There are 3 main categories of newborn brachial plexus injury.
  - *Erb palsy (Erb-Duchenne paralysis)*
    - Represents 90% of neonatal brachial plexus injuries.
    - Stretch injury of the upper cord; avulsion is rare.
    - Forty-six percent have injuries at only C5 and C6.
    - An additional 29% also have involvement of C7.
  - *Klumpke paralysis*
    - Represents about 1% of newborn brachial plexus injuries.
    - Injury to C8 and T1 roots; avulsion is more common.
  - *Total plexus injury (flail extremity)*
    - Represents 8% to 23% of newborn brachial plexus injuries.
    - Often bilateral
    - Seen almost exclusively in breech presentations and may be caused by excessive traction on both shoulders while delivering the head.
    - Diaphragmatic paralysis and Horner syndrome are more frequent with a total plexus injury than with Klumpke and Erb palsies.

Table 23-2. Brachial Plexus Terminal Nerve Injuries and Associated Deficits

Injured Nerve	Sensory Deficit	Motor Deficit
Suprascapular	None or minimal	Supraspinatus Infraspinatus
Long thoracic	None or minimal	Serratus anterior
Axillary (aka circumflex)	Shoulder joint Distal lateral shoulder	Deltoid Teres minor
Musculocutaneous	Radial forearm	Biceps brachii Brachioradialis Coracobrachialis
Radial	Most of the dorsal hand	Triceps brachii Brachioradialis Extensor carpi radialis longus and brevis Supinator Hand and finger extensors
Median	Palmar aspect and nail beds of first 3½ fingers	Abductor pollicis brevis Flexor pollicis brevis Opponens pollicis Lumbricals
Ulnar	Fifth digit and ulnar half of fourth digit	Flexor carpi ulnaris Flexor digitorum profundus Lumbricals Opponens digiti minimi Flexor digiti minimi Abductor digiti minimi interossei Adductor pollicis

Table 23-3. Risk Factors for Newborn Brachial Plexus Injuries

Maternal	Fetal	Parturitional

Fibroids
Bicornate uterus
Diabetes
Primiparity
Advanced maternal age
Grand multiparity
	Macrosomia
	Transverse lie
	Low tone
	Neonatal depression
		Abnormal presentation
		Traction on head
		Dysfunctional labor
		Prolonged second stage
		  of labor
		Assisted (eg, vacuum or
		  forceps)

SIGNS AND SYMPTOMS

- *Erb palsy (Erb-Duchenne paralysis)*
  — Weakness in shoulder abduction and external rotation, elbow flexion, forearm supination, wrist extension, and finger extension.
  — Affected neonates hold the arm in the "waiter's tip position" with the shoulder adducted and internally rotated, the elbow extended, forearm pronated, and wrist and fingers flexed (Figure 23-1).
  — Biceps reflex is absent.
  — Moro response and tonic neck reflex are asymmetric.
  — Palmar grasp reflex is intact.
  — It is unclear if there is a significant sensory deficit in affected neonates. The sensory tracts seem to have greater plasticity than the motor neurons.
- *Klumpke paralysis*
  — Characterized by weakness of the long wrist flexors and the intrinsic muscles of the hand, which leads to "claw-hand" position.
  — Grasp reflex is absent.
  — Biceps reflex is intact.
- *Total plexus injury (flail extremity)*
  — Affected neonates have no use of the affected arm, wrist, and hand.
  — All reflexes involving the affected upper extremity are absent.

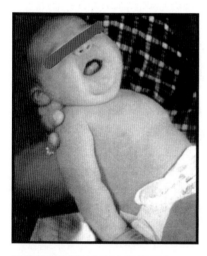

Figure 23-1. Typical posture ("waiter's tip position") of child with Erb palsy. Reproduced with permission from Griffin LY (ed): *Essentials of Musculoskeletal Care,* 3rd edition. Rosemont, IL: American Academy of Orthopaedic Surgeons; 2005.

DIFFERENTIAL DIAGNOSIS

- Distinguish from pseudoparalysis because of pain from a clavicle or humerus fracture, shoulder dislocation, septic arthritis, or osteomyelitis. If the newborn seems to be in pain (ie, grimacing) with passive arm motion or has systemic signs, radiographs, magnetic resonance imaging (MRI), and laboratory studies will help differentiate.
- Bilateral symptoms, lower extremity symptoms, or urinary retention should prompt concern for a cord injury.

MAKING THE DIAGNOSIS

- The diagnosis is made clinically.
- *Radiographs* of the clavicle and humerus should be obtained because 10% of brachial plexus injuries are associated with clavicle fracture, and another 10% with humerus fracture.
- While *electromyogram* and *somatosensory evoked potentials (SSEP)* can potentially define the degree and location of injury, the results are often confusing because of the plasticity of the newborn central nervous system.
- *Magnetic resonance imaging* can be helpful to evaluate the anatomy of the brachial plexus and surrounding structures and may identify an avulsion.
- *Magnetic resonance imaging with arthrogram* is used to evaluate for glenohumeral deformity.

TREATMENT

- During the first week, protect the arm by wrapping it close to the body.
- *Physical therapy (PT)* should begin at 7 to 10 days of life.
  — Goals of PT
    - Prevent joint contractures that are common even with complete neurologic recovery.
    - Strengthen recovering muscles.
    - Help the neonate achieve developmental milestones.
  — Most parents can be taught a simple home program of shoulder, elbow, and wrist passive range of motion.
  — Formal, supervised PT is advised for neonates who do not recover rapidly in the first month of life, or if contractures begin to develop.
- Abduction and external rotation splints may increase the risk of injury to the proximal humeral physis.
- If there is no recovery by 3 to 6 months of age, *microsurgery* to repair or reconstruct the nerves is an option.
  — Controversy remains as to the best timing for surgery.
  — Even with perfect reinnervation of affected muscles (achievement of 5/5 strength), secondary operations including soft tissue releases, tendon transfers, and osteotomies are commonly required to achieve an acceptable functional outcome.
  — Complications of microsurgery are rare; the major complication is failure to achieve the desired outcome.

EXPECTED OUTCOMES/PROGNOSIS

- Spontaneous recovery rates are as high as 90% to 95% for injuries involving only C5 and C6.
- The prognosis is worse for lower plexus injuries. Only 40% of newborns with Klumpke paralysis demonstrate some degree of recovery at 1 year of age.
- Successful recoveries begin early. Newborns who attained complete functional recovery began to recover some function in all muscle groups by 1 to 2 months of life, and 93% reach complete functional recovery by 4 months of age.

- *Predictors of poor long-term outcome* with permanent functional deficits include Horner syndrome, total plexus involvement, and failure to recover function by 3 to 6 months of life.
- More than 90% of neonates who undergo microsurgery to reconstruct the nerves will demonstrate motor improvement within 9 months after surgery; however, complete recovery is rare before age 3 years.
- For those who are left with some permanent weakness, orthopaedic procedures such as tendon transfers and osteotomies may improve function.

WHEN TO REFER

- Refer to a pediatric neurosurgeon or orthopaedic surgeon with expertise in brachial plexus injuries when
  — No spontaneous recovery by 2 to 3 months of age (Some surgeons may prefer earlier referral—know your local neurosurgeon's preferences.)
  — Total plexopathy (flail arm)
  — Associated Horner syndrome
  — Associated phrenic nerve palsy
  — Surgical referral at any point in management is appropriate if progress is unacceptable to the parents or treating physician.

PREVENTION

- Despite many advances in obstetric care and the widely accepted safety of cesarean delivery, there has been no change in the frequency of birth-related brachial plexus injury.
- Currently, there is no consensus regarding the preferred delivery method of macrosomic infants.

RELEVANT *INTERNATIONAL CLASSIFICATION OF DISEASES, NINTH REVISION, CLINICAL MODIFICATION* (ICD-9-CM) CODES

- **767.6**   Erb palsy, Klumpke paralysis, total plexus injury
- **767.7**   Phrenic nerve palsy
- **954.0**   Horner syndrome

Non-perinatal Brachial Plexus Palsy (Stingers or Burners)

INTRODUCTION/ETIOLOGY/EPIDEMIOLOGY

- Commonly called *stinger* or *burner*
- Common injury in contact sports, especially American football
- Sixty-five percent of college football players report at least one stinger during their career, with 30% suffering their first stinger in high school.

- Three mechanisms of injury are described.
  — Stretch or traction injury to the plexus
    - Commonly occurs during a direct blow to the head with lateral bending of the neck away from the affected arm. This widens the cervicothoracic angle and places tensile force on the C5 and C6 nerve roots.
  — Pinched cervical nerve roots
    - Occurs when a blow to the head causes axial loading or lateral bending toward the affected arm, most commonly pinching C5 and C6 nerve roots.
  — Direct blow to the brachial plexus causing a contusion to the nerves

SIGNS AND SYMPTOMS

- Burning pain, paresthesias, and weakness in the upper extremity after a blow to the head or neck.
- Pain usually resolves within 1 to 2 minutes, but weakness may develop hours to days following the injury and persist for several weeks.
- Weakness typically involves the muscles supplied by C5 and C6 (ie, deltoid, biceps, supraspinatus, infraspinatus).
- If mechanism of injury was a direct blow, there will be tenderness at the site of impact.
- There is no neck pain or loss of motion.

DIFFERENTIAL DIAGNOSIS

- A stinger should never cause bilateral symptoms or leg symptoms, which suggests a cord injury.
- A stinger should not cause any cervical spine tenderness or loss of neck motion, which suggests a cervical sprain, strain, or fracture.
- C7 and C8 injuries are rare with a simple stinger. Involvement suggests a more complex injury.

MAKING THE DIAGNOSIS

- Diagnosis is based on history and physical examination.
- Cervical radiographs (anteroposterior, lateral, odontoid, flexion, and extension views) should be performed if there is any suspicion of a cervical spine injury or if there is a history of more than 1 previous stinger (Figure 23-2).
  — Examine flexion and extension views for evidence of instability.
  — Examine the lateral view for evidence of *cervical stenosis*, which is associated with stingers.
  — A good screening tool for cervical stenosis is the *Torg ratio*, which is the width of the cervical canal divided by the width of the vertebral body (Figure 23-3).
  — If the Torg ratio is less than 0.8, stenosis should be suspected and an MRI should be obtained.
  — A Torg ratio should not be used as a diagnosis of cervical stenosis because false positives do occur, especially in large athletes.
  — A Torg ratio less than 0.8 is associated with a threefold increase in stingers.

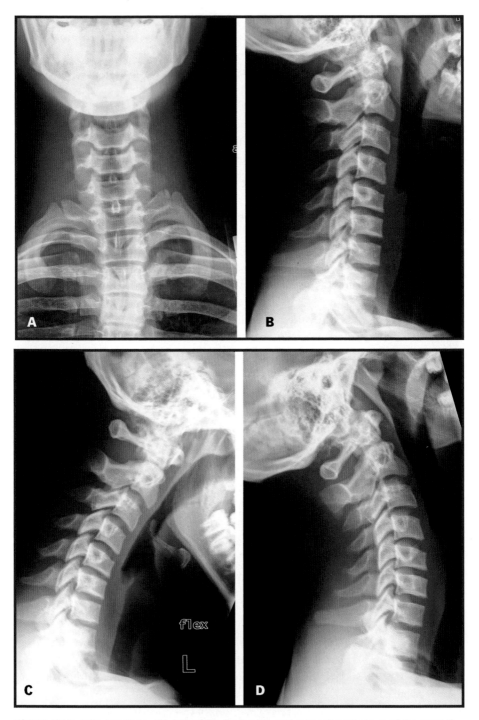

Figure 23-2. Anteroposterior (A), lateral (B), flexion (C), and extension (D) views of the normal cervical spine. Note loss of normal cervical lordosis on lateral view (B). From Metzl JD. *Sports Medicine in the Pediatric Office.* Elk Grove Village, IL: American Academy of Pediatrics; 2008.

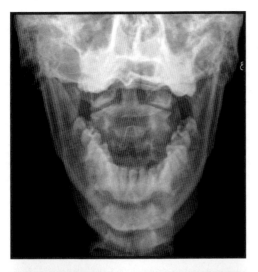

Figure 23-2e. Odontoid view of the cervical spine. From Metzl JD. *Sports Medicine in the Pediatric Office.* Elk Grove Village, IL: American Academy of Pediatrics; 2008.

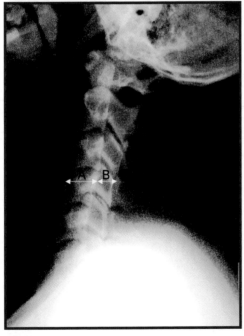

Figure 23-3. Lateral radiograph of the cervical spine. Torg or Pavlov ratio, B/A at the level of C4, is less than 0.80. From Finoff JT, Mildenberger D, Cassidy CD. Central cord syndrome in a football player with congenital spinal stenosis. *Am J Sports Med.* 2004;32:516–521. Reprinted by permission of SAGE Publications.

- If symptoms persist beyond 2 weeks, additional diagnostic studies may be performed to evaluate the extent of injury.
  - Electromyogram can identify specific nerves or segments of the plexus that have been injured.
  - Sensory nerve action potential and SSEP may also be useful in localizing the lesion.
  - Magnetic resonance imaging is now widely regarded as the best way to evaluate the brachial plexus.

TREATMENT

- Treatment is supportive. The athlete is advised to rest the upper extremity until symptoms have resolved.
- Strengthening exercises for the neck and upper extremity can be performed once weakness has started to resolve.
- Patients should not return to play until asymptomatic and strength is full and symmetrical to the uninjured side.
- Electromyogram may remain abnormal even after all weakness has resolved and should not be used as an indicator for return to play.
- Athletes with a history of more than 2 stingers or bilateral symptoms should be evaluated by a sports medicine physician for associated spine pathology before return to contact sports (Box 23-1).

Box 23-1. Return to Play Following a Brachial Plexus Injury

No contraindications
- Fewer than 3 episodes in a lifetime
- No episodes with symptoms lasting longer than 24 hours
- Full cervical range of motion
- No neurologic deficit shown in detailed examination
- No more than 1 episode of quadriparesis or quadriplegia
- No cervical radicular symptoms or other disk disease
- No cervical spine instability

Relative contraindications
- Symptoms lasting longer than 24 hours
- More than 3 previous episodes
- Two episodes of quadriparesis or quadriplegia

Absolute contraindications
- More than 2 episodes of quadriparesis or quadriplegia
- Cervical myelopathy or myelomalacia
- Continued neck discomfort
- Decreased cervical range of motion
- Neurologic deficit

EXPECTED OUTCOMES/PROGNOSIS

- The majority of simple stingers resolve without any sequelae, allowing full return to sports.
- Severe injuries (neurotmesis) are rare. These show no recovery after 3 months and are likely to be permanent. Operative intervention at 3 months may improve function in these cases.

PREVENTION

- There may be a role for extra padding over the shoulders, higher riding shoulder pad, neck rolls, and further education on proper tackling technique. However, even with these interventions, the risk of recurrence is high.

WHEN TO REFER

- Refer to a pediatric sports medicine physician
    - If symptoms are bilateral
    - If symptoms do not resolve within 2 weeks
    - If there is a history of 2 or more previous stingers

RELEVANT *ICD-9-CM* CODE

- **953.4** Brachial plexus injury

CHAPTER 24

Nursemaid Elbow (Radial Head Subluxation)

Introduction/Etiology/Epidemiology

- Annular ligament displacement may be the more appropriate name for this injury because the ligament moves into the elbow joint rather than the radial head moving away from the articulation.
- With longitudinal traction to the arm, the annular ligament slides over the radial head and becomes trapped between the capitellum and the radial head, stretching or tearing the ligament.
- In infants, the usual mechanism of injury is by rolling over and the extended arm becoming trapped beneath the body.
- In a child, the classic mechanism of injury is pulling an outstretched arm; it can also occur after a fall on an outstretched arm or as a result of a twisting injury. Injury is more likely when the forearm is pronated.
- Young children are more susceptible to this injury because of maturational anatomic differences compared with adults—the annular ligament has a smaller diameter, making it more susceptible to tearing, and the radial head and neck are more oval in shape and narrower, which allows the annular ligament to easily displace (Figure 24-1).
- Represents 15% to 27% of elbow injuries in children younger than 10 years.
- Peak incidence is between 1 and 3 years of age, but has been reported as young as 6 months and as old as 10 years.
- Slightly more common among girls

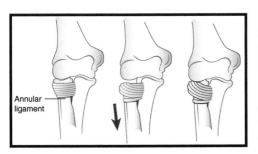

Annular ligament

Figure 24-1. Nursemaid elbow is a transient subluxation of the proximal radial head caused by pulling or yanking of a child's arm, usually inadvertently, by a parent or caregiver. From McInerny TK, Adam HM, Campbell DE, Kamat DM, Kelleher KJ, eds. *American Academy of Pediatrics Textbook of Pediatric Care.* Elk Grove Village, IL: American Academy of Pediatrics; 2009:2053

Signs and Symptoms

- The main symptom is refusal to use the arm.
- Pain is reported immediately after the injury and during any attempt to move the elbow.
- Pain is often difficult to locate precisely.
- The child is often in no distress.
- The arm is held adducted against the body, with the elbow slightly flexed and the forearm pronated (nursemaid position).
- There is usually no swelling, deformity, or ecchymosis.
- Upper extremity examination is classically normal; however, careful palpation of the anterolateral radial head may elicit mild tenderness.

Differential Diagnosis

- Differentiating features of other conditions presenting with refusal to use the arm
  — Contusions: ecchymosis and swelling
  — Upper extremity fractures: significant pain and swelling and possible deformity
  — True dislocation of the radial head: significant pain and obvious deformity (brachial plexus injury)
  — Osteosarcoma and leukemia: unremitting pain at rest
  — Necrotizing fasciitis: pain out of proportion to physical examination findings
  — Vasoocclusive crises in sickle cell disease: pain at rest
  — Although bilateral nursemaid elbow has been reported, inability to move both arms should raise suspicion of a central nervous system disorder, such as a spinal tumor.

Making the Diagnosis

- Diagnosis is clinical.
- *Radiographs*
  — Indicated for significant point tenderness, swelling, ecchymosis, or atypical history
  — Radiographs are typically normal with radial head subluxation.
  — Radiographs of the uninjured elbow can help assess injury to growth plates.
  — Consider wrist views if there is significant referred pain to the distal forearm.
- *Sonography* may demonstrate a widened space between radial head and capitellum, which represents the interposed annular ligament, but is not commonly used clinically.

Treatment

- Most cases can be successfully reduced in the pediatrician's office without sequelae.
- *Supination/flexion technique*
  — Use thumb to apply slight pressure over the radial head, then use the other hand to first supinate, then smoothly flex the elbow fully. Perform as one fluid motion.
  — There may be a palpable or audible clunk when the radial head reduces.
  — The greater the tear in the ligament, the more forceful the supination and pronation that is required to achieve successful reduction.
  — Success rates range from 69% to 86%.
- *Hyperpronation technique*
  — Place thumb over the radial head and then hyperpronatethe forearm.
  — May be less painful.
  — Success rates range from 80% to 98%.
- Observe the child after reduction until normal use of the arm is witnessed, which usually occurs within 5 to 15 minutes but may take longer in apprehensive younger children or when reduction takes place more than 4 to 6 hours after injury.
- Immobilization is not necessary after successful reduction.
- Follow-up is unnecessary unless symptoms recur.
- If a clinician reduces a nursemaid elbow successfully but the patient continues to experience severe pain, post-reduction films are warranted.
- Inability to reduce may be caused by complete disruption of the annular ligament or swelling of the ligament from edema, hematoma, or hemorrhage, or improper technique.
  — Failure is more likely if reduction is attempted 12 or more hours after the injury.
  — If 2 attempted reductions are unsuccessful, radiographs are obtained to rule out other causes of mechanical blockage, such as a loose body from a fracture.

Expected Outcomes/Prognosis

- After reduction, there are usually no long-term or permanent sequelae.
- Recurrence rates range from 5% to 39%.
- For a child with 3 or more recurrences, the elbow can be immobilized for 2 to 3 weeks to encourage stabilization of the ligament.
- Rarely, open reduction and repair or reconstruction of the ligament may be necessary.
- The incidence of annular ligament displacement decreases after 5 years of age and is exceedingly rare after 10 years of age, likely because of development of a more bulbous radial head and stronger, thicker annular ligament.

Prevention

- Avoid lifting or pulling the child up by hands or forearms.
- Avoid swinging a child by the wrists or hands.
- Lift toddlers and young children by placing the hands in the axilla and lifting gently to avoid damage to the shoulder, elbow, and wrist.

When to Refer

- If several attempts at reduction fail to result in normal use of the arm, place a posterior mold splint (see Chapter 37) with elbow flexed to 90 degrees and forearm in supination, and schedule evaluation by an orthopedist within 24 hours.

Relevant *International Classification of Diseases, Ninth Revision, Clinical Modification* Code

- **832.0**   Nursemaid elbow

CHAPTER 25

Congenital Anomalies of the Upper Extremities

General Introduction

- Upper extremity anomalies occur in approximately 1 in 626 newborns.
- May occur as an isolated finding or as a systemic condition.
- Early recognition by the pediatrician facilitates appropriate counseling, treatment, and timely referral for the infant.

NORMAL DEVELOPMENT OF THE UPPER LIMB

- Upper limb develops between the fourth and eighth weeks of gestation. Most congenital anomalies occur during this period.
- At 4 weeks, the upper limb bud grows in a proximal-to-distal pattern controlled by apical ectodermal ridge cells at its distal end.
- Finger separation is complete by 8 weeks.
- The hand initiates movement by 9 weeks.

CLASSIFICATION OF UPPER LIMB ANOMALIES

- Swanson classification of upper limb anomalies (widely used) divides upper limb anomalies into 7 categories based on the embryonic failure thought to have caused the deformity (Table 25-1).

Sprengel Deformity

INTRODUCTION/ETIOLOGY/EPIDEMIOLOGY

- Congenital elevation of the scapula
- Due to arrest of the typical caudal migration of the scapula from the embryonic limb bud to the thorax. The superior border of the scapula normally lies at the level of the seventh vertebra, with its inferior border at the sixth rib.
- In 30%, the scapula is attached to the cervical spine by cartilage, fibrous tissue, or an omovertebral bone further limiting scapulothoracic motion.
- Poses functional and cosmetic problems.

Table 25-1. International Federation of Societies for Surgeries of the Hand Embryologic Classification of Congenital Anomalies

I. Failure of formation of parts
  A. Transverse deficiencies
  B. Longitudinal deficiencies
    1. Phocomelia
    2. Radial
    3. Central
    4. Ulnar
II. Failure of differentiation
  A. Synostosis
  B. Radial head dislocation
  C. Symphalangism
  D. Syndactyly
  E. Contracture
    1. Soft tissue
      a. Arthrogryposis
      b. Pterygium
      c. Trigger
      d. Absent extensor tendons
      e. Hypoplastic thumb
      f. Clasped thumb
      g. Retroflexible thumb
      h. Camptodactyly
      i. Windblown hand
    2. Skeletal
      a. Clinodactyly
      b. Kirner deformity
      c. Delta bone

III. Duplication
  A. Thumb
  B. Triphalangism/hyperphalangism
  C. Polydactyly
  D. Mirror hand
IV. Overgrowth
  A. Limb
  B. Macrodactyly
V. Undergrowth
VI. Congenital constriction band syndrome
VII. Generalized skeletal abnormalities

Adapted from Kozin SH. Upper-extremity congenital anomalies. *J Bone Joint Surg Am.* 2003; 85-A:1564–1576. Reprinted by permission of Rockwater, Inc.

- Bilateral in 10% to 30% of cases
- Occurs more frequently in females.
- *Associated conditions and anomalies*
  — Anomalies of the clavicles, vertebrae, ribs, and shoulder musculature
  — Sprengel deformity is present in 35% of children with Klippel-Feil syndrome (a disorder of segmentation of the cervical vertebrae).
  — Patients may present with renal or pulmonary disorders.

SIGNS AND SYMPTOMS

- Shoulder asymmetry and limited shoulder abduction
- Thickened neck on the affected side
- Patients may complain of neck or shoulder pain.
- Scapula is elevated and adducted with its superior angle often palpable at base of neck.
- In mild cases, the condition may not be apparent until the child is older.

DIFFERENTIAL DIAGNOSIS

- Other causes of limited shoulder abduction include abnormal or weakened periscapular muscles.
- Other causes of shoulder and neck asymmetry include torticollis and scoliosis.

MAKING THE DIAGNOSIS

- Diagnosis is confirmed with anteroposterior (AP) radiographs of the chest and shoulders.
- Severity of the deformity varies.
- Classification by Rigault is based on the level of the scapula (Figure 25-1).
  — Grade I, the superomedial border is located between the second and fourth thoracic vertebrae.
  — Grade II, between the second thoracic and fifth cervical vertebrae
  — Grade III, above the fifth cervical vertebrae
- Cervical and thoracic spine radiographs are obtained to evaluate for associated anomalies.

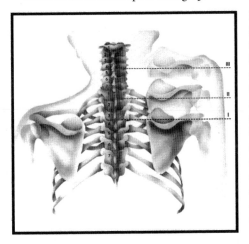

Figure 25-1. Classification of Sprengel deformity into 3 grades, according to Rigault et al. In grade I the superomedial angle of the scapula is located between the transverse apophysis of the second and the fourth thoracic vertebra. In grade II the superomedial angle is between the transverse apophysis of the second thoracic and the fifth cervical vertebra. In grade III it is located above the transverse apophysis of the fifth cervical vertebra. From Rigault P, Pouliquen JC, Guyonvarch G, Zujovic J. Congenital elevation of the scapula in childhood. *Revue de Chirurgie Orthopédique* 1976;62:5-26. © Elsevier Masson SAS. Used by permission.

TREATMENT AND EXPECTED OUTCOMES/PROGNOSIS

- Few patients require surgery.
- Grade I and most grade II deformities
  — Cause minimal functional impairment.
  — Physical therapy can improve scapula range of motion and periscapular muscle strength.
- Grade III and severe grade II deformities
  — Range of motion of the shoulder is limited, preventing abduction beyond 90 degrees.
  — Patients with significant functional deficits and cosmetic deformity may be addressed surgically, although surgical intervention for this condition is challenging.
  — Best surgical results are obtained when performed before 8 years of age.

WHEN TO REFER

- Refer patients with significant functional deficits, cosmetic deformity, or associated musculoskeletal anomalies to a pediatric orthopaedic surgeon.

RELEVANT *INTERNATIONAL CLASSIFICATION OF DISEASES, NINTH REVISION, CLINICAL MODIFICATION (ICD-9-CM)* CODE

* **755.52**   Sprengel deformity

Congenital Radioulnar Synostosis Malformation

INTRODUCTION/ETIOLOGY/EPIDEMIOLOGY

* Occurs when the radius and ulna fail to completely separate longitudinally in the seventh week of embryonic development.
* Occurs sporadically; occasionally may be inherited in an autosomal dominant fashion.
* Between 50% and 80% of cases are bilateral.
* Males are more commonly affected.
* *Associated conditions and anomalies*
  — Skeletal anomalies: developmental dysplasia of the hip, clubfeet, and deformities of the wrist and hand
  — Syndromes: fetal alcohol, Apert, Williams, and Klinefelter

SIGNS AND SYMPTOMS

* Children present with a shortened forearm held in pronation, with the inability to actively pronate and supinate the forearm.
* Pain is unusual until adolescence, when chronic radial head subluxation may cause symptoms.
* Activities of daily living such as dressing and feeding oneself may be challenging.
* Elbow flexion contracture can develop, often with concomitant radial head dislocation.
* Wrist is often hypermobile.

DIFFERENTIAL DIAGNOSIS

* Other causes of limited forearm motion include traumatic radial head subluxation or forearm fracture.

MAKING THE DIAGNOSIS

* Radiographs confirm the diagnosis (Figure 25-2).
* Classification system proposed by Cleary et al
  — Type I: fibrous synostosis with no bone involvement and a reduced radial head
  — Type II: visible osseous synostosis with a normal-appearing, reduced radial head
  — Type III: visible osseous synostosis with a hypoplastic and posteriorly dislocated radial head
  — Type IV: osseous synostosis with an anteriorly dislocated, mushroom-shaped radial head

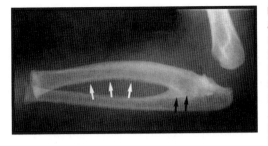

Figure 25-2. Lateral view of forearm and elbow of an infant demonstrating radioulnar stenosis. The black arrows indicate complete fusion of the proximal radius to the ulna. The white arrows show increased radial bowing. Reproduced with permission from Johnson TR, Steinbach LS (eds): *Essentials of Musculoskeletal Imaging.* Rosemont, IL: American Academy of Orthopaedic Surgeons; 2004

TREATMENT AND EXPECTED OUTCOMES/PROGNOSIS

- Few patients require surgery.
- Children with unilateral deformity and with less than 60 degrees of fixed pronation compensate for the deficit by recruiting the wrist and shoulder to perform tasks.
- Patients with bilateral deformity and those with fixed pronation greater than 60 degrees benefit from operative management.
  - — Goal of surgery is to improve the fixed rotational position of the forearm.
  - — Resecting the synostosis to allow rotational movement is not successful.

WHEN TO REFER

- Patients with functional limitations should be referred to a pediatric orthopaedic surgeon by 5 years of age, or around the time they begin school.

RELEVANT *ICD-9-CM* CODE

- **755.53**   Congenital radioulnar synostosis

Syndactyly Malformation

INTRODUCTION/ETIOLOGY/EPIDEMIOLOGY

- Failure of separation of adjacent digits during the fifth to eighth week of intrauterine development
  - — Complete: fusion of the digits up to the fingertips
  - — Incomplete: proximal interconnection only
  - — Simple: soft tissue interconnection only (Figure 25-3).
  - — Complex: osseous union

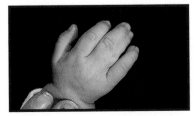

Figure 25-3. Infant with simple syndactyly of the third and fourth fingers of the right hand.

- Incidence is 1 in 2,000 live births.
- White males are more commonly affected.
- Fifty percent of cases are bilateral.
- Most cases are sporadic but familial syndactyly may occur with autosomal-dominant transmission with incomplete penetrance, commonly affecting the ring and long fingers.
- Syndactyly may be an isolated finding, associated with other anomalies, or as a component of a syndrome.
- *Associated anomalies* include concomitant polydactyly, constriction band syndrome, brachydactyly, toe webbing, and disorders of the spine and heart.
- *Associated syndromes*
  — Poland syndrome: absence or underdevelopment of the pectoralis muscle with ipsilateral syndactyly.
  — Apert syndrome (acrocephalosyndactyly): a rare autosomal-dominant disorder characterized by craniosynostosis, craniofacial anomalies, and anomalies of the hands and feet
    ▪ Syndactyly is complete, complex, and symmetrical, resembling a spade or mitten.
    ▪ In some cases all digits, including the thumb, are involved, with a single conjoined nail (synonychia).

SIGNS AND SYMPTOMS

- Webbed fingers noted at birth

DIFFERENTIAL DIAGNOSIS

- Isolated syndactyly is differentiated from syndactyly associated with other anomalies or syndromes by physical examination and family history.

MAKING THE DIAGNOSIS

- Anteroposterior radiographs of the hands distinguish simple from complex syndactyly and evaluate for other bony anomalies such as synostosis, delta phalanx, or symphalangism.

TREATMENT

- Early recognition and surgical treatment is paramount in preventing tethering and flexion contractures.
- Thumb-to-index finger syndactyly is best treated by 6 months of age, small-to-ring finger syndactyly by 1 year of age, and index-to-long as well as long-to-ring fingers by 18 months of age.

EXPECTED OUTCOMES/PROGNOSIS

- Surgical repair of isolated syndactyly produces good cosmetic and functional outcomes.
- For syndactyly associated with a syndrome, functional outcomes depend on the underlying deficits due to the syndrome, because altered hand function is often caused by more than syndactyly alone.

WHEN TO REFER

- Refer isolated syndactyly to a pediatric orthopaedic surgeon on diagnosis.
- The complex nature of associated syndromes such as Apert requires a multidisciplinary approach including pediatric orthopaedic, orthodontic, and plastic surgeons, and otolaryngologists.

RELEVANT *ICD-9-CM* CODES

- **755.11** Syndactyly, simple
- **755.12** Syndactyly, complex
- **755.55** Apert syndrome
- **756.3** Poland syndrome

Central Ray Deficiency

INTRODUCTION/ETIOLOGY/EPIDEMIOLOGY

- Failure of formation or differentiation of the central ray(s) of the hand
- The terms *cleft hand, claw hand,* and *lobster claw* have been applied to this condition, but have fallen out of favor because of their nonclinical connotations.
- Typical form (failure of differentiation)
  — Autosomal-dominant inheritance pattern with incidence of 1 in 10,000 live births
  — Associated with syndromes including de Lange and acrorenal, and cleft foot, cleft lip, cleft palate, imperforate anus, congenital heart anomalies, and deafness
- Atypical form (failure of formation)
  — Spontaneous inheritance pattern
  — Usually not associated with foot anomalies or systemic conditions. One notable association, however, is Poland syndrome, in which symbrachydactyly is associated with chest muscle and breast underdevelopment.

SIGNS AND SYMPTOMS

- Typical form
  — Usually bilateral
  — V-shaped deformity, usually with absence of the central digit(s)
  — There is often syndactyly, or occasionally polydactyly, of the digits bordering the cleft, or of the contralateral hand or feet.
  — Multiple permutations of phalangeal and metacarpal deformities can occur.
- Atypical form
  — Usually unilateral
  — U-shaped deformity that is a variant of symbrachydactyly with near absence of the index, long, and ring finger phalanges
  — Remnants of these absent digits are sometimes present.

DIFFERENTIAL DIAGNOSIS

• Differentiate typical from atypical forms via physical examination and family history

MAKING THE DIAGNOSIS

• Diagnosis can be made on physical examination.
• Hand radiographs are performed to evaluate for associated anomalies or for surgical planning.
• In the atypical form, radiographs sometimes demonstrate a transversely oriented metacarpal or phalangis within the web space, which widens the cleft.

TREATMENT AND EXPECTED OUTCOMES/PROGNOSIS

• Interestingly, most children with central ray deficiency have no functional problems. However the psychological consequences of the deformity merit operative intervention and correction.
• For the atypical form, early surgery is indicated to prevent worsening of the deformity because of a syndactyly between fingers of unequal length or transversely oriented bone in the web space. Most cases can be treated between 1 to 2 years of age.
• Cosmetic and functional surgical outcomes are generally good.

WHEN TO REFER

• Refer to a pediatric orthopaedic surgeon on diagnosis.

RELEVANT *ICD-9-CM* CODE

• **754.89**   Central ray deficiency

Polydactyly Hand Malformation

INTRODUCTION/ETIOLOGY/EPIDEMIOLOGY

• Polydactyly, or duplication of digits, along with syndactyly, is common.
• Postaxial polydactyly (ulnar or small finger) (Figure 25-4)
  — Autosomal-dominant inheritance pattern with variable penetrance
  — More common in African Americans with incidence of 1 in 143 live births versus 1 in 1,339 live births among whites
  — Associated with underlying syndromes in white populations such as chondroectodermal dysplasia or Ellis-van Creveld syndrome
  — African Americans rarely present with concomitant syndromes.
• Preaxial polydactyly (radial or thumb) (Figure 25-5)
  — Common and occurs sporadically.
  — Usually not associated with underlying syndromes. The exception is a triphalangeal thumb, which can occur along with thumb duplication. Triphalangeal thumb typically demonstrates an autosomal-dominant pattern and is associated with a number of anomalies and syndromes.

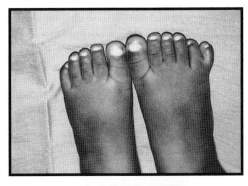

Figure 25-4. Child with postaxial polydactyly of the right foot. Reproduced with permission from Griffin LY (ed): *Essentials of Musculoskeletal Care,* 3rd edition. Rosemont, IL: American Academy of Orthopaedic Surgeons; 2005.

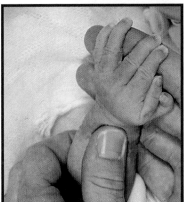

Figure 25-5. Preaxial polydactyly—infant born with supernumerary thumbs.

- Central polydactyly (index, long, or ring fingers)
  — Occurs far less frequently than preaxial or postaxial varieties.
  — Autosomal-dominant pattern with associated traits or syndromes
  — Affected children may also have toe polydactyly or concomitant syndactyly.

SIGNS AND SYMPTOMS

- Postaxial polydactyly: Classified as type A, with a well-developed supranumerary digit, or type B, with a poorly developed, pedunculated digit
- Central polydactyly: The ring finger is the most commonly duplicated digit.
- Preaxial polydactyly: Classified into 7 types, based on level of duplication and number of bones involved.
  — Type IV is the most common.
  — While most duplication is easy to identify, some type I and type II malformations only demonstrate a slightly widened nail plate.
  — Physical examination can help to observe which component is most dominated. It should be noted that neither is usually as well developed as an unaffected thumb, leading some authors to prefer the term *split thumb.*

DIFFERENTIAL DIAGNOSIS

- Screen for associated syndromes, especially with postaxial polydactyly.

MAKING THE DIAGNOSIS

- Diagnosis is based on physical examination.
- Radiographs should be performed to classify and evaluate the extent of the deformity.

TREATMENT

- Postaxial polydactyly
  — Type B malformations may be treated by tying a suture at the base of the digit. The digit will become ischemic and fall off, leaving a residual bump.
  — Type A malformations require more complex operative management. Treatment may be planned between 6 and 24 months postpartum.
- Central polydactyly
  — Treatment involves excision of the least developed digit(s).
  — Surgery should occur by the first year of life to avoid flexion contractures and deformity of the surrounding digits, which may occur with growth.
- Preaxial polydactyly
  — Type I polydactyly is often treated with observation.
  — More involved deformities benefit from operative treatment, preferably between 6 months and 1 year of age, before pinch develops. Surgical options range from ablation of the lesser component to excision of a central wedge and fusion of both components.

EXPECTED OUTCOMES/PROGNOSIS

- Preaxial types I, II, and IV have good outcomes.
- Complications from treatments of more difficult deformities include joint contractures, instability, and angulation.

WHEN TO REFER

- Refer to a pediatric orthopaedic surgeon on diagnosis.

RELEVANT ICD-9-CM CODES

- **755.01**   Polydactyly, fingers

Radial Deficiency

INTRODUCTION/ETIOLOGY/EPIDEMIOLOGY

- Radial deficiency (radial club hand) results from failure of longitudinal formation, ranging from thumb hypoplasia to complete absence of the radius.
- Rare, occurring in 1 in 30,000 live births

- Often bilateral and associated with a number of anomalies and syndromes, including Holt-Oram, thrombocytopenia absent radius (TAR), Fanconi aplastic anemia, and VACTERL.
- In these individuals, bone marrow failure does not become apparent until between 3 and 12 years of age. A chromosomal assay is therefore necessary to detect the condition prior to its onset.

SIGNS AND SYMPTOMS

- Any of a variety of radial-sided forearm, wrist, and hand deformities (Figure 25-6)

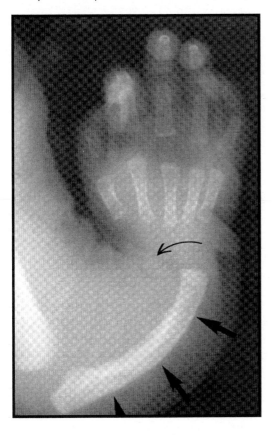

Figure 25-6. Anteroposterior view of the forearm and hand with radial club hand and complexity absence of the radius. The ulna is bowed (black arrows) and the carpus is subluxated radially on the distal ulna (curved arrow). A thumb is present. Reproduced with permission from Johnson TR, Steinbach LS (ed): *Essentials of Musculoskeletal Imaging.* Rosemont, IL: American Academy of Orthopaedic Surgeons; 2004.

DIFFERENTIAL DIAGNOSIS

- Screen for associated syndromes.

MAKING THE DIAGNOSIS

- Radial deficiency is classified by Bayne et al into 4 types based on radiographic morphology of the radius. This classification was modified by James et al to include deficiencies of the wrist and thumb (Table 25-2).

Table 25-2. Modified Classification of Radial Longitudinal Deficiency

Type	Thumb	Carpus	Distal Radius	Proximal Radius
N	Hypoplastic or absent	Normal	Normal	Normal
0	Hypoplastic or absent	Absence, hypoplasia, or coalition	Normal	Normal, radioulnar synostosis, or congenital dislocation of the radial head
1	Hypoplastic or absent	Absence, hypoplasia, or coalition	>2 mm shorter than ulna	Normal, radioulnar synostosis, or congenital dislocation of the radial head
2	Hypoplastic or absent	Absence, hypoplasia, or coalition	Hypoplasia	Hypoplasia
3	Hypoplastic or absent	Absence, hypoplasia, or coalition	Physis absent	Variable hypoplasia
4	Hypoplastic or absent	Absence, hypoplasia, or coalition	Absent	Absent

Adapted from James MA, McCarroll HR Jr, Manske PR. The spectrum of radial longitudinal deficiency: a modified classification. *J Hand Surg Am.* 1999;24:1145–1155, with permission from Elsevier.

- In addition to a radiographic examination of both upper extremities, radiographs of the spine and lower extremities, a renal ultrasound, and echocardiogram are also important components of the workup.
- Complete blood cell count and peripheral blood smears help to analyze platelet function.

TREATMENT

- Type 1 and mild type 2 deficiency can be treated with soft tissue stretching and bracing.
- More severe deficiencies require operative management.
  — Patients undergoing surgery benefit from preoperative soft tissue stretching.
  — A regimen of weekly serial casting is started in the postnatal period, and wrist centralization surgery is ideally performed around 1 year of age.
  — Surgical treatment for patients with TAR is deferred until platelet counts have approached 90,000. Platelet levels improve with age and normalize by 5 years.
  — Surgical treatment for patients with Fanconi anemia poses a more severe challenge because platelet count does not improve spontaneously and bone marrow transplant is the only cure.

EXPECTED OUTCOMES/PROGNOSIS

- Improvements in cosmetic appearance do not always enable improved function.
- Some recurrence of the angulation, as well as joint stiffness, is common postoperatively.

WHEN TO REFER

• Refer to a pediatric orthopaedic surgeon on diagnosis.

RELEVANT *ICD-9-CM* CODES

• **754.89**   Radial deficiency
• **284.09**   Fanconi aplastic anemia
• **287.5**   TAR

Bibliography

Auerbach AD, Verlander PC, Brown KE, Liu JM. New molecular diagnostic tests for two congenital forms of anemia. *J Clin Lab Anal.* 1997;11:17–22

Buck-Gramcko D. *Congenital Malformations of the Hand and Forearm.* London, England: Churchill Livingstone; 1998:xvii, 557

Cleary JE, Omer GE Jr. Congenital proximal radio-ulnar synostosis. Natural history and functional assessment. *J Bone Joint Surg Am.* 1985;67:539–545

Damore E, Kozin SH, Thoder JJ, Porter S. The recurrence of deformity after surgical centralization for radial clubhand. *J Hand Surg Am.* 2000;25:745–751

Eaton CJ, Lister GD. Syndactyly. *Hand Clin.* 1990;6:555–575

Ezaki M. Radial polydactyly. *Hand Clin.* 1990;6:577–588

Farsetti P, Weinstein SL, Caterini R, De Maio F, Ippolito E. Sprengel's deformity: long-term follow-up study of 22 cases. *J Pediatr Orthop B.* 2003;12:202–210

Flatt AE. *The Care of Congenital Hand Anomalies.* 2nd ed. St. Louis, MO: Quality Medical Publishing Inc; 1994:x, 466

Graham TJ, Ress AM. Finger polydactyly. *Hand Clin.* 1998;14:49–64

Guille JT, Miller A, Bowen JR, Forlin E, Caro PA. The natural history of Klippel-Feil syndrome: clinical, roentgenographic, and magnetic resonance imaging findings at adulthood. *J Pediatr Orthop.* 1995;15:617–626

Hoover GH, Flatt AE, Weiss MW. The hand and Apert's syndrome. *J Bone Joint Surg Am.* 1970;52:878–895

James MA, Bednar M. Deformities of the wrist and forearm. In: Green DP, ed. *Green's Operative Hand Surgery.* 5th ed. Philadelphia, PA: Elsevier/Churchill Livingstone; 2005:xv, 2313, lii

James MA, McCarroll HR Jr, Manske PR. The spectrum of radial longitudinal deficiency: a modified classification. *J Hand Surg Am.* 1999;24:1145–1155

Kozin SH. Upper-extremity congenital anomalies. *J Bone Joint Surg Am.* 2003;85-A:1564–1576

Macias CG, Bothner J, Wiebe R. A comparison of supination/flexion to hyperpronation in the reduction of radial head subluxations. *Pediatrics.* 1998;102:e10

Macias CG, Wiebe R, Bothner J. History and radiographic findings associated with clinically suspected radial head subluxations. *Pediatr Emerg Care.* 2000;16:22–25

McCarroll HR. Congenital anomalies: a 25-year overview. *J Hand Surg Am.* 2000;25:1007–1037

McDonald J, Whitelaw C, Goldsmith LJ. Radial head subluxation: comparing two methods of reduction. *Acad Emerg Med.* 1999;6:715–718

Meiner EM, Sama AE, Lee DC, Nelson M, Katz DS, Trope A. Bilateral nursemaid's elbow. *Am J Emerg Med.* 2004;22:502–503

Miura T, Nakamura R, Horii E. The position of symbrachydactyly in the classification of congenital hand anomalies. *J Hand Surg Br.* 1994;19:350–354

Miura T, Suzuki M. Clinical differences between typical and atypical cleft hand. *J Hand Surg Br.* 1984;9:311–315

Newman J. "Nursemaid's elbow" in infants six months and under. *J Emerg Med.* 1985;2:403–404

Quan L, Marcuse EK. The epidemiology and treatment of radial head subluxation. *Am J Dis Child.* 1985;139:1194–1197

Sacchetti A, Ramoska EE, Glasgow C. Non-classic history in children with radial head subluxations. *J Emerg Med.* 1990;8:151–153

Schunk JE. Radial head subluxation: epidemiology and treatment of 87 episodes. *Ann Emerg Med.* 1990;19:1019–1023

Snellman O. Subluxation of the head of the radius in children. *Acta Orthop Scand.* 1959;28:311–315

Snyder HS. Radiographic changes with radial head subluxation in children. *J Emerg Med.* 1990;8:265–269

Swanson AB. A classification for congenital limb malformations. *J Hand Surg Am.* 1976;1:8–22

Tada K, Yonenobu K, Tsuyuguchi Y, Kawai H, Egawa T. Duplication of the thumb. A retrospective review of two hundred and thirty-seven cases. *J Bone Joint Surg Am.* 1983;65:584–598

Van Heest AE. Congenital disorders of the hand and upper extremity. *Pediatr Clin North Am.* 1996;43:1113–1133

Watson BT, Hennrikus WL. Postaxial type-B polydactyly. Prevalence and treatment. *J Bone Joint Surg Am.* 1997;79:65–68

Wood VE. Congenital radioulnar synostosis. In: Buck-Gramcko D. *Congenital Malformations of the Hand and Forearm.* London, England: Churchill Livingstone; 1998:xvii, 557

Part 11: Pediatric Sports Medicine and Injuries

TOPICS COVERED

CHAPTER 26

Preparticipation Physical Evaluation

Introduction

- This chapter covers using the preparticipation physical evaluation (PPE) for musculo-skeletal evaluation and clearance. For non-musculoskeletal evaluation and clearance, refer to *Preparticipation Physical Evaluation*.
- The PPE is a tool for screening athletes before the start of training and competition.
- The goal of the PPE is to make sports participation as safe as possible.
- The primary objectives of the PPE are
  — To identify disabling or life-threatening conditions
  — To identify conditions that may predispose to injury
  — To satisfy local legal requirements
- The emphasis is not on restricting participation, but rather to facilitate participation as is medically appropriate.

Timing

- Ideal timing is 6 weeks before the start of training and competition.
  — This allows sufficient time for any necessary evaluation or treatment without interfering with participation.
- The PPE can be incorporated into well-child care visits starting at 6 years of age.

Musculoskeletal History

- The musculoskeletal history alone will identify 92% of the musculoskeletal problems affecting athletes.
- The most efficient way to obtain a complete and accurate history is to have the athlete and parent complete a comprehensive, validated questionnaire (Figure 26-1).
- The goal is to identify any chronic conditions or incompletely rehabilitated injuries.
- Ask if there is pain, instability, or limitations caused by previous injuries or surgeries.
- Any condition that has previously disqualified an athlete from competition should be reexamined in depth.

Preparticipation Physical Evaluation

HISTORY FORM

Date of Exam _____

Name _____   Sex _____ Age _____ Date of birth _____

Grade _____ School _____   Sport(s) _____

Address _____   Phone _____

Personal physician _____

In case of emergency, contact

Name _____   Relationship _____   Phone (H) _____ (W) _____

Explain "Yes" answers below.
Circle questions you don't know the answers to.

	Yes	No
1. Has a doctor ever denied or restricted your participation in sports for any reason?	☐	☐
2. Do you have an ongoing medical condition (like diabetes or asthma)?	☐	☐
3. Are you currently taking any prescription or nonprescription (over-the-counter) medicines or pills?	☐	☐
4. Do you have allergies to medicines, pollens, foods, or stinging insects?	☐	☐
5. Have you ever passed out or nearly passed out DURING exercise?	☐	☐
6. Have you ever passed out or nearly passed out AFTER exercise?	☐	☐
7. Have you ever had discomfort, pain, or pressure in your chest during exercise?	☐	☐
8. Does your heart race or skip beats during exercise?	☐	☐

9. Has a doctor ever told you that you have (check all that apply):
☐ High blood pressure ☐ A heart murmur
☐ High cholesterol ☐ A heart infection

	Yes	No
10. Has a doctor ever ordered a test for your heart? (for example, ECG, echocardiogram)	☐	☐
11. Has anyone in your family died for no apparent reason?	☐	☐
12. Does anyone in your family have a heart problem?	☐	☐
13. Has any family member or relative died of heart problems or of sudden death before age 50?	☐	☐
14. Does anyone in your family have Marfan syndrome?	☐	☐
15. Have you ever spent the night in a hospital?	☐	☐
16. Have you ever had surgery?	☐	☐
17. Have you ever had an injury, like a sprain, muscle or ligament tear, or tendinitis, that caused you to miss a practice or game? If yes, circle affected area below:	☐	☐
18. Have you had any broken or fractured bones or dislocated joints? If yes, circle below:	☐	☐
19. Have you had a bone or joint injury that required x-rays, MRI, CT, surgery, injections, rehabilitation, physical therapy, a brace, a case, or crutches? If yes, circle below:	☐	☐

Head	Neck	Shoulder	Upper arm	Elbow	Forearm	Hand/fingers	Chest
Upper back	Lower back	Hip	Thigh	Knee	Calf/shin	Ankle	Foot/toes

	Yes	No
20. Have you ever had a stress fracture?	☐	☐
21. Have you been told that you have or have you had an x-ray for atlantoaxial (neck) instability?	☐	☐
22. Do you regularly use a brace or assistive device?	☐	☐
23. Has a doctor ever told you that you have asthma or allergies?	☐	☐

	Yes	No
24. Do you cough, wheeze, or have difficulty breathing during or after exercise?	☐	☐
25. Is there anyone in your family who has asthma?	☐	☐
26. Have you ever used an inhaler or taken asthma medicine?	☐	☐
27. Were you born without or are you missing a kidney, an eye, a testicle, or any other organ?	☐	☐
28. Have you had infectious mononucleosis (mono) within the last month?	☐	☐
29. Do you have any rashes, pressure sores, or other skin problems?	☐	☐
30. Have you had a herpes skin infection?	☐	☐
31. Have you ever had a head injury or concussion?	☐	☐
32. Have you been hit in the head and been confused or lost your memory?	☐	☐
33. Have you ever had a seizure?	☐	☐
34. Do you have headaches with exercise?	☐	☐
35. Have you ever had numbness, tingling, or weakness in your arms or legs after being hit or falling?	☐	☐
36. Have you ever been unable to move your arms or legs after being hit or falling?	☐	☐
37. When exercising in the heat, do you have severe muscle cramps or become ill?	☐	☐
38. Has a doctor told you that you or someone in your family has sickle cell trait or sickle cell disease?	☐	☐
39. Have you had any problems with your eyes or vision?	☐	☐
40. Do you wear glasses or contact lenses?	☐	☐
41. Do you wear protective eyewear, such as goggles or a face shield?	☐	☐
42. Are you happy with your weight?	☐	☐
43. Are you trying to gain or lose weight?	☐	☐
44. Has anyone recommended you change your weight or eating habits?	☐	☐
45. Do you limit or carefully control what you eat?	☐	☐
46. Do you have any concerns that you would like to discuss with a doctor?	☐	☐

FEMALES ONLY

	Yes	No
47. Have you every had a menstrual period?	☐	☐

48. How old were you when you had your first menstrual period? _____

49. How many periods have you had in the last 12 months? _____

Explain "Yes" answers here:

_____
_____
_____
_____
_____
_____
_____
_____

I hereby state that, to the best of my knowledge, my answers to the above questions are complete and correct.

Signature of athlete _____ Signature of parent/guardian _____ Date _____

Figure 26-1. Preparticipation physical evaluation history form from *Preparticipation Physical Evaluation,* 3rd Edition, with musculoskeletal, diet, and menstrual questions highlighted.

* Previous surgery should be documented in detail (eg, "ACL reconstruction" rather than "knee surgery").
  — Inquire whether the surgeon has prescribed specific activity restrictions, a brace or support, protective equipment, or modifications for sports, and whether postoperative rehabilitation has been completed.
* Use of a supportive brace or device may be prescribed by a treating physician for return to play or indicate a self-treated or unresolved injury.
  — Further questioning and examination of the specific joint may be necessary to determine whether additional treatment is required and whether the brace is appropriate.
  — Inspect braces for proper fit and integrity before each season.
* For any athlete with a history of stress fracture
  — Dietary and menstrual history should be reviewed in detail (see " Female Athlete Triad" in Chapter 29 on page 308).
  — Training errors should be corrected and improper equipment (eg, shoes) replaced.
  — Examination should focus on identifying risk factors such as muscle weakness, pes planus, pes cavus, or over-pronation that can be addressed through rehabilitation or supportive orthoses (see Chapter 29).

Musculoskeletal Examination

* Goals of the musculoskeletal examination
  — Evaluate for recovery from previous injuries (Box 26-1).
  — Identify any modifiable risk factors for reinjury (eg, muscle weakness or inflexibility, pes planus).
  — Identify any asymmetries in joint motion or muscle strength or size that may indicate an underlying musculoskeletal condition.
* The orthopaedic screening examination (Figure 26-2) is sufficient in the asymptomatic athlete with no history of prior injury.
* The orthopaedic screening examination should be supplemented with a comprehensive examination of the affected area(s) for patients with
  — History of previous injury
  — Pain, instability, locking, limited range of motion, weakness, or atrophy noted in the history or on the screening examination
* Referral to a sports medicine physician is recommended when the required comprehensive examination is beyond the examiner's expertise.

Box 26-1. Criteria for Clearance to Play After a Sprain, Strain, Dislocation, or Overuse Injury

Full, pain-free range of motion of the injured joint or joints controlled by the injured muscle

Minimal or no swelling

Near-normal muscle strength (at least 85%–90% of the uninjured side) (If a supportive brace or taping is required to achieve, that is acceptable.)

No pain or instability with sports-specific activities (eg, running, jumping, cutting)

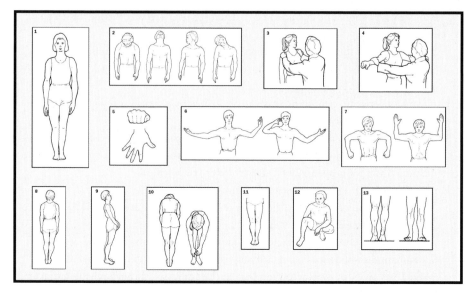

Figure 26-2. Orthopaedic screening examination. See Web site for detailed notes about each screening step. Available at: mediwire.healingwell.com/main/Default.aspx?P=Content&Article ID=197811. Accessed March 2, 2010.

Clearance

- General guidelines for clearance after sprains, strains, dislocations, and overuse injuries are listed in Box 26-1.
- For fractures, clearance should be determined by the treating physician.
  - In some cases, return to play may be allowed in a padded cast or splint, depending on patient comfort, the risk for further injury, and rules of the sports organization.
- For developmental conditions and deformities, activity modifications may be necessary based on symptoms or physical abilities.
- Clearance falls into 1 of 4 categories (Box 26-2) and should be individualized based on the following:
  - Does participation place the athlete at risk for serious injury or illness?
  - Does participation place other participants at risk for injury or illness?
  - Can the athlete safely participate while being treated (eg, rehabilitation program, brace)?
    - In some cases a protective brace, padding, or taping may provide the stability or protection needed for clearance.
    - Whether a specific brace or padding technique is allowed is determined by the rules of the specific sports organization, and the final decision is usually made by the sporting event's officials.
  - Can limited participation be allowed while treatment is being completed?
    - For example, a baseball pitcher with an elbow injury may be able to safely bat and play first base.
    - Determine which strength and conditioning activities are safe so that the athlete can maintain fitness during recovery.

— If clearance is denied only for certain sports, in what activities can the athlete safely participate?
  - For example, an athlete with an upper extremity injury may be able to safely participate in soccer or cross-country running.
- Referral to a sports medicine physician is recommended if there are any questions or uncertainty regarding clearance.
- Medical decisions to permanently restrict sports participation are best done in a consensus manner with subspecialty consultation and discussion with the athlete and family.

Box 26-2. Clearance Categories

Cleared without restrictions

Cleared with recommendations for further evaluation

Not cleared pending further evaluation, treatment, or rehabilitation

Not cleared for certain activities or not cleared for any activity

Legal Issues

- By the high school level all states except Rhode Island require some type of PPE.
- Legislative requirements vary by state for the timing and content of the evaluation and qualifications of the examiner.
  - In a number of states, nurses, physician assistants, and chiropractors are allowed to complete the PPE.
- Health Insurance Portability and Accountability Act guidelines allow a physician to communicate to the school only that the athlete is cleared or not cleared.
  - Discussion of the details of the PPE or the reason an athlete is not cleared is not permitted without the athlete and parents' consent.
- It is in the athlete's best interest to have relevant medical information available to the team's athletic trainer.
  - Athletic trainers are frequently the first responders at sporting events.
  - Athletic trainers can supervise rehabilitation protocols and communicate with physicians about the athlete's progress or ability to perform sports-specific exercises.

Athletes With Special Needs

- The Rehabilitation Act of 1973 and the Americans With Disabilities Act of 1990 mandate equal opportunity to anyone wishing to participate in athletics.
- For athletes with special needs, the PPE should be more comprehensive.
  - An evaluation of braces, prosthetic devices, or specialized equipment such as wheelchairs should be included in the PPE.
  - Input from physical or occupational therapists about functional abilities is helpful.
  - Clearance for athletes with trisomy 21 or atlantoaxial instability is discussed in Chapter 65.

CHAPTER 27

Strains, Sprains, and Dislocations

Muscle Strains

INTRODUCTION/ETIOLOGY/EPIDEMIOLOGY

- Tear of some or all of the fibers in a muscle
- Caused by a sudden, forceful change in the length of the muscle-tendon unit, most commonly an eccentric contraction against a significant load
- Less frequently, strains result from a rapid or forceful stretch to a muscle, or from repetitive overuse.
- Athletes who sprint, jump, leap, or kick are most susceptible.
- Strains usually occur at the musculotendinous junction.
- Most commonly affect muscles in the lower extremity, and those that cross 2 joints (ie, hamstrings, rectus femoris, gastrocnemius).
- The hamstrings are the most frequently strained muscle in the lower extremity and can lead to significant disability.

SIGNS AND SYMPTOMS

- Acute onset muscle pain during activity
- Some report a pop or tearing sensation.
- Weight bearing is usually painful.
- Physical examination reveals some or all of the following:
  — Muscle tenderness
  — Edema or ecchymosis
  — Pain and weakness with contraction of the injured muscle
  — Pain with passive stretch of the injured muscle

DIFFERENTIAL DIAGNOSIS

* Apophyseal avulsion fracture
  — Frequently mistaken for a muscle strain in the skeletally immature athlete
  — If there is any bony tenderness or if pain is at the proximal or distal aspect of the muscle, rather than the midsubstance, radiographs should be performed to rule out an avulsion fracture.

MAKING THE DIAGNOSIS

* The diagnosis is made clinically
* Strains are graded into 3 categories (Box 27-1).
* Magnetic resonance imaging (MRI) may be performed to confirm location and degree of injury.

TREATMENT

* Initial treatment includes rest, ice, compression, and elevation (RICE).
  — Ice can be applied for 10 to 15 minutes every few hours.
  — Heat and vigorous stretching or massage should be avoided during the initial injury period.
* Crutches may be necessary until weight bearing is comfortable.

Box 27-1. Common Grading of Strains and Sprains

Strains	
Grade 1	Stretch injury Some individual fibers are torn, but comprises only a small percentage of overall muscle. No loss of strength or motion
Grade 2	Partial tear of the muscle Some degree of ecchymosis or swelling Some loss of strength or motion
Grade 3	Complete rupture of the muscle Major hemorrhage and complete loss of function
Sprains	
Grade 1	Stretching of ligament fibers Minimal to no swelling Stress tests demonstrate pain but no laxity.
Grade 2	Partial tear of one or more ligaments Moderate pain and swelling Some laxity on stress test
Grade 3	Complete disruption of the ligament fibers Significant pain, swelling, and bruising Inability to ambulate Gross laxity on stress test of ligament

- Use of nonsteroidal anti-inflammatory drugs (NSAIDs) is controversial.
  — Studies demonstrate that NSAIDs can reduce inflammation in the short term but may impair muscle repair process in the long term, resulting in decreased muscle tensile strength and force production.
- A rehabilitation program of progressive stretching and strengthening exercises should be initiated as soon as pain begins to subside because early mobilization can help facilitate recovery.

EXPECTED OUTCOMES/PROGNOSIS

- Return to play ranges from 2 to 3 days for mild strains to 3 to 12 weeks for severe strains.
- Hamstring strains have a high rate of recurrence (12%–31%) and can lead to prolonged disability if rehabilitation is inadequate or return to play is rushed.
- Hip adductor strains (groin pulls) take longer to heal and are also prone to reinjury.

WHEN TO REFER

- Rarely, muscle strains require management by a sports medicine physician or orthopaedic surgeon.
  — Severe strains with significant loss of motion, strength, or function
  — Large, tense, painful hematomas, which may be aspirated to reduce pain

PREVENTION

- Warming up (5–10 minutes of light jogging or calisthenics) before physical activity may reduce the risk for muscle strains by increasing blood flow to muscles, making them more pliable.

RELEVANT *INTERNATIONAL CLASSIFICATION OF DISEASES, NINTH REVISION, CLINICAL MODIFICATION (ICD-9-CM)* CODES

- **843.8** Hip or thigh muscle strain (eg, hamstring, rectus femoris, hip adductors)
- **844.9** Calf muscle strain (eg, gastrocnemius)

Joint Sprains

INTRODUCTION/ETIOLOGY/EPIDEMIOLOGY

- Sprains are the most common injuries in sports for all age groups.
- Radiographs are frequently necessary to rule out fracture.
- Severity is graded into 3 categories (Box 27-1).

PRINCIPLES OF TREATMENT

- Protection, rest, ice, compression, elevation, and mobilization (PRICEM)
  - Protection
    - Crucial for early ligament healing
    - Provides needed stability for moderate and severe sprains.
    - Protection is continued until
      - Weight bearing is pain-free for lower extremity injuries.
      - Functional motion is pain-free for upper extremity injuries.
  - Rest
    - Reduce activities to a pain-free level.
  - Ice
    - Fifteen to 20 minutes at a time
    - Can be done as frequently as once an hour.
    - Heat should be avoided because it will worsen swelling.
  - Compression
    - An elastic bandage should be wrapped distal to proximal.
    - Remove for sleeping.
  - Elevation
    - Above the heart as much as possible
  - Mobilization
    - Early mobilization, which is appropriate for most mild and moderate sprains, can help facilitate recovery.
    - For all but the mildest of sprains, a rehabilitation program to restore range of motion, flexibility, strength, and proprioception will speed recovery and should be initiated as early as tolerated by the athlete.
- Nonsteroidal anti-inflammatory drugs
  - Reduce pain and inflammation, which may shorten recovery time by allowing rehabilitation to progress more quickly.
  - May increase early ligament strength.
  - Ibuprofen 3 times a day or naproxen twice a day for 7 to 10 days
- Criteria for return to sports
  - Little to no pain
  - Full range of motion
  - Near-normal strength
  - Able to perform sports-specific drills without any pain or instability
    - A functional brace or taping technique may be used to achieve this.

Ankle Sprains

- Ankle sprains account for up to 28% of all sports-related injuries.
- Athletes between 15 and 19 years of age are most frequently affected.
- Basketball, soccer, football, and volleyball are the most common sports.
- Eighty-five percent are lateral (Figure 27-1a,b).
  — The anterior talofibular (ATF) and calcaneofibular (CF) ligaments are the most frequently injured.
  — Usual mechanism is excessive inversion of a plantar flexed ankle.
- Ten percent are syndesmotic (high ankle sprains) (Figure 27-1).
  — Injury to the syndesmosis complex (interosseous membrane and inferior tibiofibular ligaments)
  — Usual mechanism is excessive external rotation on a dorsiflexed ankle.

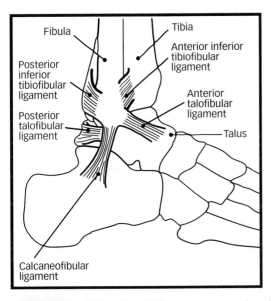

Figure 27-1a. Lateral ankle ligaments (PTF, ATF, and CF) and inferior tibiofibular ligaments. Available at: www.niams.nih.gov/Health_Info/Sprains_strains/default.asp.

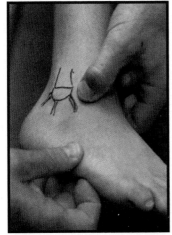

Figure 27-1b. Palpation of lateral ankle ligaments. From Sullivan JA, Anderson SJ, eds. *Care of the Young Athlete.* Rosemont, IL: American Academy of Orthopaedic Surgeons and American Academy of Pediatrics; 2000.

- Five percent are medial.
  — Injury to deltoid ligament
  — Mechanism is excessive eversion, usually from a high impact.
  — More commonly associated with fibula

SIGNS AND SYMPTOMS

- Pain after a twisting injury to the ankle
- Some report a pop at the time of injury.
- Weight bearing is painful.
- Swelling and bruising may be mild or severe.
- Range of motion is often limited because of pain.
- The injured ligament is tender to palpation (see Figure 27-1b).
- *Anterior drawer test* (see Figure 4-39) and *talar tilt tests* (Figure 27-2)
  — Can confirm the diagnosis of lateral ankle sprain and grade injury severity.
  — Sensitivity (96%) and specificity (84%) for detecting a ligament tear is best at 5 days after the injury.
  — Less reliable during the acute phase because patient guarding can cause false negatives
- *Reverse talar tilt test*
  — Grades severity of medial ankle sprains.
- *External rotation test*
  — Forced external rotation of the ankle
  — Painful with syndesmotic sprains, but also with fractures
- *Squeeze test*
  — Compression of tibia and fibula at mid-calf
  — Causes pain at the ankle with syndesmosis sprains, but also with fractures.

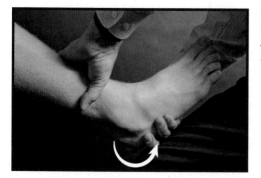

Figure 27-2. Talar tilt test. From Anderson SJ, Harris SS, eds. *Care of the Young Athlete.* 2nd ed. Elk Grove Village, IL: American Academy of Pediatrics; 2010.

DIFFERENTIAL DIAGNOSIS

- *Ankle fracture*
  — Skeletally immature patients with tenderness over the physis but normal radiographs should be treated for a *Salter-Harris type 1 injury* (see Chapter 35).
  — *Avulsion fracture of the fifth metatarsal*
    - Caused by same mechanism as a lateral ankle sprain
    - There will be tenderness at base of fifth metatarsal.
    - Radiographs of foot (anteroposterior [AP], lateral, oblique) are required for diagnosis.
- *Peroneal tendon subluxation*
  — Subluxation can be reproduced with active ankle eversion.

MAKING THE DIAGNOSIS

- The diagnosis of a lateral ankle sprain can be made clinically.
  — Radiographs (AP, lateral, mortise) should be performed to rule out fracture if there is bony tenderness or inability to bear weight immediately after the injury and for 4 steps in the clinic/emergency department.
- Radiographs should be performed for all medial and syndesmosis sprains.
  — Medial sprains are more commonly associated with fractures.
  — Syndesmosis sprains require radiographs to grade severity.
    - The clear space between the tibia and fibula 1 cm above the joint line should be less than 5 to 6 mm on AP and mortise views (Figure 27-3).
      - Grade 1: no widening of clear space
      - Grade 2: clear space widened, but less than 10 mm
      - Grade 3: clear space wider than 10 mm

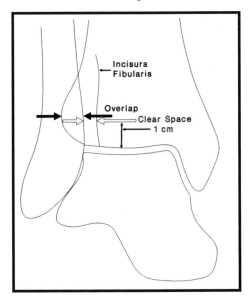

Incisura
Fibularis

Overlap

Clear Space
1 cm

Figure 27-3. Clear space between tibia and fibula. Reproduced with permission from Lutter LD, Mizel MS, Pfeffer GB (eds). *Orthopaedic Knowledge Update: Foot and Ankle.* Rosemont, IL: American Academy of Orthopaedic Surgeons;1994:241–253.

TREATMENT

- Initial treatment includes RICE and weight bearing as tolerated.
- Ice should be applied for 15 to 20 minutes every 2 to 4 hours.
- Heat should be avoided.
- An air stirrup is preferred over a compression wrap because it also provides protection and support, which is helpful in promoting earlier weight bearing.
- Athletes with more severe sprains may require use of crutches or a walking boot until weight bearing is more comfortable.
- Nonsteroidal anti-inflammatory drugs are recommended during the first 7 to 10 days after injury.
  — They reduce pain and inflammation, which may shorten recovery time by allowing rehabilitation to progress more quickly.
  — Studies also show they may increase early ligament strength.
- Prolonged immobilization weakens the ligaments, while early mobilization decreases adhesions and increases ligament strength.
- Rehabilitation to restore range of motion, flexibility, strength, and proprioception speeds recovery and should be initiated as early as tolerated by the athlete.

EXPECTED OUTCOMES/PROGNOSIS

- *Lateral ankle sprains*
  — Average time to return to sports
    ▪ Grade 1: 8 days
    ▪ Grade 2: 15 days
    ▪ Grade 3: 28 days
  — After an initial sprain the risk for reinjury is up to 5 times higher.
  — An estimated 20% to 40% of athletes suffer from chronic instability.
  — Very few require surgical stabilization.
  — The most common reason for persistent pain is inadequate rehabilitation.
  — Severe and repetitive ankle sprains increase the risk for osteoarthritis.
- *Medial ankle sprains*
  — Recovery takes twice as long as for lateral ankle sprains.
- *Syndesmosis sprains*
  — Average time to return to sports is 6 weeks.
  — Grade 3 injuries usually require surgical stabilization.
  — Recurrent instability is less common than with lateral ankle sprains.
  — Heterotopic ossification in the syndesmosis is a possible complication.

WHEN TO REFER

- To a sports medicine physician
  — Lateral or medial ankle sprains that remain symptomatic despite a comprehensive rehabilitation program
- To an orthopaedic surgeon who specializes in sports injuries
  — Grade 2 and 3 syndesmosis sprains

PREVENTION

- Strategies proven to reduce the risk of recurrent ankle sprains
  - A rehabilitation program that includes proprioception training
  - A semirigid ankle brace or athletic tape during athletic activities

RELEVANT *ICD-9-CM* CODES

- **845.00**   Ankle sprain
- **845.01**   Medial ankle sprain
- **845.02**   Lateral ankle sprain (CF)
- **845.09**   Lateral ankle sprain (ATF or PTF)
- **845.03**   Syndesmosis sprain

Acromioclavicular Joint Sprain

INTRODUCTION/ETIOLOGY/EPIDEMIOLOGY

- Also called a shoulder separation
- Rare before 13 years of age
- Most are grade 1 injuries involving only the acromioclavicular (AC) ligament.
- Grade 2 injuries involve the AC ligament and one of the coracoclavicular (CC) ligaments (Figure 27-4).
- Grade 3 injuries involve the AC ligament and both of the CC ligaments.
- Usual mechanism is a blow to the side or top of shoulder.
- Usually occur in collision sports (eg, football, hockey).
- Five to 10 times more common in males

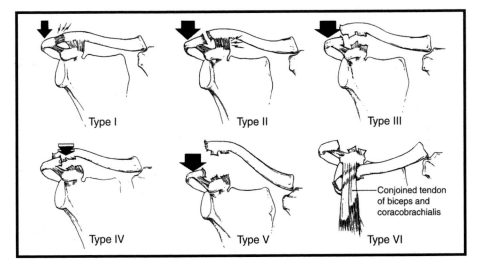

Figure 27-4. Classification of acromioclavicular separations. Adapted with permission from Rockwood CA Jr: Subluxation and dislocations about the shoulder, in Rockford CA Jr, Green DP (eds): *Rockwood and Green's Fractures in Adults,* ed 3. Philadelphia, PA: JB Lippincott; 1988.

SIGNS AND SYMPTOMS

- Pain and tenderness at the injured ligaments
- There may be slight swelling.
- For grade 2 and 3 sprains, the distal clavicle may be visibly elevated.
- Bruising is uncommon and usually indicates a fracture.
- Crossover test is positive.
  — Arm adduction across body causes pain.
- Piano key sign is positive in grade 2 and 3 injuries.
  — Ability to depress the distal end of clavicle

DIFFERENTIAL DIAGNOSIS

- Clavicle fracture
- Shoulder dislocation or subluxation

MAKING THE DIAGNOSIS

- The diagnosis is based on clinical and radiographic findings
- Severity is graded by degree of displacement on radiographs.
  — Ten-degree cephalad view of the AC joint (Zanca view) (Figure 27-5)
  — Comparison is made to uninjured side.

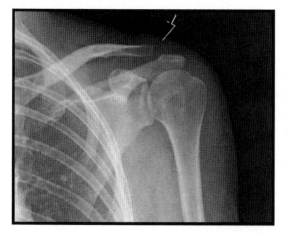

Figure 27-5. Acromioclavicular (AC) separation (type II)—anteroposterior (AP) view. AP view of the left shoulder shows minimal displacement (grade 2) of the AC joint (black arrow). Reproduced with permission from Johnson TR, Steinbach LS (eds): *Essentials of Musculoskeletal Imaging.* Rosemont, IL: American Academy of Orthopaedic Surgeons; 2004.

TREATMENT

- Rest, ice, compression, and elevation
- Nonsteroidal anti-inflammatory drugs
- A sling should be used for comfort.
- Rehabilitation is helpful if the arm has been immobilized for more than 5 to 7 days.

EXPECTED OUTCOMES/PROGNOSIS

- Prognosis for return to high-level sports, even throwing, is excellent with non-operative treatment.
- Average time to return to sports depends on injury severity.
  — Grade 1: 3 days to 2 weeks
  — Grade 2: 2 to 4 weeks
  — Grade 3: 6 to 12 weeks
- Surgical stabilization is very rarely needed.
- There may be some discomfort at the joint for up to 6 months after the injury.
- In grade 2 and 3 sprains, the distal clavicle will remain visibly elevated.
- There is an increased risk of AC joint osteoarthritis.

WHEN TO REFER

- To an orthopaedic surgeon who specializes in sports injuries or shoulder surgery
  — Significant displacement on radiographs
  — Limited improvement with nonoperative treatment

PREVENTION

- Several taping techniques and braces are available, but there is no evidence that they can reduce the risk for AC joint injury.

RELEVANT *ICD-9-CM* CODES

- **840.0**   AC ligament sprain
- **840.1**   CC ligament sprain

Multidirectional Instability of the Shoulder

INTRODUCTION/ETIOLOGY/EPIDEMIOLOGY

- Shoulder pain or subluxation or dislocation episode(s) due to multidirectional (anterior, posterior, inferior) ligamentous laxity
- Multidirectional instability (MDI) is an important risk factor for rotator cuff impingement or tendinopathy in adolescents (see Chapter 29).
- Equally common in males and females
- May be bilateral.
- Between 25% and 100% also have generalized ligamentous laxity (generalized joint hypermobility), isolated or associated with connective tissue disorder such as Ehlers-Danlos syndrome.
- Multidirectional instability can also result from repetitive microtrauma, such as with repetitive overhead arm motions in sports like tennis, volleyball, swimming, and baseball.

SIGNS AND SYMPTOMS

- Patients may report one or all of the following symptoms:
  — Shoulder pain
  — Feelings of instability, popping, or shifting in the shoulder
  — One or more episodes of subluxation or dislocation, often with minimal to no trauma, such as rolling over in bed or reaching forward or overhead
  — Ability to voluntarily dislocate or sublux the shoulder
  — Radiating paresthesias are occasionally reported.
  — Activities such as swimming, carrying bags, and overhand throwing may reproduce or aggravate symptoms.
- Common physical examination findings
  — *Positive sulcus test* (see Figure 4-16) indicating inferior laxity is the hallmark of multidirectional instability.
  — *Load and shift maneuver* (see Figure 4-15) is positive for anterior and posterior laxity.
  — There is often weakness with resisted testing of the rotator cuff muscles (see Figure 4-18).
  — *Scapular dyskinesis* (asymmetrical scapular movement) may be prominent.
  — *Apprehension and relocation tests* (see figures 4-17 and 4-18) may be positive.
  — There is often tenderness along the anterior shoulder, medial scapular border, and rhomboid and levator scapulae muscles.
  — Beighton score (see Figure 4-2) may reveal generalized ligamentous laxity.

DIFFERENTIAL DIAGNOSIS

- Other causes of shoulder pain and popping can be distinguished from MDI by their absence of multidirectional laxity on examination and other features specific to the diagnosis (Table 27-1).

Table 27-1. Causes of Shoulder Pain and Popping Distinguishable From Multidirectional Instability

Cause	Differentiating Feature(s)
Traumatic shoulder dislocation/subluxation	• Usually caused by significant trauma • Examination demonstrates laxity in only one direction, usually anterior.
Glenoid labral tear	• Can result from acute subluxation or dislocation or repetitive microtrauma. • Painful catching is common symptom. • MRI with arthrogram can identify.
Rotator cuff impingement/ tendinopathy	• May result from MDI. • Positive impingement signs on examination • MRI can identify.
Cervical spine disorders	• Pain radiates from neck or is reproduced with neck ROM • Spurling test may be positive.

MRI, magnetic resonance imaging; MDI, multidirectional instability; ROM, range of motion.

MAKING THE DIAGNOSIS

- The diagnosis is made clinically.
- Neck examination should be performed to evaluate for possible cervical etiology.
- *Radiographs* in MDI are normal but are indicated to evaluate for other pathology if any of the following are present:
  — Pain persisting longer than a month
  — Nighttime pain
  — Acute trauma with limited range of motion
  — History of multiple instability episodes
  — Radiographic series should include AP view in internal rotation, axillary view, and scapular-Y view.
- For patients failing to respond to conservative treatment, *MRI* of the shoulder can evaluate for other causes, such as rotator cuff tendinopathy or labral pathology.
- *Magnetic resonance imaging with arthrogram* is necessary to rule out a labral tear.

TREATMENT

- A physical therapy program focused on strengthening of the rotator cuff, deltoid, and scapular stabilizing muscles (middle and lower trapezius, rhomboids, levator scapulae, and serratus anterior)
- Advise patients to avoid irritating activities while undergoing rehabilitation to reduce symptoms more quickly and facilitate recovery.
- Nonsteroidal anti-inflammatory drugs may be used in the early phase of treatment to control pain or if there is concomitant rotator cuff impingement or tendinopathy.

EXPECTED OUTCOMES/PROGNOSIS

- Most patients will experience a decrease in their symptoms with nonoperative management, but this may take 3 to 6 months.
- Outcomes after surgery are not much better than with conservative management; even though the ligaments can be tightened surgically, over time the collagen fibers eventually stretch out again and laxity returns.
- Surgery for comorbid conditions, such as a labral tear, is associated with better outcomes.

WHEN TO REFER

- For patients with unsatisfactory improvement in symptoms after 3 to 6 months of conservative treatment and activity modification, referral to a sports medicine physician or orthopaedic surgeon specializing in sports or shoulder surgery is recommended.
- For patients with generalized ligamentous laxity who have signs or symptoms that suggest a connective tissue disorder (eg, extensible skin, poor wound healing, easy bruising, Marfan stigmata), referral to a geneticist specializing in connective tissue disorders may be helpful.

PREVENTION

- Maintaining balanced strength in the rotator cuff and scapular stabilizing muscles can reduce the frequency of and morbidity from recurrent subluxation or dislocation episodes.
- Shoulder stabilizing braces are available (Figure 27-6).
  — Because they significantly limit shoulder abduction and external rotation, they are not practical for use in most sports, except for football linemen.
  — Patients who sublux or have pain while sleeping may benefit from wearing a brace at night.

RELEVANT *ICD-9-CM* CODE

- **718.81**   Shoulder laxity

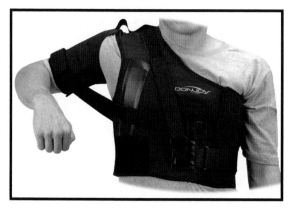

Figure 27-6. Shoulder stabilizing brace. Courtesy DJO, LLC.

Traumatic Shoulder Subluxation or Dislocation

INTRODUCTION/ETIOLOGY/EPIDEMIOLOGY

- About 20% occur in children and adolescents between 10 and 20 years of age.
- Less than 2% occur in children younger than 10 years.
- Ninety-five percent are *anterior dislocations,* tearing the anterior inferior glenohumeral ligament.
  — Most are associated with a Bankart lesion (detachment of the capsule from the anterior glenoid).
  — Most occur in contact or collision sports.
  — The usual mechanism of injury is a blow to an abducted and externally rotated shoulder.
  — Less commonly results from a fall on an outstretched arm.
- *Posterior dislocation*
  — Uncommon
  — May occur in collision sports such as football and hockey.
  — The usual mechanism of injury is posteriorly directed force to an arm that is adducted and internally rotated.

— Reported following seizures and electric shocks

  ▪ Mechanism is sudden vigorous contraction of internal rotators.

— Often associated with MDI of the shoulder.

SIGNS AND SYMPTOMS

- Patients report feeling that their shoulder popped out.
- There is pain at rest or with attempted movement of the arm.
- Physical examination findings if evaluation is performed before reduction
  — Visible deformity with prominent lateral acromion and loss of normal rounded contour of the deltoid
  — With an anterior dislocation, the arm is held in a slightly externally rotated position.
  — With a posterior dislocation, the arm is held in an internally rotated position.
  — Up to 30% of patients have temporary axillary nerve dysfunction, with numbness or paresthesias of the skin overlying the deltoid or deltoid weakness.
- Physical examination findings if evaluation is performed after reduction
  — Range of motion may be limited for several weeks following the injury.
  — Rotator cuff strength is often diminished secondary to pain (see Figure 4-18).
  — Load and shift test reveals anterior or posterior laxity (see Figure 4-15).
  — Positive *apprehension test* (see Figure 4-17) can be performed in supine position or standing.
    ▪ Examiner abducts, then externally rotates the arm with gentle force placed on the posterior shoulder.
    ▪ Test result is positive if patient reports apprehension that the shoulder will dislocate.
  — A *relocation test* (see Figure 4-18) result may also be positive.
    ▪ Test is performed with patient in the supine position.
    ▪ Immediately after eliciting a positive apprehension test, examiner applies gentle posteriorly directed pressure on the anterior shoulder.
    ▪ Test result is positive if this maneuver relieves the patient's apprehension.

DIFFERENTIAL DIAGNOSIS

- Shoulder subluxation
  — If the spontaneous reduction happens quickly, a dislocation may be difficult to distinguish from a subluxation. Treatment is the same, but risk for recurrent instability may be lower after a subluxation.
- Scapular or humerus fracture
  — Swelling and bruising
  — Significant point tenderness
  — Radiographs are positive.
- Rotator cuff tear
  — Uncommon in adolescents
  — Apprehension test is negative.
  — Rotator cuff weakness is significant.

- Multidirectional instability
  — Reported trauma is usually minimal.
  — Positive sulcus sign
  — Bilateral symptoms

MAKING THE DIAGNOSIS

- The diagnosis can be made clinically, but pre-reduction radiographs are commonly performed to determine the direction of dislocation and evaluate for fracture.
- Post-reduction films should always be performed to confirm the humeral head is reduced and evaluate for associated fractures.
- Radiographic findings after shoulder dislocation may include
  — Hill-Sachs defect (Figure 27-7a)
    ▪ Impaction injury to the posterior lateral humeral head
    ▪ Reported in 38% to 90% of patients with an anterior dislocation.
    ▪ If moderately sized, can contribute to recurrent instability.
  — Fractures of the greater tuberosity and glenoid rim: uncommon in pediatric patients (Figure 27-7b)
- Radiographic series should consist of
  — True AP view
    ▪ Normally there should be no overlap of the humerus and glenoid.
  — Anteroposterior with shoulder in internal rotation
    ▪ Best for identifying a Hill-Sachs defect
  — Axillary and scapular-Y views
    ▪ Confirm humeral head is located in glenoid.
    ▪ Axillary view may be difficult to obtain pre-reduction.
- Magnetic resonance imaging is not necessary in the acute setting.
- Magnetic resonance imaging with arthrogram is the preferred imaging study for surgical planning.

TREATMENT

- Reduction may be performed immediately on-site by an athletic trainer or a physician experienced in shoulder dislocations.
- In the emergency department setting, adequate sedation, analgesics, and muscle relaxants are recommended before performing reduction because muscle spasm and pain can make reduction difficult.
- Immobilize in a sling for comfort, usually for 3 to 4 weeks.
- Nonsteroidal anti-inflammatory drugs, analgesics, and ice are used as needed to control pain.
- Comprehensive physical therapy program
  — Begin with gentle passive range of motion exercises.
  — Progress to strengthening the rotator cuff and scapular stabilizing muscles.

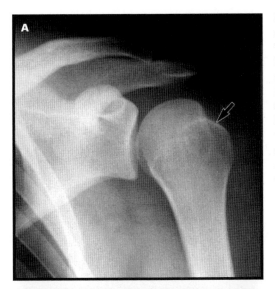

Figure 27-7a. Hill-Sachs lesion—anteroposterior (AP) internal rotation view. AP internal rotation view of the left shoulder shows a superolateral compression fracture, or Hill-Sachs lesion (arrow), which is characteristic of an anterior dislocation of the humeral head. Reproduced with permission from Johnson TR, Steinbach LS (eds): *Essentials of Musculoskeletal Imaging.* Rosemont, IL: American Academy of Orthopaedic Surgeons; 2004.

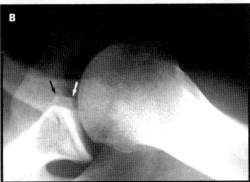

Figure 27-7b. Axillary view showing erosion of the glenoid rim (arrows) associated with anterior glenohumeral instability. Reproduced with permission from Griffin LY (ed): *Essentials of Musculoskeletal Care,* 3rd edition. Rosemont, IL: American Academy of Orthopaedic Surgeons; 2005.

— Usually takes 2 to 4 months for return to sports.
- Shoulder stabilizing brace (Figure 27-6) is recommended if practical for athlete's sport or position.
- The athlete must understand there is a significant risk of recurrence.
- Indications for surgical stabilization
— Recurrent dislocations
— Some physicians advocate surgical stabilization after a first-time dislocation for athletes in high physical contact sports such as football because the re-dislocation rate is so high.

EXPECTED OUTCOMES/PROGNOSIS

- Recurrence rates after a first-time shoulder dislocation are between 80% and 85% in patients younger than 20 years.
- More than 70% of these recur in the first 2 years after the initial event.
- Recurrence rates are 10% to 20% after arthroscopic stabilization.

WHEN TO REFER

• All patients with a shoulder dislocation should be referred to an orthopaedic surgeon specializing in sports medicine or shoulder surgery to discuss treatment options.

PREVENTION

• Maintaining balanced strength in the rotator cuff and scapular stabilizing muscles may reduce the risk for recurrent subluxation or dislocation.
• Shoulder stabilizing braces (Figure 27-6) may be helpful but are practical only for some sports and positions.

RELEVANT *ICD-9-CM* CODES

• **831.01**   Anterior dislocation, shoulder
• **831.02**   Posterior dislocation, shoulder

CHAPTER 28

Traumatic Muscle Injuries

Muscle Contusions

- Second most common type of muscle injury, next to strains
- Caused by direct, non-penetrating blows to the muscle belly, which leads to bleeding into the muscle and hematoma formation
- Most common locations are the quadriceps (anterior or lateral thigh) and brachialis (upper arm).
- They occur most frequently in contact sports such as football, rugby, soccer, and martial arts.
- Almost all resolve with rest, ice, compression, and elevation (RICE) followed by rehabilitation exercises. Because quadriceps contusions are the most common muscle contusion and are most likely to develop complications, they are highlighted as follows.

Quadriceps Contusion

INTRODUCTION/ETIOLOGY/EPIDEMIOLOGY

- Quadriceps are the most common location for muscle contusion.
- Knee to the thigh is most common mechanism.

SIGNS AND SYMPTOMS

- Pain and swelling in anterior or lateral thigh that is worse with movement; bruising may be visible.
- The patient may complain of knee stiffness and difficulty bearing weight.
- Physical examination findings include tenderness, edema, ecchymosis, weakness, and pain with passive stretch of the quadriceps muscle.
- A palpable mass will be present if the intramuscular hematoma is significant.
- Active straight leg raise will be painful and may be impossible for patient to perform.
- In more severe cases a knee effusion may be seen.

- Contusion severity is based on the degree of active knee flexion post-injury.
  — Mild: active knee flexion greater than 90 degrees
  — Moderate: active knee flexion between 45 and 90 degrees
  — Severe: active knee flexion less than 45 degrees

DIFFERENTIAL DIAGNOSIS

- Quadriceps strain
- Femur fracture
- Bony/soft tissue tumor
- Hip pointer

MAKING THE DIAGNOSIS

- The diagnosis can usually be made clinically.
- If the history is unclear or atypical, imaging may be helpful.
- *Radiographs* can identify a fracture or tumor.
- *Ultrasound* may be used to measure hematoma size to help determine if surgical evacuation should be considered in a high-level athlete.
- *Magnetic resonance imaging* can confirm or rule out muscle injury and provide detailed characterization of the lesion; it is especially helpful in identifying small hematomas deep within the muscle belly, when ultrasound is inconclusive or when patients fail to respond to early treatment.

TREATMENT

- Rest, ice, compression, and elevation
- Immobilization of the knee in moderate flexion for the first 24 hours facilitates healing, reduces the risk of complications by limiting the size of hematoma formation, and results in faster return to sports and activities.
- For the athlete who does not present immediately, the thigh should be wrapped in maximally tolerable knee flexion.
- After 24 to 48 hours, active quadriceps stretching and isometric strengthening should begin in a pain-free range.
- Crutches should be used until there is at least 90 degrees of knee flexion and no limp.
- The athlete may *return to play* when knee flexion is full and pain-free, and quadriceps size and strength are equal to the uninjured side.
- Athletes should wear a modified thigh pad to prevent reinjury.

EXPECTED OUTCOMES/PROGNOSIS

- Prognosis is excellent if treatment is begun promptly.
- Following the protocol of immediate immobilization in knee flexion, the average time to return to play was 3.5 days compared with 18 days when immobilization was delayed and 47 days when the thigh was wrapped with the knee in extension.

- *Complications* are more likely when treatment is delayed.
  — Myositis ossificans, a benign proliferation of bone and cartilage at the site of the hematoma, is the most common complication (Figure 28-1).
    - It should be suspected if a patient is not improving after 4 to 5 days of treatment or if symptoms, especially knee flexion, worsen 2 to 3 weeks after initial injury.
    - It can be detected on radiographs within 3 to 6 weeks after initial injury.
    - Myositis ossificans may delay rehabilitation and return to play for up to a year.
    - The lesion should be excised once it shows decreased activity on bone scan (6–12 months).
  — Acute compartment syndrome caused by large hematoma occurs less frequently.
  — Nerve palsy can result when the hematoma compresses a nerve, or rarely if the nerve itself is damaged from the initial impact.

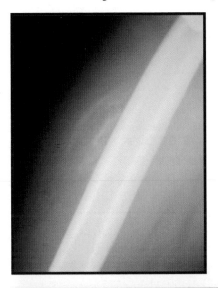

Figure 28-1a. Radiograph of the femur showing myositis ossificans in the quadriceps muscle.

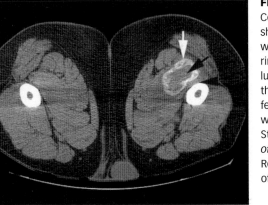

Figure 28-1b. Myositis ossificans. Computed tomography scan showing well-circumscribed mass with a sharply marginalized ossified rim (white arrow) and a central lucent area (black arrow). Note that there is no contact with the femur (arrowhead). Reproduced with permission from Johnson TR, Steinbach LS (eds): *Essentials of Musculoskeletal Imaging.* Rosemont, IL: American Academy of Orthopaedic Surgeons; 2004.

PREVENTION

- Wearing thigh pads during contact sports will help protect from injury, but they are not currently commonplace in activities like rugby and marital arts.
- Animal studies have shown contracted muscle requires a greater force to impart injury; therefore, some suggest teaching athletes to "tighten up" before impact occurs. However, not all impact is predictable and this theory has never been tested clinically.
- Early immobilization in flexion decreases the risk of myositis ossificans.
- While selective COX-2 inhibitors and indomethacin have been shown to protect against heterotopic ossification following total hip arthroplasty, they have not been studied with quadriceps contusion.

WHEN TO REFER

- Severe swelling or pain at rest warrants immediate referral to an emergency department for compartment pressure testing and possible decompression surgery.
- Refer to a pediatric orthopaedic surgeon
  — In the case of a large hematoma, when surgical evacuation may be considered
  — If functional improvement is not dramatic once treatment is initiated
  — If complications such as myositis ossificans develop

RELEVANT *INTERNATIONAL CLASSIFICATION OF DISEASES, NINTH REVISION, CLINICAL MODIFICATION (ICD-9-CM)* CODES

- **924.00**   Quadriceps contusion
- **728.12**   Myositis ossificans

Hip Pointer

INTRODUCTION/ETIOLOGY/EPIDEMIOLOGY

- Iliac crest contusion that results in a subperiosteal hematoma
- Caused by a direct blow or fall onto the hip
- Most commonly occurs in football.

SIGNS AND SYMPTOMS

- Pain and swelling over the iliac crest
- Point tenderness, ecchymosis, and muscle spasm
- Pain with contraction of abdominal muscles

DIFFERENTIAL DIAGNOSIS

- Hip fracture
- Avulsion fracture
- Muscle contusion
- Muscle strain

MAKING THE DIAGNOSIS

- The diagnosis is made clinically, but radiographs should be performed to rule out a fracture or avulsion.

TREATMENT

- Rest with hip in position of comfort.
- Crutches until pain-free ambulation
- Reduce pain and swelling with ice, nonsteroidal anti-inflammatory drugs, and compression with an elastic bandage or compression shorts.
- Physical therapy for stretching or strengthening of core muscles
- Injection of local anesthetic may be considered in the highly competitive athlete to expedite return to play but is usually reserved for adult patients.
- Return to play is possible once there is no pain with jogging or activation of abdominal muscles.

EXPECTED OUTCOMES/PROGNOSIS

- Prognosis is excellent; most can return to their previous level of sports participation within days to weeks, depending on the severity of the contusion.
- Hematoma formation can lead to compression of the lateral femoral cutaneous nerve (meralgia paraesthetica), which is the main potential complication.

PREVENTION

- For return to contact sports, a hip pad should be worn to protect the area.

WHEN TO REFER

- Refer to pediatric sports medicine specialist or pediatric orthopaedic surgeon for symptoms of meralgia paraesthetica, such as a burning, tingling, or stabbing sensation in the anterolateral thigh.

RELEVANT *ICD-9-CM* CODES

- **924.01**   Hip pointer
- **355.1**   Meralgia paraesthetica

Pelvic Avulsion Fractures

INTRODUCTION/ETIOLOGY/EPIDEMIOLOGY

- Occur when a forceful muscle contraction or elongation causes separation of the apophysis from the pelvic bone (Figure 28-2a–d). Figure 28-3 shows an anterior view of the pelvis labeled with apophyses.
- Most common mechanisms are sprinting, kicking, or performing leaps or splits in gymnastics or cheerleading.

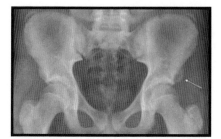

Figure 28-2a. Anterior inferior iliac spines avulsion fracture.

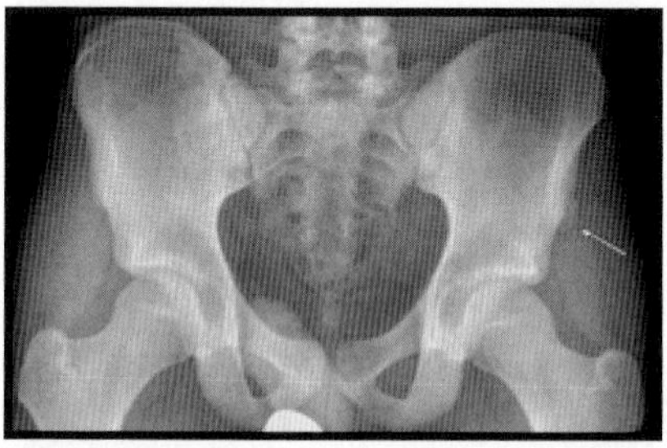

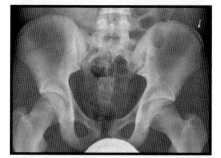

Figure 28-2b. Anterior superior iliac spines avulsion fracture.

Figure 28-2c. Iliac crest avulsion fracture.

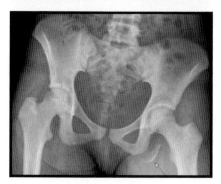

Figure 28-2d. Ischial tuberosity avulsion fracture.

- Less often, there is gradual onset of pain when the fracture results from repetitive loading during these activities over time.
- The most common locations are the ischial tuberosity, anterior superior iliac spines (ASIS), and anterior inferior iliac spines (AIIS), but avulsions can also occur at the lesser trochanter, iliac crest, and pubic symphysis (Figure 28-2).
- Eighty percent are sports related, and 70% to 90% occur in boys.

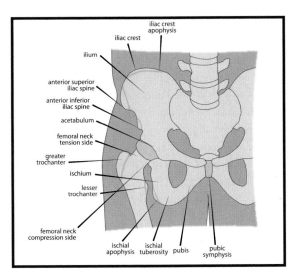

Figure 28-3. Apophyses of the pelvis. From Metzl JD. *Sports Medicine in the Pediatric Office.* Elk Grove Village, IL: American Academy of Pediatrics; 2008.

- Peak incidence is between 14 and 18 years of age.
  — During adolescence, the pelvic apophyses are weaker than the attached musculotendinous units, so a forceful contraction is more likely to cause an avulsion fracture than a muscle strain in this age group.
  — Ischial tuberosity avulsions occur at an average age of 19 years because of the later age of formation of this apophysis.

SIGNS AND SYMPTOMS

- Patients typically report a sudden, painful pop in the anterior or lateral hip or buttock.
- Weight bearing is painful.
- Local swelling and ecchymosis may be noted.
- The injured apophysis will be tender, but the attached muscle is usually non-tender.
- There will be pain with active contraction or passive stretch of the attached muscle and often decreased flexibility and strength.

DIFFERENTIAL DIAGNOSIS

- Muscle strain
- Pelvic apophysitis
- Bony or soft tissue tumor
- Hip pointer

MAKING THE DIAGNOSIS

- *Radiographs* are required for diagnosis and will reveal a displaced bony fragment at the involved site.
  — Anteroposterior view of the pelvis will show most avulsions (Figure 28-2a–d).
  — Oblique view of the pelvis allows better visualization of the AIIS and ASIS and may be helpful for diagnosing these avulsions.

TREATMENT

- Most pelvic avulsion fractures heal with nonoperative treatment.
- During the initial post-injury period, athletes should use ice and remain non-weight bearing on crutches until ambulation is no longer painful, which usually takes 2 to 4 weeks.
- Heat, massage, and vigorous stretching should be avoided during this period.
- Once weight bearing is no longer painful, rehabilitation may begin, initially concentrating on gentle flexibility exercises and later strengthening.
- Once there is full, pain-free range of motion and near-normal strength, the athlete may start a gradual, stepwise return to sporting activities, starting with jogging, then running, then sport-specific drills before full return to play .
- Repeat radiographs are not necessary unless symptoms persist beyond the expected healing time.

EXPECTED OUTCOMES/PROGNOSIS

- Time to return to sports varies depending on the site and severity of injury.
  — Anterior superior iliac spine, AIIS, and iliac crest: 6 to 8 weeks
  — Ischial tuberosity and pubic symphysis: 3 to 4 months
- Premature return to activities can result in re-rupture and prolonged recovery.
- Chronic pain and nonunion are possible complications in cases of delayed or inadequate treatment.
- Acute-onset meralgia paresthetica has been reported with ASIS avulsions.

PREVENTION

- Adolescent athletes should be counseled to seek treatment for any lingering muscle strain of the hip or thigh because it may represent an apophysitis that could predispose to avulsion fracture if not identified and treated.

WHEN TO REFER

- Refer to a pediatric sports medicine specialist
  — If assistance is needed for supervision of rehabilitation or clearance to return to play
- Refer to a pediatric orthopaedic surgeon
  — Avulsions with more than 2 cm of separation
  — Persistent pain beyond expected time for recovery and inability to resume prior level of sports participation
  — Chronic nonunions

RELEVANT ICD-9-CM CODE

- **808.41**   Pelvic avulsion fractures

CHAPTER 29

Overuse Injuries

Overuse injuries occur when an anatomic structure is subjected to repetitive stress, resulting in forces beyond what that structure can withstand. Young athletes can sustain overuse injuries to bones, growth centers, tendons, and fascia. Rapid increases in training and long-term, high-level training, particularly in a single sport, are the most common causes of overuse injuries. Other contributing factors include suboptimal equipment, poor training surfaces or a sudden change in training surface, poor technique, imbalances in muscle strength or flexibility, and variants of normal anatomic alignment such as pes planus or pes cavus.

Overuse injuries involving the growth plates (physes and apophyses) are unique to children and adolescents. Unlike bone and tendon, which are composed of a strong extracellular matrix designed to withstand compressive and tensile loads, growth plates are composed mainly of cartilage cells, so they have little resistance to stress. Injuries to the apophyses are most common. These areas of secondary ossification, where muscle-tendon units attach to bone, are the weakest point in the biomechanical chain.

Little League Shoulder

INTRODUCTION/ETIOLOGY/EPIDEMIOLOGY

- Many terms have been used to describe this injury, including osteochondrosis, epiphysiolysis, rotation stress fracture, and Salter-Harris I injury to the proximal humeral epiphysis.
- Results from repetitive overhead activity, which causes microtrauma to the proximal humeral physeal plate
- Can occur in any sport with repetitive overhead activity, including swimming, tennis, volleyball, and gymnastics.
- Most common in high-level pitchers between 10 and 14 years of age.

SIGNS AND SYMPTOMS

- Shoulder pain with insidious onset, exacerbated by throwing or other overhead athletic activity
- Loss of throwing velocity or accuracy
- Tenderness with palpation of the proximal lateral humerus
- May have painful or decreased shoulder range of motion.
- Usually have pain with resisted shoulder elevation or external rotation.

DIFFERENTIAL DIAGNOSIS

- Rotator cuff tendonitis, impingement, or subacromial bursitis
- Proximal humeral fracture
- Biceps tendonitis
- Glenohumeral instability
- Labral tear
- Bone tumor

MAKING THE DIAGNOSIS

- Diagnosis can be made clinically.
- *Plain radiographs* (anteroposterior [AP] view in internal and external rotation, and a scapular Y-view) are often normal but may show classic finding of widening of the proximal humeral epiphysis when compared with the opposite shoulder (Figure 29-1). There may also be fragmentation, sclerosis, or demineralization of the epiphysis or metaphysis.
- *Magnetic resonance imaging (MRI)* is not usually indicated unless there is suspicion for alternative pathology. In Little League shoulder, MRI will demonstrate edema at the physis.

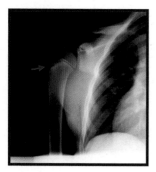

Figure 29-1. Anteroposterior view of the shoulder showing widening of the proximal humeral physis consistent with Little League shoulder (proximal humeral epiphysitis). From Metzl JD. *Sports Medicine in the Pediatric Office.* Elk Grove Village, IL: American Academy of Pediatrics; 2008.

TREATMENT

- Rest from throwing and other overhead activities is necessary to allow the physis to heal.
- Nonsteroidal anti-inflammatory drugs (NSAIDs) do not speed the healing process and are rarely needed because rest from throwing is usually enough to relieve pain.
- Range of motion and strengthening exercises are begun when they can be performed without pain.
- Once the athlete has full pain-free range of motion and strength, return to throwing begins with light tosses over a short distance and progresses gradually over 4 to 6 weeks to maximum effort pitching from regulation distance.

EXPECTED OUTCOMES/PROGNOSIS

- The average time from initial treatment to return to competitive activity is 3 months.
- Because this is a growth plate injury, symptoms resolve with skeletal maturity.
- Athletes who do not seek medical attention early in the course of their injury may be forced to stop overhead activity because of pain and impaired performance.

WHEN TO REFER

- Refer to a pediatric sports medicine specialist
  — Pain that persists despite 4 to 6 weeks of rest from overhead activities
  — Pain at rest, instability, or significant weakness

PREVENTION

- Pitchers should follow published guidelines for pitch count maximums and number of rest days between pitching appearances (tables 29-1 and 29-2).
- Breaking pitches (eg, curveballs, sliders) may increase risk for Little League shoulder, so they should be avoided until skeletal maturity (Tanner stage IV or V, or approximately 14 years of age).
- Throwing mechanics should be reviewed by a knowledgeable coach.
- Cardiovascular fitness and core strength should be maintained year-round.
- Children in sports involving repetitive overhead activity should be encouraged to report any discomfort in the upper extremity immediately. Such complaints should be promptly evaluated.

RELEVANT *INTERNATIONAL CLASSIFICATION OF DISEASES, NINTH REVISION, CLINICAL MODIFICATION (ICD-9-CM)* CODE

- **732.1**   Osteochondrosis, upper extremity (Little League shoulder)

Table 29-1. Pitch Count Maximums by Age

League Age	Maximum Pitches Per Day
17–18 y	105
13–16 y	95
11–12 y	85
9–10 y	75
7–8 y	50

Pitch count limits pertain to pitches thrown in games only. These limits do not include throws from other positions, instructional pitching during practice sessions, and throwing drills, which are important for the development of technique and strength. Backyard pitching practice after a pitched game is strongly discouraged. Adapted with permission from Little League Baseball, Inc. Available at: www.littleleague.org/Assets/forms_pubs/media/PitchingRegulationChanges_BB_11-13-09.pdf. Accessed March 3, 2010.

Table 29-2. Rest Days by Age

For Pitchers Aged 14 Years and Younger	
Pitches in a Day	Rest Time
66 or more	4 days
51–65	3 days
36–50	2 days
21–35	1 day
1–20	0 days
For Pitchers Aged 15 to 18 Years	
Pitches in a Day	Rest Time
76 or more	4 days
61–75	3 days
46–60	2 days
31–45	1 day
1–30	0 days

Adapted with permission from Little League Baseball, Inc. Available at www.littleleague.org/Assets/forms_pubs/media/PitchingRegulationChanges_BB_11-13-09.pdf. Accessed March 3, 2010.

Rotator Cuff Tendonitis/Impingement

INTRODUCTION/ETIOLOGY/EPIDEMIOLOGY

* Inflammation and thickening of rotator cuff tendons or subacromial bursa cause them to become impinged under the coracoacromial arch when the arm is elevated.
* Commonly occurs in overhead sports such as tennis, baseball, softball, volleyball, and swimming.
* In young athletes, rotator cuff tendonitis or impingement is usually caused by shoulder ligamentous laxity or muscle imbalance, rather than actual narrowing of the subacromial space, as seen in adults.
* Additional etiologic factors include improper throwing technique and excessive pitching, oversized tennis rackets, and use of hand paddles and drag suits in the pool.
* Tears of the rotator cuff due to overuse are rare in pediatric and adolescent athletes.

SIGNS AND SYMPTOMS

* Pain with overhead activity that does not improve with warm-up
* May progress to pain with activities of daily living, pain at rest, or nighttime pain.
* Patients may report diminished strength with overhead activities.
* There is tenderness with palpation of the rotator cuff tendons in the subacromial space.
* Shoulder range of motion, especially elevation, and strength may be limited.
* Resisted strength testing of the individual rotator cuff muscles may reproduce symptoms.
* Neer or Hawkins impingement test may be positive (see Figure 4-19).

DIFFERENTIAL DIAGNOSIS

- Little League shoulder
- Biceps tendonitis
- Glenohumeral instability
- Acromioclavicular sprain
- Proximal humeral fracture
- Labral tear
- Thoracic outlet syndrome

MAKING THE DIAGNOSIS

- Diagnosis can be made clinically. Imaging is usually not necessary.
- When the diagnosis is uncertain, *plain radiographs* may be helpful to rule out bony injury such as Little League shoulder.
- *Magnetic resonance imaging* may be useful in cases refractory to conservative management or if there is concern for other injuries.
  — In most cases of rotator cuff tendonitis or impingement, MRI demonstrates inflammation or thickening of the rotator cuff tendons or subacromial bursa.
- If there is concern for a labral tear, *MRI with arthrogram* is the diagnostic study of choice.

TREATMENT

- Temporary rest from overhead activities
- Nonsteroidal anti-inflammatory drugs can reduce inflammation and are recommended when there is pain with activities of daily living or at rest.
- The most important aspect of treatment is a *physical therapy program* to correct the muscle imbalance. A comprehensive program focusing on range of motion, rotator cuff strengthening, and periscapular stabilization should be initiated as soon as possible.
- Sport-specific technique and equipment should be evaluated.
- Surgical intervention is rarely needed in the pediatric and adolescent athlete. In cases unresponsive to nonoperative management, shoulder arthroscopy may be helpful for identification of additional pathology or debridement of chronically inflamed and injured rotator cuff tendons.

EXPECTED OUTCOMES/PROGNOSIS

- Response to nonoperative management is usually excellent, resulting in return to full participation in previous activities.
- Return to sports depends on the severity of symptoms, ranging from 2 to 4 weeks to 4 to 6 months.
- Symptoms are likely to progress if the underlying muscle imbalance and joint instability are not corrected. This may ultimately lead to inability to participate in the inciting activity.
- If biomechanical or equipment issues are not addressed, or if proper muscular balance is not maintained, symptoms may recur.

WHEN TO REFER

- Refer to a pediatric sports medicine specialist when there has been no response to rest and physical therapy.

PREVENTION

- Pitchers should follow published guidelines for pitch count maximums and number of rest days between pitching appearances (tables 29-1 and 29-2).
- High-velocity pitching (over 80 miles per hour) and breaking pitches (eg, curveballs, sliders) should be avoided until skeletal maturity (Tanner stage IV or V, or approximately 14 years of age).
- Children and adolescents should not throw competitively for more than 9 months out of the year.
- All overhead athletes should be encouraged to pay close attention to correct technique. Throwing mechanics should be reviewed by a knowledgeable coach.
- Cardiovascular fitness and core strength should be maintained year-round.
- Initiating a rotator cuff strengthening program in at-risk athletes before the onset of problems may be helpful.
- Continuing a rotator cuff maintenance program after recovery can help prevent recurrent episodes.
- Children in sports involving repetitive overhead activity should be encouraged to report any discomfort in the upper extremity immediately. Such complaints should be promptly evaluated.

RELEVANT *ICD-9-CM* CODE

- **726.11**   Rotator cuff tendonitis

Little League Elbow (Medial Epicondyle Apophysitis)

INTRODUCTION/ETIOLOGY/EPIDEMIOLOGY

- Most common cause of medial elbow pain in young pitchers
- Caused by the repetitive valgus force at the elbow that occurs with the pitching motion. The valgus force causes tension stress on the medial side of the elbow and compression stress on the lateral side.
- While classic Little League elbow refers to an apophysitis of the medial epicondylar growth plate, the term is often used more broadly to describe a constellation of overuse pitching injuries to the immature elbow, including medial epicondyle apophysitis, osteochondritis dissecans of the capitellum, and olecranon apophysitis.
- Annual incidence of elbow pain in baseball pitchers between 9 and 12 years of age has been reported to be 20% to 40%.
- Other activities that put skeletally immature athletes at risk include football quarterback, non-pitching throwing in baseball, gymnastics, and tennis.

SIGNS AND SYMPTOMS

- Medial elbow pain during or after pitching
- There may be stiffness, swelling, limited elbow extension, and occasionally, mechanical symptoms such as locking and popping.
- Impaired performance including loss of pitching accuracy and reduced velocity may be reported.
- Patients have localized tenderness over the medial epicondyle (see figures 4-22a and 29-2).
- Medial elbow swelling or effusion may be present.
- If symptoms have been long-standing, there may be lack of full elbow extension.

DIFFERENTIAL DIAGNOSIS

- Medial epicondyle avulsion fracture
- Flexor-pronator tendonitis
- Ulnar collateral ligament sprain or tear
- Ulnar nerve injury or neuritis
- Neoplasm
- Pain referred from the neck or shoulder

MAKING THE DIAGNOSIS

- Diagnosis can be made clinically.
- *Radiographs* are often negative in the early stages of the injury.
  — Anteroposterior, lateral, and oblique views of both elbows should be obtained for comparison.
  — Positive findings may include medial epicondyle physeal widening, enlargement, fragmentation, or avulsion of the medial epicondyle (Figure 29-3).
- *Magnetic resonance imaging* is helpful to evaluate for other conditions, such as osteochondritis dissecans of the capitellum, ulnar collateral ligament injury, or flexor-pronator tendonitis.

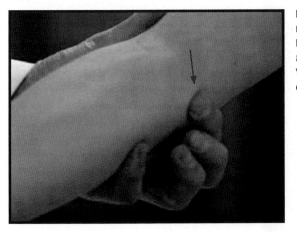

Figure 29-2. Palpation of the medial epichondyle. From Metzl JD. *Sports Medicine in the Pediatric Office.* Elk Grove Village, IL: American Academy of Pediatrics; 2008.

TREATMENT

- Initial treatment is complete rest from throwing until pain and tenderness resolve (usually 4 to 6 weeks).
- Ice and NSAIDs are rarely needed because pain typically only occurs with throwing, but they may be helpful when swelling is present.
- As symptoms improve, a rehabilitation program is initiated, beginning with stretching and range of motion exercises followed by progressive strengthening for upper body and core muscles.
- Once the athlete has no tenderness and full, pain-free range of motion and strength, return to throwing begins with light tosses over a short distance and progresses gradually over 4 to 6 weeks to maximum effort pitching from regulation distance.
- The athlete should work with an experienced coach to evaluate and correct any underlying errors in throwing or pitching technique.

EXPECTED OUTCOMES/PROGNOSIS

- If treated properly and early in the course, most athletes can return to pitching.
- The average time from initial treatment to return to competitive activity is 8 to 12 weeks.
- Some may not be able to return to their previous level of play, even with timely, proper treatment.
- Athletes who continue to throw with pain and disregard recommendations for treatment are at risk for long-term, possibly permanent, sequelae.
  — Complications may include growth disturbance around the elbow; joint stiffness including flexion contracture; chronic, progressive medial elbow pain; and bony deformity including premature elbow arthrosis.

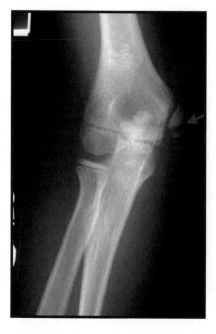

Figure 29-3. Anteroposterior radiograph of the elbow showing widening at the medial epicondylar apophysis. In this case, radiograph findings indicate that the problem is more advanced. If patients complain of medial pain with throwing, radiograph may be normal in appearance and show no evidence of widening. From Metzl JD. *Sports Medicine in the Pediatric Office.* Elk Grove Village, IL: American Academy of Pediatrics; 2008.

WHEN TO REFER

- Refer to a pediatric sports medicine specialist
  — No improvement in symptoms after 6 to 8 weeks of rest
  — When guidance is needed for supervision of physical therapy or clearance for return to throwing
- Refer to a pediatric orthopaedic surgeon
  — Widening or displacement of the medial epicondyle apophysis of more than 5 mm, which may require surgical fixation (see Chapter 35)

PREVENTION

- Pitchers should follow published guidelines for pitch count maximums and number of rest days between pitching appearances (tables 29-1 and 29-2).
- High-velocity pitching (over 80 miles per hour) and breaking pitches (eg, curveballs, sliders) should be avoided until skeletal maturity (Tanner stage IV or V, or approximately 14 years of age).
- Children and adolescents should not throw competitively for more than 9 months a year.
- All overhead athletes should be encouraged to pay close attention to correct technique. Throwing mechanics should be reviewed by a knowledgeable coach.
- Cardiovascular fitness and core strength should be maintained year-round.
- Children in sports involving repetitive overhead activity should be encouraged to report any discomfort in the upper extremity immediately. Such complaints should be promptly evaluated.

RELEVANT *ICD-9-CM* CODE

- **732.1**   Little League elbow

Osgood-Schlatter Disease

INTRODUCTION/ETIOLOGY/EPIDEMIOLOGY

- Traction apophysitis, or osteochondrosis, of the tibial tuberosity caused by repetitive, forceful contraction of the quadriceps muscle
- Onset usually associated with a period of rapid growth combined with activity
- Affects males between 10 and 15 years of age and females between 8 and 13 years of age.
- The incidence has been higher among boys, a trend which is changing as more and more girls participate in organized sports.
- Bilateral in 25% to 50% of patients
- Most commonly seen in running and jumping sports such as basketball, soccer, and gymnastics
- Intrinsic risk factors include tight rectus femoris (see Figure 4-6), tight hamstrings (see Figure 4-5), patella alta, and external tibial rotation (see Figure 22-1), all of which increase the traction stress on the tibial tubercle from the patellar tendon.

SIGNS AND SYMPTOMS

- Pain at the tibial tubercle that is worse with activity and improves with rest
- Onset of symptoms is usually gradual but can sometimes be acute, such as during a sprint or a jump, or after direct impact to the tubercle.
- Localized tenderness over the tibial tuberosity (see figures 4-28a and 29-4a)
- Bony prominence and soft tissue swelling may be present.
- Resisted knee extension is typically painful.
- Tight quadriceps and hamstrings, external tibial rotation, or patella alta may be noted.
- There may be pain with an active straight leg raise test. Inability to perform an active straight leg raise, or inability to maintain a straight leg during this test, suggests a disruption of the extensor mechanism, such as a tibial tubercle avulsion fracture.

DIFFERENTIAL DIAGNOSIS

- Characteristic tenderness over the tibial tuberosity with an otherwise normal knee examination will usually rule out other causes of knee pain.
- Patellofemoral pain syndrome
- Sinding-Larsen-Johansson syndrome
- Patellar tendonitis
- Stress fracture of the proximal tibia
- Osteochondritis dissecans
- Referred pain from the hip
- Rarely, bony neoplasm or infection

MAKING THE DIAGNOSIS

- Diagnosis can be made clinically. Imaging is not usually necessary.
- *Plain radiographs*
  - Only indicated to rule out other pathology in patients with atypical signs and symptoms or those who do not respond to usual treatment.
  - Most patients with Osgood-Schlatter disease (OSD) will have normal radiographs.
  - Elevation, irregularity, and fragmentation of the tibial tubercle apophysis are normal variants of ossification and do not indicate OSD.
  - Soft tissue swelling anterior to the tibial tubercle is suggestive of OSD (Figure 29-4b).
- *Magnetic resonance imaging* is not necessary unless another diagnosis is suspected.

TREATMENT

- While some level of activity modification may be helpful initially, complete cessation of activity is not usually required.
- Activity that causes significant pain or altered gait should be avoided. Discomfort that occurs only after activity should not preclude participation.
- A patellar strap (Figure 29-5) may reduce pain with activity.
- Anti-inflammatory medications should not be used before activity because they may mask pain indicating a worsening injury.

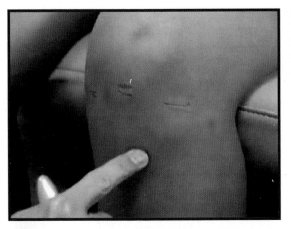

Figure 29-4a. Palpation of tibial tuberosity. From Metzl JD. *Sports Medicine in the Pediatric Office.* Elk Grove Village, IL: American Academy of Pediatrics; 2008.

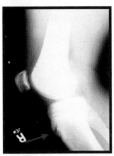

Figure 29-4b. Lateral view of the knee showing Osgood-Schlatter disease with soft tissue swelling overlying the tibial apophysis. From Metzl JD. *Sports Medicine in the Pediatric Office.* Elk Grove Village, IL: American Academy of Pediatrics; 2008.

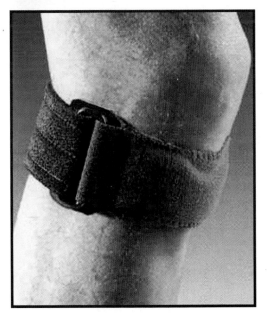

Figure 29-5. Patellar strap. ©BSN medical Inc. Used by permission.

- A protective pad over the tibial tuberosity will protect against direct trauma.
- Ice can help reduce pain (apply for 15–20 minutes, 2 or 3 times a day, not immediately before activity)
- Quadriceps and hamstring stretching are recommended to reduce tension at the tibial tubercle.
- Corticosteroid injection is not recommended because it may result in complications such as subcutaneous atrophy.

EXPECTED OUTCOMES/PROGNOSIS

- Symptoms generally resolve with time, before or concurrent with closure of the tibial tubercle apophysis.
- Many will have residual prominence of the tubercle into adulthood.
- Occasionally, pain persists following closure of the growth plate.
- Persistent discomfort with kneeling into adulthood may indicate the presence of a residual ossicle(s). These can be surgically removed.
- Tibial tubercle avulsion is a rare complication.
- Genu recurvatum (tibial forward curvature resulting in hyperextension of the knee) has been noted as a rare but serious complication of OSD, resulting from premature closure of the anterior portion of the proximal tibial epiphyseal plate.

WHEN TO REFER

- Refer to a pediatric sports medicine specialist
  — No improvement after several weeks of rest and nonoperative treatment
- Refer to a pediatric orthopaedist
  — Concern for tibial tubercle avulsion (unable to perform a straight leg raise or significant widening or displacement of tubercle on lateral radiographs).

PREVENTION

- Maintain quadriceps strength and flexibility, particularly during periods of rapid growth.

RELEVANT *ICD-9-CM* CODE

- **732.4**   OSD

Sinding-Larsen-Johansson Syndrome

INTRODUCTION/ETIOLOGY/EPIDEMIOLOGY

- Apophysitis of the inferior pole of the patella caused by repetitive traction from the patellar tendon
- In skeletally mature athletes, this same mechanism leads to patellar tendonitis (jumper knee).
- Affects children 8 to 13 years of age, with an average age of 12 years in boys and 9 years in girls.
- Patients are usually involved in athletic activities requiring running, jumping, or kicking.
- Symptoms may develop after repetitive microtrauma or begin following an episode of acute trauma such as a fall onto the knee or a kick or jump that causes a sudden increase in symptoms.
- Affected children are usually in a period of rapid growth, resulting in tight quadriceps.

SIGNS AND SYMPTOMS

- Anterior knee pain localized to the inferior pole of the patella, which worsens during activities such as running, jumping, and climbing stairs
- Localized tenderness at the inferior pole of the patella
  — With the knee relaxed in full extension, apply gentle downward pressure to the superior pole of the patella to elevate the inferior pole, allowing for direct palpation of the apophysis.
- Patients may have a positive Ely test, indicating tight rectus femoris (see Figure 4-6).

DIFFERENTIAL DIAGNOSIS

- Patellofemoral pain syndrome
- Osteochondritis dissecans
- Patellar tendonitis
- Stress fracture

MAKING THE DIAGNOSIS

- Diagnosis can be made clinically. Imaging is not necessary.
- *Radiographs*
  — May be helpful to evaluate for other causes of anterior knee pain in patients with chronic, recurrent, or unusual symptoms.
  — Most patients with Sinding-Larsen-Johansson (SLJ) syndrome will have normal radiographs, but some may demonstrate fragmentation, calcification, or a small avulsion of the inferior pole of the patella (Figure 29-6a, b).

TREATMENT AND PREVENTION

- Treatment and prevention are the same as for OSD.

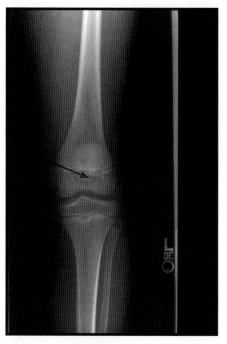

Figure 29-6a. Anteroposterior view of the knee with Sinding-Larsen-Johansson disease. From Metzl JD. *Sports Medicine in the Pediatric Office.* Elk Grove Village, IL: American Academy of Pediatrics; 2008.

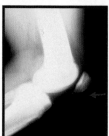

Figure 29-6b. Lateral view of the knee showing chronic avulsion of the distal pole of the patella consistent with Sinding-Larsen-Johansson disease. From Metzl JD. *Sports Medicine in the Pediatric Office.* Elk Grove Village, IL: American Academy of Pediatrics; 2008.

EXPECTED OUTCOMES/PROGNOSIS

- Symptoms resolve with time, before or concurrent with closure of the apophysis.
- Prognosis is excellent, without residual symptoms or sequelae.

WHEN TO REFER

- Refer to a pediatric sports medicine specialist
  — No improvement after several weeks of rest and nonoperative treatment
- Refer to a pediatric orthopaedist
  — Removal of symptomatic fragments or a necrotic area of the tendon, if present, may be helpful in chronic cases.

RELEVANT *ICD-9-CM* CODE

- **732.4**   SLJ syndrome

Sever Disease (Calcaneal Apophysitis)

INTRODUCTION/ETIOLOGY/EPIDEMIOLOGY

- Caused by repetitive traction from the Achilles tendon or repetitive impact on the heel
- Affects children between 7 and 15 years of age, at an average age of 12 years for boys and 9 years for girls.
- More common in boys
- Bilateral in just more than 60% of patients
- Typically occurs in running or jumping sports such as soccer, basketball, or gymnastics.

SIGNS AND SYMPTOMS

- Activity-related heel pain that is worse on hard surfaces or in shoes with cleats
- Onset is usually insidious, but may also be triggered by acute trauma.
- May cause a limp.
- Swelling is rare.
- Tender with mediolateral compression of the calcaneus or at the Achilles tendon insertion
- Frequently, the calf muscles are tight (see Figure 4-4) and ankle dorsiflexors are weak.
- More than 25% of patients have pes planus (flatfoot) or subtalar over-pronation (see Figure 4-36).

DIFFERENTIAL DIAGNOSIS

- Sever disease can be distinguished from most other conditions affecting the heel by location of pain, age of patient, and absence of other symptoms.
- Swelling and erythema are unusual with Sever disease and should prompt evaluation for other causes of heel pain such as
  — Calcaneal stress fracture
  — Plantar fasciitis
  — Retrocalcaneal bursitis
  — Achilles tendonitis
  — Heel contusion
  — Heel fat pad syndrome
  — Bone cyst
  — Infection, tumor, and systemic disease such as ankylosing spondylitis or juvenile rheumatoid arthritis

MAKING THE DIAGNOSIS

- Sever disease is a clinical diagnosis.
- Imaging studies are helpful only to rule out other causes of heel pain.
  — *Radiographic findings* such as fragmentation, sclerosis, and widening of the apophysis may occur with normal apophyseal development.
  — *Magnetic resonance imaging findings* include bone bruising and edema in the calcaneal apophysis or metaphysis.

TREATMENT

- Activity that causes significant pain or altered gait should be avoided. Discomfort that occurs only after activity should not preclude participation.
- Heel cups (Figure 29-7) are often helpful in reducing pain to allow resumption of activity but should be discontinued when asymptomatic, because long-term use can promote calf muscle tightness.
- Calf muscle stretching (Figure 29-8a, b)
- Ice can reduce pain (apply for 15–20 minutes, 2 or 3 times a day).
- Nonsteroidal anti-inflammatory drugs may be helpful if rest, ice, heel cups, and stretching do not relieve the pain.
- Custom-molded shoe inserts may be helpful for those with pes planus or subtalar over-pronation.
- Limit training time on hard surfaces and in cleated shoes, which can concentrate stress over the posterior heel.

EXPECTED OUTCOMES/PROGNOSIS

- Most are able to return to their previous level of activity within 2 months.
- Symptoms may recur but all will resolve with time, before or concurrent with closure of the calcaneal apophysis at about 12 years of age in girls and 15 years of age in boys.
- Long-term sequelae and complications into adulthood have not been reported.

WHEN TO REFER

- Refer to a pediatric sports medicine specialist
  — If no improvement with this treatment in 6 to 8 weeks, a brief period (2–4 weeks) of non-weight bearing in a short-leg cast may be helpful.

PREVENTION

- Maintain calf flexibility and ankle dorsiflexion strength, especially during periods of rapid growth.
- Limit use of cleated shoes and running time on hard surfaces.

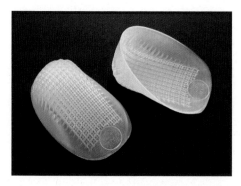

Figure 29-7. Heel cups. TuliGel Heavy Duty Heel Cups, TuliGel, and Tuli's are trademarks of Medi-Dyne Healthcare Products, Ltd., Colleyville, TX.

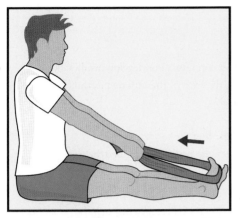

Figure 29-8a. Calf muscle stretch using a towel. Used with permission from Children's Memorial Hospital, Chicago, IL.

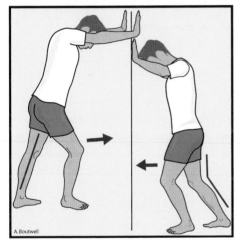

Figure 29-8b. Standing calf stretches should be performed with knee straight (for gastrocnemius muscle) and with knee bent (for soleus muscle). Used with permission from Children's Memorial Hospital, Chicago, IL.

RELEVANT *ICD-9-CM* CODE

- **732.5** Sever disease

Iselin Disease (Lateral Foot Pain)

INTRODUCTION/ETIOLOGY/EPIDEMIOLOGY

- Uncommon apophysitis of fifth metatarsal base caused by repetitive traction of the peroneus brevis tendon
- Children aged 12 to 18 years are most at risk; however, it can occur as early as 8 years of age in girls and 10 years of age in boys.
- Most common in sports that stress the forefoot such as roller-skating and ballet.

SIGNS AND SYMPTOMS

- Lateral foot pain that is worse with activity
- Friction from shoes can exacerbate the pain.
- Onset may be acute (after an acute ankle inversion injury) or develop insidiously.
- Tenderness, and often a bony prominence, at the base of the fifth metatarsal (see Figure 4-38)
- There may be mild erythema and edema.
- The patient may walk on the medial side of the foot.
- Resisted ankle eversion and passive ankle inversion usually reproduce the pain.

DIFFERENTIAL DIAGNOSIS

- Iselin syndrome should be distinguished from an acute fracture through the base of the fifth metatarsal (Figure 29-9).
- Less common etiologies of lateral foot pain are infection and tumor.

MAKING THE DIAGNOSIS

- Iselin syndrome is a clinical diagnosis.
- Imaging studies are only helpful to evaluate for other causes of lateral foot pain in cases where the diagnosis is uncertain, or to rule out a fracture in cases of acute trauma.
  — Radiographs should include AP, lateral, and oblique views of both feet.
  — Sclerosis, widening, and fragmentation are all consistent with normal apophyseal development.

TREATMENT

- Treatment is similar to Sever disease.
- Activity that causes significant pain or altered gait should be avoided. Discomfort that occurs only after activity should not preclude participation.
- Stretches should target peroneal muscles as well as gastroc-soleus complex.
- Taping to support the midfoot may reduce mild pain with activity.
- During recovery, the athlete may continue sport-specific activities that do not cause pain.

EXPECTED OUTCOMES/PROGNOSIS

- Duration of symptoms is highly varied and depends on age at onset and the inciting sport or activity.
- Symptoms may resolve after a few months or persist for years. The fifth metatarsal apophysis closes at about 18 years of age.
- Complications into adulthood are rare.
  — Ossicles may rupture from the tubercle and persist after symptoms resolve.
  — Bony overgrowth at the site is a fairly common finding.
  — Neither of these conditions is likely to cause persistent problems.

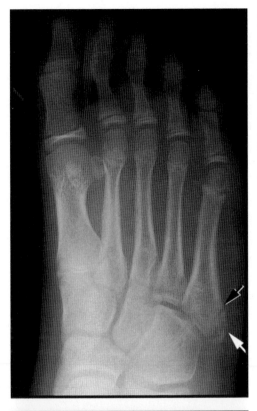

Figure 29-9a. Anteroposterior view of the foot of a skeletally immature patient shows a fifth metatarsal apophysis. The longitudinally oriented line is indicated by the black arrow; the white arrow indicates slight fragmentation at the base of the fifth metatarsal, signs of an apophysitis. Reproduced with permission from Johnson TR, Steinbach LS (eds): *Essentials of Musculoskeletal Imaging.* Rosemont, IL: American Academy of Orthopaedic Surgeons; 2004.

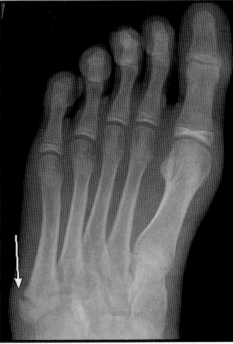

Figure 29-9b. Acute fracture through the base of the fifth metatarsal. Note fracture line is transversely oriented, unlike apophysis, which is longitudinally oriented.

WHEN TO REFER

- Refer to a pediatric sports medicine specialist
  - — Persistent pain or inability to return to activities despite treatment

PREVENTION

- Prevention is similar to Sever disease.
- Shoe size should be checked frequently during periods of rapid growth.

RELEVANT *ICD-9-CM* CODE

- **732.5**   Iselin syndrome

Stress Fractures

INTRODUCTION/ETIOLOGY/EPIDEMIOLOGY

- Stress fractures are caused by repetitive loading of a bone.
- Under normal amounts of stress and loading, bone resorption results and is followed by adequate new bone formation, resulting in strong bone in areas of high stress.
- When stress on a bone is persistent or excessive, bone formation cannot keep up with resorption, resulting in a weaker microtrabecular network, which then fails under the persistent load.
- The tibia and lesser metatarsals are the most common sites of stress fractures in the young athlete.
- Stress fracture of the fifth metatarsal is a less common but more problematic injury because of propensity for delayed union or nonunion.
- The highest incidence rates of stress fractures are seen in long-distance runners.
- Other high-risk sports are those that require repetitive running and jumping such as track and field, basketball, gymnastics, and soccer.
- The most common cause is a sudden increase in frequency, intensity, or duration of training.
- Other contributing factors include improper footwear, hard or irregular training terrain, pes plano valgus, pes cavus, leg-length discrepancy, and lower extremity weakness or inflexibility.
- Stress fractures may be preventable (Box 29-1).

Metatarsal Stress Fractures

INTRODUCTION/ETIOLOGY/EPIDEMIOLOGY

- The second and third metatarsals account for more than 80% of metatarsal stress fractures.
- Runners and ballet dancers are most at risk.

Box 29-1. Prevention of Stress Fractures

Avoid rapid increases in mileage and intensity of training. Do not increase by more than 10% per week.

Running shoes should fit well and be replaced every 300 to 500 miles.

Irregular and hard terrain (concrete) should be avoided when possible.

Do not run through persistent pain.

Pain should be evaluated promptly so that contributing factors can be addressed and treatment initiated before serious injury develops.

Female athletes involved in at-risk sports should be screened carefully for components of the female athlete triad, which could put them at risk for stress fractures.

SIGNS AND SYMPTOMS

- Patients report dorsal foot pain that is worse with activity and resolves with rest.
- Initially, the pain may only occur at the end of activity. As the injury worsens, the pain starts occurring earlier into the run and eventually hurts at rest.
- There is usually a history of a recent change in training, shoes, or running surface.
- Patients can usually localize the pain to a specific area of the foot by pointing with one finger.
- There will be localized bony tenderness, sometimes associated with soft tissue swelling.
- Pain can often be elicited with axial loading of the affected metatarsal or with mediolateral compression of the metatarsals.

DIFFERENTIAL DIAGNOSIS

- Interdigital neuroma
- Metatarsalgia
- Plantar fasciitis
- Freiberg infraction
- Infection
- Tumor

MAKING THE DIAGNOSIS

- *Radiographs* (AP, lateral, oblique) may show evidence of stress fracture if symptoms have been present for 4 to 6 weeks.
  — Findings may include periosteal reaction or elevation, narrowing of the medullary canal, longitudinal cortical thickening, sclerosis, or fracture line (Figure 29-10a, b).
  — If radiographs are normal but suspicion for stress fracture is high, the athlete can be treated presumptively and radiographs repeated in 3 to 4 weeks.
- If immediate confirmation of the diagnosis is needed, MRI is recommended (Figure 29-11).

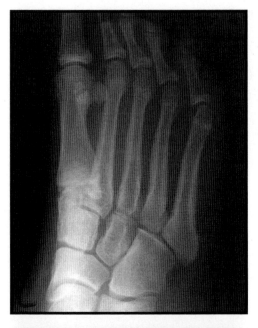

Figure 29-10a. Stress fracture of the metatarsal (early)—medial oblique view. Anteroposterior view of the foot in a patient who reported a 2-day history of pain in the second metatarsal does not show an obvious fracture. Reproduced with permission from Johnson TR, Steinbach LS (eds): *Essentials of Musculoskeletal Imaging.* Rosemont, IL: American Academy of Orthopaedic Surgeons; 2004.

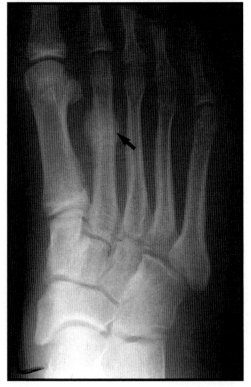

Figure 29-10b. Stress fracture of the metatarsal (late)—anteroposterior (AP) view. AP view of the same patient in Figure 29-10a 3 weeks later shows callus formation at the site of the stress fracture (black arrow). Reproduced with permission from Johnson TR, Steinbach LS (eds): *Essentials of Musculoskeletal Imaging.* Rosemont, IL: American Academy of Orthopaedic Surgeons; 2004.

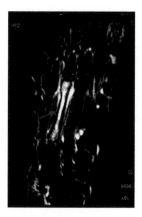

Figure 29-11. Magnetic resonance imaging showing metatarsal stress fracture. From Metzl JD. *Sports Medicine in the Pediatric Office.* Elk Grove Village, IL: American Academy of Pediatrics; 2008.

TREATMENT

- Decrease weight-bearing activity to a pain-free level.
- Use of a cast shoe or walker boot may allow for pain-free weight bearing.
- If the patient is still having pain with ambulation in a walker boot, crutches may be used until walking is pain-free.
- When ambulation is no longer painful and tenderness is resolved, a progressive return to activity is initiated. Patients can usually resume running in 4 to 6 weeks.
- Return to running should begin slowly and follow a program of gradually increasing mileage and intensity.
- Repeat radiographic studies are reserved for cases that do not respond to conservative management. In these cases, computed tomography (CT) can be used to evaluate the presence of bony healing or nonunion. Magnetic resonance imaging is not useful in these cases because it can remain positive for up to 12 months after the original injury.

EXPECTED OUTCOMES/PROGNOSIS

- The natural history of an untreated stress fracture is progressive pain with activity and eventually at rest.
- With adequate rest, monitoring, and gradual return to activity, complete recovery can be expected.
- Stress fractures of the proximal fifth metatarsal at the diaphyseal-metaphyseal junction (Jones fractures) are more prone to nonunion because of their location in a vascular watershed area (Figure 29-12a, b).

WHEN TO REFER

- Stress fractures of the proximal fifth metatarsal at the diaphyseal-metaphyseal junction (Jones fractures) require referral to an orthopaedic surgeon.
  — Treatment options include prolonged cast immobilization and non–weight-bearing or surgical fixation.
  — Surgery may allow for a quicker return to play.

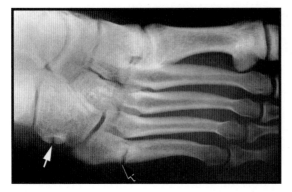

Figure 29-12a. Jones fracture with bipartite os peroneum—anteroposterior (AP) view. AP view of the foot shows a transverse, incomplete fracture line with intact medial border at the metaphyseal-diaphyseal junction (black arrow), a location characteristic of a Jones fracture. A bipartite os peroneum (white arrow) is also present. Reproduced with permission from Johnson TR, Steinbach LS (eds): *Essentials of Musculoskeletal Imaging.* Rosemont, IL: American Academy of Orthopaedic Surgeons; 2004.

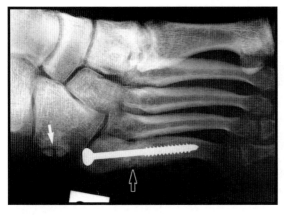

Figure 29-12b. Same patient in 29-12a. The fracture required open reduction and internal fixation. The fracture appears to have healed (black arrow). The bipartite os peroneum (white arrow) is seen again. Reproduced with permission from Johnson TR, Steinbach LS (eds): *Essentials of Musculoskeletal Imaging.* Rosemont, IL: American Academy of Orthopaedic Surgeons; 2004.

RELEVANT *ICD-9-CM* CODE

- **733.94**   Stress fracture, metatarsal

TIBIAL STRESS FRACTURES

Introduction/Etiology/Epidemiology

- Most are found at the posteromedial cortex of the tibia.
- Stress fracture of the anterior tibial cortex is a less common but more problematic injury, referred to as the "dreaded black line" on radiographs.

Signs and Symptoms

- Shin pain that is worse with activity and resolves with rest
- Initially, the pain may only occur at the end of activity, and as the injury worsens, the pain starts occurring earlier into the run, and eventually hurts at rest.
- There is usually a history of a recent change in training, shoes, or running surface.

- Patients can usually localize the pain to a specific area of the tibia by pointing with one finger.
- There will be localized bony tenderness, sometimes associated with soft tissue swelling.
- Pain can often be elicited with single leg jumping (positive hop test).

Differential Diagnosis

- *Shin splints* (medial tibial stress syndrome or tibial periostitis) are more likely to be bilateral and demonstrate diffuse tenderness that is most pronounced at the medial border of the tibia at the muscle-bone junction (Figure 29-13). Patients often report the pain decreases after a warm-up and worsens when they stop activity. This is in contrast to stress fractures, which usually demonstrate persistent pain that worsens after the warm-up and only decreases when activity stops.
- Other less common etiologies of shin pain include chronic exertional compartment syndrome, infection, and tumor.

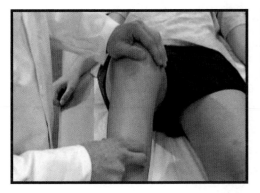

Figure 29-13. Palpation of the medial border of the tibia. From Metzl JD. *Sports Medicine in the Pediatric Office.* Elk Grove Village, IL: American Academy of Pediatrics; 2008.

Making the Diagnosis

- Same as for metatarsal stress fractures, except that radiographs may not be positive even after 4 to 6 weeks. As a result, MRI is recommended for diagnosis when stress fracture is suspected but radiographs are negative (Figure 29-14a, b).

Treatment

- Similar to metatarsal stress fractures
- Use of a pneumatic leg brace during the initial rest period may allow for more rapid return to activity (Figure 29-15).
- Physical therapy
  — Often necessary to regain muscle strength after a period of non-weight bearing.
  — Can address underlying intrinsic risk factors such as muscle strength or flexibility imbalances.
- Patients can usually resume running in 6 to 8 weeks if tenderness has resolved.

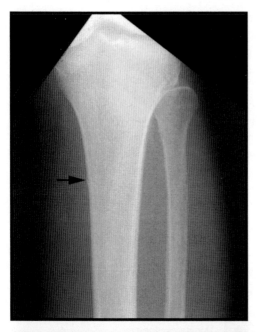

Figure 29-14a. Anteroposterior view of left tibia in a patient training for a marathon shows subtle cortical irregularity in the proximal medial tibial diaphysis (arrow). This is the area of maximal tenderness. Reproduced with permission from Johnson TR, Steinbach LS (eds): *Essentials of Musculoskeletal Imaging.* Rosemont, IL: American Academy of Orthopaedic Surgeons; 2004.

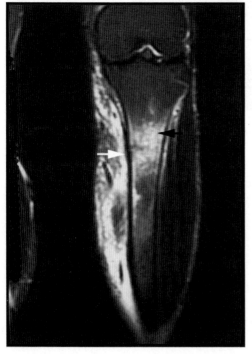

Figure 29-14b. Coronal fat-suppressed T2-weighted magnetic resonance imaging shows marrow edema (black arrow) and a transverse stress fracture in the proximal medial tibial diaphysis (white arrow). Reproduced with permission from Johnson TR, Steinbach LS (eds): *Essentials of Musculoskeletal Imaging.* Rosemont, IL: American Academy of Orthopaedic Surgeons; 2004.

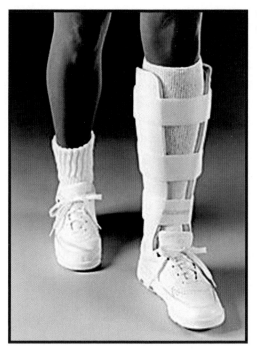

Figure 29-15. Pneumatic leg brace. Courtesy of DJO, LLC.

Expected Outcomes/Prognosis

* The natural history of an untreated stress fracture is progressive pain with activity and eventually at rest.
* With adequate rest, monitoring, and gradual return to activity, complete recovery can be expected.
* Anterior cortical injuries have a high risk of progression to complete fracture with continued activity.

When to Refer

* Stress fractures of the anterior tibial cortex are difficult to treat and require referral to an orthopaedic surgeon.
  — These injuries involve the tension-bearing side of the bone and are considered high risk because of the possibility of progression to an acute transverse fracture.
  — Treatment options include prolonged cast immobilization and non–weight-bearing or intramedullary rodding. Rodding will generally allow for a quicker return to play.

Relevant ICD-9-CM Code

* **733.93** Tibial stress fracture

FEMORAL NECK STRESS FRACTURES

Introduction/Etiology/Epidemiology

- Femoral neck stress fractures occur most frequently in runners and dancers.
- Stress fractures on the lateral aspect of the neck are on the tension side and are subject to distraction forces. Athletes with stress injuries in this location are at increased risk for progression to complete fracture.
- Stress injuries to the inferomedial aspect of the femoral neck are subject to compressive forces and may heal with more conservative treatment.

Signs and Symptoms

- Presenting symptoms are often vague.
- Patients complain of hip or groin pain during or after activity.
- Pain may radiate to the anterior thigh or medial knee.
- If symptoms have been present for several weeks, the athlete may have aching hip pain at rest or at night.
- Because physical examination findings in femoral neck stress fractures are nonspecific, have a high index of suspicion for this injury in any runner with anterior hip pain.
- The most common finding is painful and decreased range of motion, particularly with internal and external rotation.
- There may be tenderness in the inguinal region, but more often there is no tenderness to palpation.
- There may be an antalgic gait, and if not, the pain can often be elicited with hopping on the affected side.

Differential Diagnosis

- Hip muscle strain
- Iliopsoas bursitis
- Internal snapping hip syndrome
- Inguinal or sports hernia
- Transient synovitis of the hip
- Slipped capital femoral epiphysis
- Legg-Calve-Perthes disease
- Infection (eg, septic arthritis, osteomyelitis)
- Neoplasm
- Testicular pathology may also cause groin pain.

Making the Diagnosis

- *Radiographs* (AP and frog lateral views of the hip) may show sclerosis, periosteal reaction, or cortical disruption (Figure 29-16).
- Because radiographs are often normal, if history and examination suggest femoral neck stress fracture, a bone scan, MRI, or CT should be obtained.

- Because of its high sensitivity, *MRI* is considered the gold standard for evaluating femoral neck stress fractures and will reveal increased signal consistent with bone marrow edema as well as cortical disruption if present (Figure 29-17).
- *Bone scan* is also a highly sensitive test and in some cases may be preferable because of cost and availability (Figure 29-16b).
- *Computed tomography* can help localize the injury to the tension or compression side.

Treatment

- Most compression-side fractures can be treated nonoperatively with 6 to 8 weeks of non–weight-bearing or activity restriction to a pain-free range.
- Tension-side fractures are usually managed by percutaneous screw fixation followed by restricted weight bearing postoperatively.
- Physical therapy
  — Often necessary to regain muscle strength after a period of non-weight bearing.
  — Can address underlying intrinsic risk factors such as muscle strength or flexibility imbalances.

Expected Outcomes/Prognosis

- Most athletes with compression-side fractures can expect to return to their previous level of activity after appropriate treatment.
- Tension-side fractures are at significant risk for progression to a complete break with displacement, avascular necrosis of the femoral head, nonunion, and varus deformity.

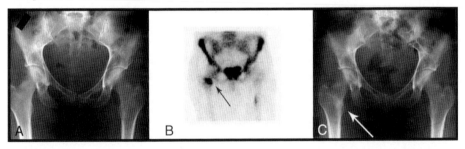

Figure 29-16. Stress fracture of the femoral neck. A, Initial anteroposterior radiography shows no apparent sign of fracture. B, Bone scan showing markedly increased uptake at site of femoral neck fracture (arrow). C, Subsequent radiograph shows sclerosis in femoral neck. Reproduced with permission from Griffin LY (ed): *Essentials of Musculoskeletal Care,* 3rd edition. Rosemont, IL: American Academy of Orthopaedic Surgeons; 2005.

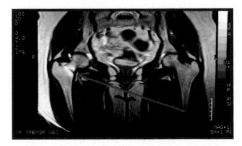

Figure 29-17. Magnetic resonance imaging of the hip showing compression side femoral neck stress fracture in a 17-year-old runner. From Metzl JD. *Sports Medicine in the Pediatric Office.* Elk Grove Village, IL: American Academy of Pediatrics; 2008.

When to Refer

- Patients with confirmed or suspected femoral neck stress fracture are immediately made non-weight bearing on crutches and promptly referred to an orthopaedist or pediatric sports medicine specialist for management because of the risk for progression to a complete break, especially fractures on the tension side.

Relevant ICD-9-CM Code

- **733.95**   Femoral stress fracture

Female Athlete Triad

INTRODUCTION/ETIOLOGY/EPIDEMIOLOGY

- Female athlete triad is a syndrome consisting of 3 related conditions—disordered eating behaviors, amenorrhea, and low bone mineral density.
- While the exact prevalence of the triad is unknown, up to 62% of female athletes report disordered eating, up to 79% report abnormal menses, and 10% to 50% have low bone mineral density.
- While amenorrhea is the menstrual condition listed in the original statements about the female athlete triad, this is the endpoint on a continuum of menstrual irregularities. In the future, the term *menstrual irregularity* will likely be used so conditions such as oligomenorrhea, anovulation, and luteal suppression are also included.
- While the documented number of athletes meeting all 3 criteria is low, those with 2 of the conditions, in particular the combination of disordered eating and menstrual dysfunction, is much higher.
- Female athlete triad occurs most commonly in sports where a lean physique is believed to provide a competitive advantage, such as cross-country running, gymnastics, figure skating, diving, and ballet.
- Although true osteoporosis may not develop, low bone mineral density puts these athletes at increased risk for stress fractures.

SIGNS AND SYMPTOMS

- A history of amenorrhea or altered menstrual cycles is often the first abnormality detected.
- Some athletes are diagnosed with the triad only after presenting with a stress fracture, prompting further questioning and bone health investigation.
- Rarely, decreasing athletic performance may be the only symptom reported.
- Athletes may not be forthcoming with their eating habits. Disordered eating includes pathogenic weight control measures such as food restriction, vomiting, use of laxatives, diuretics, or appetite suppressants, or failure to meet the energy demands of exercise.
- Athletes with symptoms such as cold intolerance, light-headedness, constipation, and sore throat are likely to have a clinical eating disorder (ie, anorexia nervosa, bulimia nervosa).
- Physical examination is generally normal in female athlete triad.

DIFFERENTIAL DIAGNOSIS

- *Diagnostic and Statistical Manual of Mental Disorders,* 4th Edition criteria will differentiate disordered eating from a clinical eating disorder.
- Differential diagnosis of amenorrhea is broad, including but not limited to pregnancy, thyroid disease, pituitary disease or tumor, polycystic ovarian syndrome, Turner syndrome, and premature ovarian failure.

MAKING THE DIAGNOSIS

- Any female athlete with a stress fracture should be evaluated for female athlete triad with a comprehensive menstrual, diet, and athletic history, including attitude about body image and weight, any decrease in athletic performance, and body mass index (BMI) calculation.
- Bone density assessment with dual energy x-ray absorptiometry is recommended for any athlete with history of stress fracture, amenorrhea for 12 months or more, BMI less than 18 or the fifth percentile for age, or weight less than the fifth percentile for age.

TREATMENT

- Treatment of female athlete triad often requires a multidisciplinary approach, including a physician, mental health professional, and nutritionist who are experienced with treating eating disorders.
- Athletes should be encouraged to include coaches, trainers, and parents in the treatment plan.
- The goal of treatment is spontaneous resumption of regular menstrual cycles. This often requires a decrease in activity or increase in caloric intake to correct the energy imbalance and allow for normal menses.
- There are no prospective studies on the benefit of hormone replacement therapy in the treatment of amenorrhea in athletes.
- Athletes should be counseled on adequate calcium (1,200–1,500 mg per day) and vitamin D (400–800 IU per day) intake.

EXPECTED OUTCOMES/PROGNOSIS

- Although little data exist on the natural history of this disorder, it is likely that without intervention, many of these components will continue for the duration of the patient's athletic career and possibly beyond.
- Athletes with untreated bulimia or anorexia nervosa are at risk for significant morbidity and mortality.
- There is evidence that irreversible bone loss occurs after 3 years of amenorrhea.

WHEN TO REFER

- Those with prolonged, severe, or worsening signs or symptoms should be referred to a local center specialized in the care of eating disorders.

PREVENTION

- The preparticipation physical evaluation is an ideal time to screen young women with a menstrual, a diet, and an exercise history. Amenorrhea, whether primary or secondary, should be addressed and investigated rather than dismissed as a normal consequence of athletic activity.
- Athletes involved in high-risk activities should be given nutritional information and guidance about maintaining proper balance between caloric intake and energy expenditure.
- Female athletes should be educated about the detrimental effects of disordered eating and amenorrhea, stressing the negative effects these conditions can have on their athletic success.
- Coaches and parents should be made aware of the triad and the effect it can have on young women.

RELEVANT *ICD-9-CM* CODES

- **626.0**   Amenorrhea
- **733.90**   Osteopenia
- **783.22**   Underweight
- **783.21**   Weight loss

CHAPTER 30

Patellofemoral Disorders

Patellofemoral Pain Syndrome

INTRODUCTION/ETIOLOGY/EPIDEMIOLOGY

- Patellofemoral pain syndrome (PFPS) is one of the most common knee disorders.
  — Affects 10% of young female athletes and 7% of young male athletes.
  — Also common in those who do not participate in sports
- Pain comes from mechanical strain or stress on the medial or lateral retinaculum or subchondral bone.
- The mechanism is often multifactorial and involves some combination of direct trauma, overuse, and abnormal patellar tracking.
  — The most frequent causes of abnormal patellar tracking are quadriceps weakness and tight muscle-tendon units that result from periods of active growth.
  — Less frequently, anatomic variants such as femoral anteversion or external tibial torsion cause abnormal patellar tracking (see Chapter 22).
- Patellofemoral pain syndrome should be distinguished from chondromalacia, which is not a diagnosis, but rather a surgical finding of softening or fibrillation of the patellar articular cartilage.
  — Many people with PFPS do not have chondromalacia, and many with chondromalacia do not have PFPS.
  — In those with chondromalacia and PFPS symptoms, no correlation exists between severity of chondromalacia and severity of symptoms.
- Patellofemoral pain syndrome is seen in 20% to 27% of patients with chronic anterior cruciate ligament (ACL) deficiency, and in 48% of patients with chronic posterior cruciate ligament deficiency.
- Patellofemoral pain syndrome is reported by 32% of patients after ACL reconstruction.

SIGNS AND SYMPTOMS

- Anterior knee pain that is worse with activity, especially running and jumping
  — Patients are usually unable to localize pain to one specific location and frequently use the "grab sign" (patient grabs the entire front of the knee) to show where the pain is felt.
- Pain is frequently bilateral.
- Pain is usually worse with stairs (especially descending), kneeling, and after prolonged sitting (theatre sign).
- There may be mild swelling or grinding, popping, or cracking around the patella with knee extension or flexion.
- Some report a "giving way" sensation. This is caused by pain inhibiting the quadriceps muscle, resulting in knee collapse without joint instability.
- In most cases the physical examination is normal.
- In some cases, one or more of the following findings may be noted:
  — Infrapatellar swelling or mild effusion
  — Tenderness along the patellar facets or retinaculum (Figure 30-1)
  — Pain with compression of patella
  — Crepitus felt under patella with knee extension (Note that crepitus is a common finding in normal knees that does not require treatment in the absence of pain.)
- Usually one or more of the following risk factors are also present:
  — Weak quadriceps
  — Weak hip external rotators or hip abductors
  — Tight lateral retinaculum (lateral patellar tilt)
  — Tight quadriceps (see Figure 4-6)
  — Tight gastrocnemius (see Figure 4-4)
  — Excessive lateralization of the tibial tubercle, such as from external tibial rotation
  — Hypermobile patella (Patella can be displaced in either direction more than 25%–50% of its width.)
  — Miserable malalignment—internal femoral rotation, knee valgus, and pes planus.

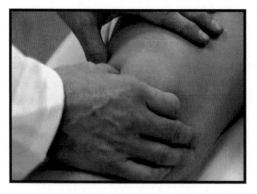

Figure 30-1. Palpation of medial and lateral patellar facets. From Metzl JD. *Sports Medicine in the Pediatric Office.* Elk Grove Village, IL: American Academy of Pediatrics; 2008.

DIFFERENTIAL DIAGNOSIS

- Patellar tendonitis
- Osgood-Schlatter disease
- Sinding-Larsen-Johanssen syndrome
- Iliotibial band friction syndrome
- Patella dislocation or subluxation
- Osteochondritis dissecans
- Meniscus tear
- Hip conditions such as *Perthes* or *slipped capital femoral epiphysis* can produce vague anterior knee pain in the setting of a normal physical examination.
- Inflammatory arthropathy
- Infection

MAKING THE DIAGNOSIS

- The diagnosis can be made clinically.
- *Imaging studies* and *laboratory tests* are normal in patients with PFPS, but may be necessary to rule out other causes of anterior knee pain (see Differential Diagnosis above).
  - *Radiographs of the knee* (anteroposterior [AP], lateral, notch, and sunrise views) should be the first step in the evaluation for alternate causes of knee pain suggested by history or examination.
    - History of direct trauma
    - Significant bruising, swelling, or effusion
    - Restricted motion
    - Pain at rest
    - Mechanical symptoms (catching, locking, or giving way)
    - Focal tenderness not around the patella (eg, femoral condyle or joint line)
    - Patients younger than 10 years
    - A bipartite patella is seen in less than 2% of the population and is rarely a cause of patellofemoral pain.
  - *Advanced imaging studies* such as magnetic resonance imaging (MRI) may be necessary to identify conditions that typically do not produce findings on plain radiographs (eg, osteochondritis dissecans, meniscus tear, osteomyelitis).
  - *Hip radiographs* are indicated if there is tenderness around the hip or if hip range of motion is reduced or painful.

TREATMENT

- Painful activities should be avoided.
  - Athletes should be encouraged that activity restriction is temporary and return to activities without knee pain is the goal of treatment.
  - Effort should be made to identify a list of non-painful activities that the athlete can continue.

- Nonsteroidal anti-inflammatory drugs (NSAIDs) and ice may reduce pain that persists with activities of daily living.
- When pain is acute or severe, a short period in a knee immobilizer may be helpful.
- A comprehensive rehabilitation program of quadriceps and hip strengthening is the key to successful treatment.
  — Improvements in iliotibial band, hip flexor, and hamstring flexibility can also reduce patellofemoral pain.
  — Painful rehabilitation exercises should be avoided.
  — Patellar taping may reduce pain to allow for progression of strengthening exercises.
- Patients with pes planus may benefit from custom-molded shoe inserts.
- For some patients, a patellar stabilizing brace (Figure 30-2) may reduce pain with sports and activities.

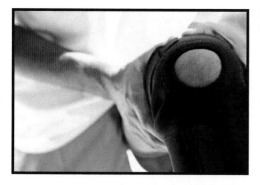

Figure 30-2. Patellar stabilizing brace. Courtesy of DJO, LLC.

EXPECTED OUTCOMES/PROGNOSIS

- The natural history of PFPS in adolescence is for spontaneous resolution over time as skeletal maturity evolves and growth slows.
- Nonoperative treatment is successful in reducing symptoms for most patients.
- Prognosis for patients with miserable malalignment is fair.
  — Many continue to have pain into adulthood, and there is some evidence they may be at increased risk for early osteoarthritis.
  — Realignment procedures may be recommended for the rare patient with severe malalignment whose symptoms limit functional activities of daily living.

WHEN TO REFER

- Refer to a sports medicine physician when there is no improvement in symptoms despite compliance with comprehensive rehabilitation program

PREVENTION

- Avoid rapid increases in activity.
- Maintaining lower extremity strength, especially in the quadriceps, hip abductors, and hip external rotators, and flexibility in hamstrings and iliotibial band may prevent recurrent pain.

RELEVANT *INTERNATIONAL CLASSIFICATION OF DISEASES, NINTH REVISION, CLINICAL MODIFICATION (ICD-9-CM)* CODE

- **719.46**   PFPS

Patellar Subluxation or Dislocation

INTRODUCTION/ETIOLOGY/EPIDEMIOLOGY

- *Acute, traumatic patellar dislocations*
  - — Most common in patients between 10 and 17 years of age, when rapid growth results in tight muscle-tendon units and relative ligamentous laxity
  - — Incidence is estimated at 43 per 100,000 children and is similar for boys and girls.
  - — The usual mechanism of injury is a sudden internal rotation of the femur or valgus stress on the knee while the foot is fixed, tearing the medial patellar femoral ligament (MPFL), which is the primary restraint to lateral displacement.
  - — Forty percent to 72% of acute patellar dislocations result in an osteochondral fracture of the patella (medial or middle facet) or femur (lateral aspect of trochlea) (Figure 30-3).
- *Chronic patellar instability* (recurrent subluxations or dislocations)
  - — May develop after an acute, traumatic patellar dislocation in a previously normal knee, but is more often caused by one or more of the following intrinsic risk factors:
    - Ligamentous laxity
    - Femoral trochlear dysplasia (flattening of the sulcus)
    - Patella alta
    - Tight lateral patellar supporting structures (iliotibial band, lateral hamstrings, lateral retinaculum)
  - — Patients with intrinsic risk factors often experience instability with minimal trauma, such as standing from a seated position or pivoting while walking.

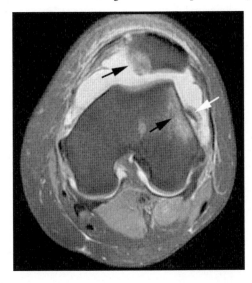

Figure 30-3. Patellar dislocation (postreduction)—axial magnetic resonance imaging (MRI). Axial T2-weighted, fat-suppressed MRI scan shows increased signal intensity indicating marrow edema in the lateral femoral condyle and the medial patella (black arrows), consistent with impaction injury. Note the joint effusion with an osteocartilaginous fragment in the lateral joint space (white arrow). Reproduced with permission from Johnson TR, Steinbach LS (eds): *Essentials of Musculoskeletal Imaging.* Rosemont, IL: American Academy of Orthopaedic Surgeons; 2004.

SIGNS AND SYMPTOMS

- Most report a popping or tearing sensation and feeling the patella shift out of place.
- Most (90%) reduce spontaneously when the knee is extended.
- Those that do not reduce spontaneously will present with visible lateral displacement of the patella and prominent femoral condyles.
- A hemarthrosis usually develops within a few hours after injury.
  — A large, tense hemarthrosis is often associated with an osteochondral fracture.
- There is limited range of motion and difficulty bearing weight.
- There may be tenderness around the patella, especially over the medial facet, medial retinaculum, and adductor tubercle of the medial femoral epicondyle.
- A *patellar apprehension test* (see Figure 4-35) is usually positive.
- After recurrent episodes
  — Signs and symptoms may be less pronounced than after the initial injury.
  — There is greater likelihood of identifying one or more intrinsic risk factors.
    ▪ Hypermobile patella (Can be displaced laterally or medially more than 25% of its width.)
    ▪ Tight iliotibial band, tight hamstrings (see figures 4-6 and 4-7), or tight lateral retinaculum (Downward pressure on medial border of patella does not significantly elevate lateral patella border. The lateral rectinoculum is tight. This is called positive lateral patellar tilt.)
    ▪ Beighton score (see Figure 4-2) greater than 4, indicating generalized ligamentous laxity

DIFFERENTIAL DIAGNOSIS

- Patellofemoral pain syndrome (PFPS)
  — Can cause a "giving way" sensation because of pain inhibiting the quadriceps muscle, resulting in knee collapse without instability.
- Ligament sprain
  — Injury mechanism, signs, and symptoms are similar to ACL injury, so Lachman test should be performed on all patients with suspected patella dislocation.
- Osteochondritis dissecans
- Meniscus tear
- Fracture

MAKING THE DIAGNOSIS

- The diagnosis can be made clinically.
- Pre- and post-reduction radiographs (AP, lateral, oblique, and sunrise views) are performed to evaluate for associated osteochondral fracture.
  — After successful reduction, mild lateral patella subluxation or tilt may be seen on the sunrise view (Figure 30-4).
  — Patella alta or a shallow trochlea may be noted.

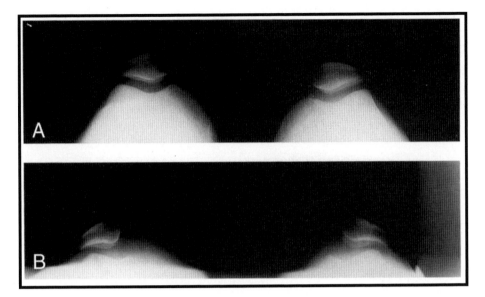

Figure 30-4. Bilateral axial patellofemoral radiographs (sunrise view). A, Patellae well aligned in the femoral groove. B, Bilateral patellar subluxation and lateral patellar tilt. Reproduced with permission from Griffin LY (ed): *Essentials of Musculoskeletal Care,* 3rd edition. Rosemont, IL: American Academy of Orthopaedic Surgeons; 2005.

- Magnetic resonance imaging is not necessary in the acute period.
  - For patients with persistent pain or mechanical symptoms (locking, catching) during rehabilitation, MRI is useful to evaluate for an osteochondral or chondral injury that may have been missed on initial radiographs (see Figure 30-3).
  - Magnetic resonance imaging can also assess for subtle chondral injuries and the location and degree of injury to the medial patellofemoral ligament, which helps with surgical planning for patients with recurrent instability.
  - Trochlear dysplasia is more accurately assessed on an MRI than on radiographs.

TREATMENT

- For dislocations that do not reduce spontaneously, prompt reduction is performed using adequate analgesia or sedation.
  - With the athlete supine and knee extended to relax the hamstrings, reduction is performed by gently applying a medial force to the lateral side of the patella.
  - If reduction is difficult because the patella is locked on the lateral femoral condyle, a downward force is applied first, followed by a medial force.
  - Radiographs are performed before and after reduction.
    - Any loose bodies will eventually require arthroscopy for fixation or removal.

- Following reduction
  — A compression wrap is applied and the knee is immobilized in extension using a commercial knee immobilizer.
  — If there is a large hemarthrosis, aspiration can reduce patient discomfort and facilitate early rehabilitation.
  — Ice and NSAIDs are recommended to reduce pain and swelling.
- After 7 to 10 days of immobilization and non-weight bearing
  — Transition from a knee immobilizer to a functional patella stabilizing brace (Figure 30-2) or taping (Figure 30-5). After recurrent dislocations, this may be possible within a few days of the injury.
  — Comprehensive rehabilitation program begins with early mobilization and isometric quadriceps strengthening, followed by progressive core and lower extremity strengthening.
  — *Return to sports* is allowed when there is normal range of motion and adequate strength, balance, coordination, and endurance. This typically takes 8 to 12 weeks. A patella stabilizing brace is recommended during sports and to reduce risk for recurrence.
  — Activity modification should be considered for patients with recurrent symptoms despite compliance with a comprehensive rehabilitation program and use of patella stabilizing brace.
- Operative treatment
  — Generally reserved for patients with recurrent dislocations despite compliance with several months of an aggressive, comprehensive rehabilitation program.
  — Primary repair of the MPFL in the first couple of weeks after injury is occasionally recommended for high-level athletes.
  — Patients with frequent dislocations despite compliance with several months of comprehensive rehabilitation may benefit from surgical reconstruction of the MPFL. If intrinsic risk factors are present, a realignment procedure may also be performed.
  — Postsurgical rehabilitation is the same as for nonoperative treatment.
  — Return to sports after surgery usually is possible in 4 to 6 months.

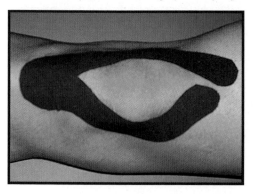

Figure 30-5. Patellar taping, which usually can be done after 7 to 10 days of immobilization using a brace. Available at: www.automailer.com/tws/pics/knee_taping.jpg.

EXPECTED OUTCOMES/PROGNOSIS

- After nonoperative treatment, prognosis is fair.
  — Recurrence rates range from 15% to 44%.
  — Recurrence is more likely with
    - Younger age
    - Intrinsic risk factors
    - Inadequate rehabilitation
    - Failure to maintain good lower extremity strength
    - Participation in high-risk sports and activities
  — Thirty percent to 50% will experience chronic patellofemoral pain.
- After operative treatment
  — Prognosis is variable but generally better than nonoperative treatment for preventing recurrent instability, although many patients continue to have patellofemoral pain that can limit sports participation.
  — Potential complications after a realignment procedure include
    - Excessive lateral retinacular release, causing medial patellar instability
    - Genu recurvatum may develop after a tibial tubercle transfer in a skeletally immature patient.

WHEN TO REFER

- To an orthopaedic surgeon
  — Osteochondral fracture or loose body
  — High-level athlete with acute complete tear of the MPFL
- To a sports medicine physician
  — Persistent symptoms despite compliance with a comprehensive rehabilitation program

PREVENTION

- Strategies shown to reduce the risk for recurrent pain and instability
  — Using a functional patellar stabilizing brace during activity (see Figure 30-2)
  — Maintaining good strength in the lower extremities, especially in the quadriceps, hip abductors, and hip external rotators

RELEVANT *ICD-9-CM* CODES

- **836.3**   Acute patellar dislocation
- **718.36**   Recurrent patellar dislocation or subluxation

CHAPTER 31

Internal Derangement of the Knee (Knee Injury)

Anterior Cruciate Ligament Sprains

INTRODUCTION/ETIOLOGY/EPIDEMIOLOGY

- Anterior cruciate ligament (ACL) injuries occur most commonly in basketball, soccer, football, and downhill skiing.
- Typical injury mechanism is a valgus or rotational force to the knee with the foot planted, or a hyperextension.
- More than 70% of ACL injuries occur without body contact (noncontact mechanism).
  — Landing from a jump
  — Decelerating quickly
  — Changing direction suddenly
- Anterior cruciate ligament injuries are being diagnosed in patients younger than 11 years with increasing frequency because of increased awareness, better diagnostic tools, and more children participating in high-intensity sports training at younger ages.
  — Children may experience an intrasubstance ACL tear or an avulsion injury of the tibial attachment of the ACL (see Tibial Eminence Fracture on page 326). The diagnosis and treatment of each is markedly different.
- After 11 years of age, the incidence increases steadily with age and skill level, with an overall incidence of 1 in 100 high school athletes.
- Girls who play sports that involve running and cutting are 2 to 8 times more likely to injure their ACL than boys, probably because of any of the following factors:
  — Increasing ACL laxity due to an increase in estrogen
  — The tendency for females to have a smaller intercondylar notch, smaller ACL, higher incidence of generalized ligamentous laxity, knee valgus, femoral internal rotation, and greater strength imbalances in the lower extremities
  — *Poor neuromuscular control of knee motion during landing and cutting appears to be the most important risk factor.*
    - Reduced activation of the hamstring muscles
    - Reduced knee and hip flexion
    - Greater dynamic knee valgus

SIGNS AND SYMPTOMS

- Sensation of a painful pop, followed by immediate swelling, feeling of instability, and difficulty bearing weight
- Physical examination reveals a significant effusion and limited range of motion.
  — About 67% of acute hemarthroses in children are caused by an ACL tear, but a hemarthrosis may not occur in children younger than 10 years with an ACL rupture.
- There may not be any tenderness unless associated injuries are present.

DIFFERENTIAL DIAGNOSIS

- Sprain of the posterior cruciate ligament (PCL) or collateral ligaments
- Meniscal tear
- Chondral injury
- Distal femoral or proximal tibia fracture
- Patellar sleeve avulsion
- Tibial eminence fracture
- Patellar subluxation
- "Giving way" due to patellofemoral pain

MAKING THE DIAGNOSIS

- The diagnosis is made clinically by demonstrating a positive Lachman test (see Figure 4-29).
- Posterior drawer test, varus and valgus stress tests, and Apley and McMurray tests should be performed to evaluate for other ligament or meniscus injuries (Table 31-1) (figures 4-30–4-34).
- Radiographs (anteroposterior [AP], lateral, skyline, and tunnel views) should be performed to rule out other injuries.
  — Anteroposterior view may reveal a small fleck of bone avulsed from the lateral tibia (Segond fracture) (Figure 31-1), which is pathognomonic for ACL injury.

Table 31-1. History and Physical Examination Findings of Acute Knee Injuries

Injured Structure	Mechanism of Injury	Physical Examination Test
ACL	Hyperextension, twisting	Lachman test; anterior drawer
MCL	Valgus force	Valgus laxity
Patellar dislocation	Direct blow to the patella or twisting injury to the extended knee	Apprehension test
PCL	Posterior force to tibia or hyperextension	Sag sign Posterior drawer test Quadriceps active test
Meniscus	Twisting	McMurray test Apley test

ACL, anterior cruciate ligament; MCL, medial collateral ligament; PCL, posterior cruciate ligament.

- Magnetic resonance imaging (MRI) may be performed to evaluate for associated soft tissue injuries as suggested by history and physical examination. Magnetic resonance imaging is also helpful to confirm ACL injury (Figure 31-2), especially when surgery is being considered.

TREATMENT

- *Initial treatment* consists of protection, rest, ice, elevation, and mobilization (PRICEM).
  — Protection is provided with crutches or a knee immobilizer.
  — Nonsteroidal anti-inflammatory drugs are helpful for control of pain and swelling.
  — If there is a large hemarthrosis, aspiration can improve patient comfort and facilitate early rehabilitation.

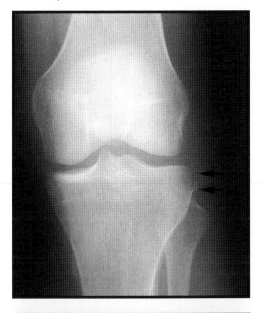

Figure 31-1. Segond fracture, anteroposterior view. Black arrows point to a small avulsion (flake) fracture of the lateral tibia just below the articular surface of the tibia. Reproduced with permission from Johnson TR, Steinbach LS (eds): *Essentials of Musculoskeletal Imaging.* Rosemont, IL: American Academy of Orthopaedic Surgeons; 2004.

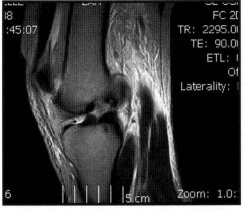

Figure 31-2. Sagittal magnetic resonance imaging demonstrating anterior cruciate ligament tear, noted by absence of blank fibers running from anterior tibia to posterior femur. Reproduced with permission from Johnson TR, Steinbach LS (eds): *Essentials of Musculoskeletal Imaging.* Rosemont, IL: American Academy of Orthopaedic Surgeons; 2004

- A rehabilitation program, starting with early weight-bearing and range of motion exercises, is initiated as soon as possible after the pain begins to subside, usually within 5 to 7 days of the injury.
- Whether to pursue nonoperative or operative treatment is a complex decision that depends on the patient's age, symptoms, degree of laxity on examination, associated injuries, and future sports demands. An orthopaedic surgeon or pediatric sports medicine physician can provide information to help the patient and family choose the most appropriate treatment.
- *Nonoperative treatment*
  — Consists of a comprehensive rehabilitation program to build lower extremity and core strength, balance, and endurance, which can take 6 to 12 weeks.
  — After nonoperative treatment, patients are advised to avoid high-demand sports (Table 31-2) because of the risk for recurrent instability and secondary meniscal injuries.
  — Appropriate for patients who do not intend to pursue high-demand sports
  — Often recommended as a temporizing treatment for skeletally immature athletes who intend to pursue high-demand sports in the future but must delay surgical treatment until their physes have closed.
- *Operative treatment*
  — Operative treatment is recommended for
    - Patients with an associated meniscus tear or other ligament injury
    - Skeletally mature athletes who intend to pursue high-demand sports

Table 31-2. Anterior Cruciate Ligament Demands of Various Sports

High demand	Football
	Soccer
	Ice hockey
	Field hockey
	Basketball
	Lacrosse
	Gymnastics
	Wrestling
	Volleyball
Moderate demand	Baseball
	Softball
	Track (non-jumping field events)
	Tennis (doubles)
Low demand	Swimming
	Jogging
	Crew

Adapted from Dorizas JA, Stanitski CL. Anterior cruciate ligament injury in the skeletally immature. *Orthop Clin North Am.* 2003;34:355–363

— A variety of arthroscopic techniques and graft types are available for reconstructing the ACL.
   ■ Bone-patellar-bone and hamstring autografts have been used with equal success; choice is surgeon dependent.
   ■ Patellar tendon allografts are being used with increasing frequency. Advantages over autograft include
      ◆ Less pain in the immediate postoperative period
      ◆ No disruption of the patient's patellar tendon, which may reduce the risk of patellofemoral pain in the future
— After surgery, rehabilitation follows the same protocol as for nonoperative treatment, but takes longer to complete.
— Return to sports typically takes 6 to 8 months.
• *Treatment for skeletally immature athletes with isolated ACL injuries is controversial.*
   — Surgical treatment using standard techniques creates a risk of growth disturbance. The tunnel site for the new ligament would traverse the tibial and femoral physis.
   — Physeal-sparing techniques may be used to allow very young athletes to return to high-demand sports.
      ■ Long-term stability after these modified procedures is unpredictable. Many eventually require ACL reconstruction when skeletally mature.
   — Most often, skeletally immature patients are encouraged to avoid high-demand sports until they reach skeletally maturity, at which time the ACL is reconstructed using standard techniques.

EXPECTED OUTCOMES/PROGNOSIS

• Despite disparity in injury rates, treatment outcomes are similar for females and males.
• After nonoperative treatment
   — An ACL-deficient knee is prone to episodes of instability and the risk for secondary meniscus tears.
   — Twenty percent to 27% develop patellofemoral pain.
• After ACL reconstruction, patellofemoral pain is reported by 32% of patients.
   — Risk factors are persistent quadriceps weakness and knee flexion contracture after rehabilitation, and use of a patellar tendon autograft.
• After surgical treatment for an ACL tear, many athletes are able to return to their previous level of competition.
   — Recurrence rate after surgery (graft rupture) is approximately 9% to 10%.
• Unfortunately, regardless of treatment, an ACL sprain is associated with a tenfold increased risk for osteoarthritis later in life. This is probably because of intra-articular damage suffered at the time of the injury and the neuromuscular deficits that follow.
• Partial tears, especially in the skeletally immature athlete, may have better outcomes after nonoperative treatment than complete tears.
   — Some partial tears may heal sufficiently to provide knee stability for high-demand sports.

WHEN TO REFER

- Patients with ACL sprains should be referred to an orthopaedic surgeon with expertise in pediatric sports injuries or a pediatric sports medicine physician to evaluate and discuss treatment options.

PREVENTION

- Neuromuscular training programs that improve strength and balance and teach safe landing mechanics have been shown to reduce the risk for ACL injury among female adolescent soccer and basketball athletes by up to 88%.
- A functional knee brace (Figure 31-3) can provide a subjective sense of improved stability, but there is no evidence that it reduces the risk of recurrent ACL sprains.

RELEVANT *INTERNATIONAL CLASSIFICATION OF DISEASES, NINTH REVISION, CLINICAL MODIFICATION (ICD-9-CM)* CODE

- **844.2**   Sprain or rupture of cruciate ligament of knee

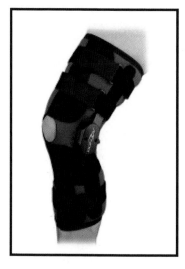

Figure 31-3. Hinged knee brace.
Courtesy of DJO, LLC.

Tibial Eminence Fracture

INTRODUCTION/ETIOLOGY/EPIDEMIOLOGY

- The tibial eminence is where the ACL inserts.
- Tibial eminence fractures occur in children between 8 and 14 years of age.
- The usual mechanism is hyperextension of the knee with or without valgus or rotational stress.
- In the past, these injuries were most commonly reported after a fall from a bike.
- More recently, tibial eminence fractures are being seen with increasing frequency in other sports as a result of the growing number of children participating in high-intensity sports training at younger ages.

SIGNS AND SYMPTOMS

- Sensation of a painful pop, followed by immediate swelling, feeling of instability, and difficulty bearing weight
- Physical examination reveals significant effusion and limited range of motion.
- A Lachman test may be positive and may be also painful.

DIFFERENTIAL DIAGNOSIS

- Same as for ACL sprain

MAKING THE DIAGNOSIS

- Radiographs (AP and lateral views) will demonstrate the fracture (Figure 31-4).
- Injury severity is graded based on the amount of displacement of the avulsed fragment on the lateral radiograph.
  — Type I: minimal displacement (<2 mm)
  — Type II: moderate displacement
  — Type III: significant displacement

TREATMENT

- Type I fractures
  — Immobilization in a long-leg cast with the knee in 20 to 30 degrees of flexion, which minimizes tension in the ACL
  — Isometric quadriceps exercises are initiated while in the cast.
  — Length of immobilization varies from 2 to 3 weeks for older children to 6 to 8 weeks for younger children.
  — A progressive rehabilitation program follows.
  — Return to play is usually possible after about 6 weeks of rehabilitation.

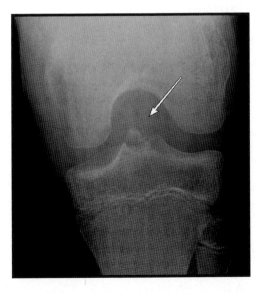

Figure 31-4. Radiograph of tibial eminence fracture.

- Type II and III fractures
  — Controversy exists with regard to treatment.
    - Some recommend surgical fixation for all type II and III injuries.
    - Others recommend surgical fixation only if immediate closed reduction with hyperextension is unsuccessful. However, there is a lack of consensus as to what constitutes successful closed reduction.
    - One study comparing surgical fixation with closed reduction found no differences in clinical healing.

EXPECTED OUTCOMES/PROGNOSIS

- Tibial eminence fractures have an excellent prognosis, despite the fact that 40% will demonstrate residual laxity with Lachman test even after the fracture is healed.
  — Laxity is caused by an associated partial tear or elongation of the ACL at the time of injury.
  — Short-term studies show no correlation between residual laxity and functional instability.
- Regardless of reduction method, studies show most patients are able to return to their previous level of activity.

WHEN TO REFER

- Tibial eminence fractures should be referred to a pediatric orthopaedic surgeon (types II and III) or pediatric sports medicine physician (type I) for treatment.

RELEVANT *ICD-9-CM* CODE

- **823.0**   Tibial eminence fracture

Medial Collateral Ligament Sprain

INTRODUCTION/ETIOLOGY/EPIDEMIOLOGY

- The medial collateral ligament (MCL) is the most commonly sprained ligament in the knee.
- Medial collateral ligament sprains can occur in isolation or in conjunction with ACL and meniscus injuries.
- The most common mechanism is a valgus stress to the knee with the foot fixed, and is usually associated with contact with another player.

SIGNS AND SYMPTOMS

- Sharp, medial knee pain after a valgus stress, followed by immediate swelling, feeling of instability, and difficulty bearing weight
- Physical examination reveals limited range of motion, with localized swelling or effusion, and significant tenderness along the medial aspect of the knee.

- A positive *valgus stress test* (see Figure 4-31) confirms the diagnosis and determines injury severity.
  — Perform first with the knee in full extension.
    - Laxity with the knee in full extension suggests a grade III MCL injury or an associated ACL tear.
  — Repeat at 30 degrees of flexion, which isolates the MCL.
    - Grade I: pain but no laxity
    - Grade II: pain and some laxity, but definite end point
    - Grade III: significant laxity with no end point; may not be painful
  — *A valgus stress test should not be performed on a skeletally immature athlete until after radiographs have ruled out a physeal fracture.*

DIFFERENTIAL DIAGNOSIS

- Physeal fracture
- Patellar subluxation
- Meniscus tear
- Anterior cruciate ligament or PCL injury

MAKING THE DIAGNOSIS

- The diagnosis can be made clinically using the valgus stress test.
- Radiographs (AP, lateral, skyline, and tunnel views) are performed to rule out a fracture and are required before performing valgus stress test in a skeletally immature patient.
- Magnetic resonance imaging is recommended if associated injuries are suspected.
- On MRI, an MCL injury is indicated by increased signal within the ligament or discontinuity of the fibers (Figure 31-5).

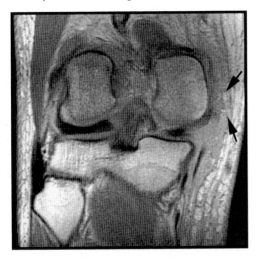

Figure 31-5. Coronal proton-density-weighted magnetic resonance imaging scan showing complete disruption of the fibers of the medial collateral ligament (black arrows), consistent with a severe tear. Reproduced with permission from Johnson TR, Steinbach LS (eds): *Essentials of Musculoskeletal Imaging.* Rosemont, IL: American Academy of Orthopaedic Surgeons; 2004.

TREATMENT

- Initial treatment consists of PRICEM and weight bearing as tolerated.
  — Protection is afforded through the use of crutches or a knee immobilizer or functional hinged knee brace (see Figure 31-3).
  — Early mobilization and progressive rehabilitation are initiated as soon as possible after the pain begins to subside, usually within 5 to 7 days of the injury.
- Isolated MCL sprains, even grade III injuries, do not require surgical treatment.
- Surgical reconstruction may be considered for grade III MCL sprains that are associated with ACL injuries.

EXPECTED OUTCOMES/PROGNOSIS

- Almost all athletes are able to return to their previous level of competition.
- Return to sports varies depending on the severity of injury.
  — Two to 4 weeks for grade I and II injuries
  — Six to 12 weeks for grade III injuries
- Recurrent instability after an isolated MCL sprain is rare, even for grade III injuries.

WHEN TO REFER

- To an orthopaedic surgeon with expertise in treating pediatric sports injuries
  — When associated injuries are present
- To a pediatric sports medicine physician
  — When symptoms persist despite completion of a comprehensive rehabilitation program

PREVENTION

- A functional hinged knee brace (see Figure 31-3) may reduce the risk for reinjury during sports and is recommended for those with grade II and III sprains.

RELEVANT *ICD-9-CM* CODE

- **844.1**   Sprain or rupture of MCL

Posterior Cruciate Ligament Injury

INTRODUCTION/ETIOLOGY/EPIDEMIOLOGY

- Posterior cruciate ligament sprains are uncommon.
- The mechanism is a posterior-directed force to the proximal tibia (eg, fall onto a flexed knee, impact with the dashboard in a motor vehicle accident) or hyperextension.
- Forty-seven percent are associated with other ligament injuries.
- Sports-related PCL sprains are less common than those associated with high-energy trauma but are more likely to be isolated injuries.

SIGNS AND SYMPTOMS

- Unlike with ACL injuries, patients usually do *not* report a pop and are often able to continue playing their sport.
- Symptoms are often nonspecific and may include
  — Vague posterior knee pain
  — Pain with knee flexion or squatting
  — Mild swelling
  — Instability
- Physical examination may reveal mild effusion and limited range of motion.
- Tests for PCL injury include
  — *Sag sign:* With patient supine, knees and hips flexed to 90 degrees, examiner holds heels and looks for sagging of tibia relative to uninjured side.
  — *Posterior drawer test* (see Figure 4-30): Tibia will sag posteriorly in this position when the PCL is injured, so it is first pulled anteriorly before assessing posterior translation.
    - Grade I sprain: 0 to 5 mm
    - Grade II sprain: 5 to 10 mm
    - Grade III sprain: more than 10 mm
  — *Quadriceps active test:* The knee is flexed to 90 degrees and the foot stabilized while the anterior surface of the tibial plateau is palpated. The patient is asked to extend the knee. Anterior translation of the tibia is abnormal, indicating PCL tear.
- Posterior cruciate ligament injury may produce a false-positive Lachman test result.

DIFFERENTIAL DIAGNOSIS

- Anterior cruciate ligament sprain
- Fracture
- Patellar subluxation
- Meniscus tear

MAKING THE DIAGNOSIS

- The diagnosis can be made clinically, but because PCL sprains may be associated with other injuries, imaging is recommended.
- Radiographs (AP, lateral, skyline, and tunnel views) are recommended to rule out a fracture.
- Magnetic resonance imaging is 99% sensitive for identifying acute PCL injuries.
- On MRI, a PCL injury is indicated by increased signal within the ligament or discontinuity of the fibers (Figure 31-6).

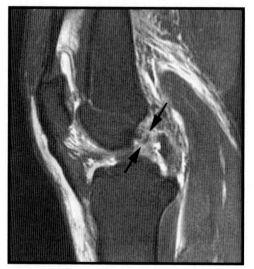

Figure 31-6. Posterior cruciate ligament (PCL) tear. Sagittal T2-weighted, fat-suppressed magnetic resonance imaging scan shows disruption and edema at the femoral attachment of the PCL (black arrows), diagnostic of a PCL tear. Reproduced with permission from Johnson TR, Steinbach LS (eds): *Essentials of Musculoskeletal Imaging*. Rosemont, IL: American Academy of Orthopaedic Surgeons; 2004.

TREATMENT

- Initial treatment consists of PRICEM and weight bearing as tolerated.
  - Protection is afforded through the use of crutches or a knee immobilizer or functional hinged knee brace (see Figure 31-3) if needed for pain control or stability with ambulation.
  - Early mobilization and progressive rehabilitation are initiated as soon as possible.
  - Return to sport is possible when there is full range of motion, good strength and endurance, and no instability with functional movements. This typically takes 4 to 8 weeks.
- There is no strong evidence that surgical management of grade I and II injuries significantly improves outcomes.
- Indications for surgical reconstruction
  - Grade III sprains
  - Associated injuries
    - Return to sport after operative treatment may take 9 to 12 months.

EXPECTED OUTCOMES/PROGNOSIS

- The prognosis for return to previous level of sport is good for most grade I and II injuries.
- Long-term prognosis
  - Forty-eight percent of patients with chronic PCL deficiency develop patellofemoral pain syndrome.
  - Increased risk for meniscus and articular cartilage injury and arthritis has been reported.
  - Individual outcomes are difficult to predict because they do not seem to correlate with degree of laxity on examination.

WHEN TO REFER

- To an orthopaedic surgeon with expertise in treating pediatric sports injuries
  — When associated injuries are present
- To a pediatric sports medicine physician
  — When symptoms persist despite completion of a comprehensive rehabilitation program

RELEVANT *ICD-9-CM* CODE

- **844.1**   Sprain or rupture of cruciate ligament of knee

Meniscus Tears

INTRODUCTION/ETIOLOGY/EPIDEMIOLOGY

- The menisci are 2 semilunar-shaped pieces of fibrocartilage between the femoral condyles and tibial plateau that dissipate impact forces to the knee and contribute to rotatory stability.
- The peripheral 20% to 30% of the medial meniscus and 10% to 25% of the lateral meniscus are vascularized and capable of healing after a tear.
- *Tears in patients younger than 14 years are uncommon* and are usually associated with a discoid meniscus.
- Tears in adolescents are more often associated with ligament injuries of the knee.
- The medial meniscus, because it is less mobile, is more commonly torn than the lateral meniscus.
- Typical mechanism of injury is twisting or pivoting while running or jumping.

SIGNS AND SYMPTOMS

- Most report a painful pop during a twisting injury to the knee.
- For isolated meniscus tears, swelling is usually delayed and may be minimal.
- Additional symptoms include snapping, catching, locking, or limited motion.
- Physical examination findings may include some or all of the following:
  — Effusion
  — Joint-line tenderness
  — Decreased range of motion
  — Positive Apley compression test (see Figure 4-34)
  — Positive McMurray test (see Figure 4-33)
  — Pain with squatting or duckwalking (walking in a full-squat position)

DIFFERENTIAL DIAGNOSIS

- Osteochondritis dissecans (OCD)
- Osteochondral fracture
- Ligament sprain
- Tibial eminence fracture
- Discoid meniscus
- Patellofemoral pain syndrome
- Patella subluxation
- Popliteal tendonitis
- Plica

MAKING THE DIAGNOSIS

- Radiographs are performed to rule out other etiologies such as OCD or fracture.
- Magnetic resonance imaging is the best imaging study for identifying meniscus tears (Figure 31-7).
  — Sensitivity is 67% to 79%.
  — Specificity is 83% to 91%.
  — Increased signal from normal vasculature in the posterior menisci of children and adolescents may be mistaken for a tear, so clinical correlation is important.

TREATMENT

- Meniscal tears will require surgical treatment on an elective basis.
  — Surgical options include repair with sutures or bioabsorbable implants, or partial or total removal of the torn part of the meniscus.
- Small, peripheral tears in younger patients may be initially treated with a short period of immobilization and non-weight bearing followed by rehabilitation and rest from impact activities.

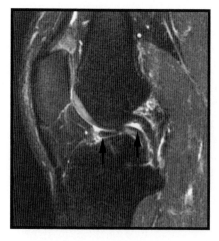

Figure 31-7. Meniscal (bucket handle) tear. Sagittal T2-weighted, fat-suppressed magnetic resonance imaging scan showing an area of meniscal signal intensity in the region of the intercondylar notch (black arrows), consistent with a displaced bucket handle tear. Reproduced with permission from Johnson TR, Steinbach LS (eds): *Essentials of Musculoskeletal Imaging.* Rosemont, IL: American Academy of Orthopaedic Surgeons; 2004.

EXPECTED OUTCOMES/PROGNOSIS

* For small, peripheral tears that heal with nonoperative treatment, long-term prognosis is good.
* For tears requiring surgery, early osteoarthritis is a common sequela and is more likely with a partial or total removal of the torn meniscus.

WHEN TO REFER

* All patients with meniscus tears should be referred to an orthopaedic surgeon with expertise in treating pediatric sports injuries.
  — Urgent referral is required for the displaced meniscus tear that is locked between the tibia and the femur and prevents the patient from straightening the knee.

RELEVANT *ICD-9-CM* CODES

* **836.1**   Meniscus tear, lateral
* **836.2**   Meniscus tear, medial

Discoid Meniscus (Snapping Knee Syndrome)

INTRODUCTION/ETIOLOGY/EPIDEMIOLOGY

* A circular-shaped meniscus that develops as an anatomic variant, probably congenital
* Present in 1.5% to 15.5% of the population, with a higher prevalence in Asian populations
* Bilateral in 20%
* Almost exclusively affects the lateral meniscus.
* More prone to injury than a normal meniscus
* Three types
  — The third type is inherently unstable because there is no tibial attachment, so the meniscus may sublux in and out of the intercondylar notch as the knee is flexed and extended.

SIGNS AND SYMPTOMS

* Usually asymptomatic, unless an unstable type or there is an associated tear.
* When symptomatic, common complaints include pain, swelling, snapping, catching, locking, or limited motion.
* There may or may not be a history of trauma.
* Physical examination findings may be normal or include effusion, joint-line tenderness, decreased range of motion, a pop with extension of the knee, positive McMurray or Apley compression test (see figures 4-33 and 4-34), and quadriceps atrophy.

DIFFERENTIAL DIAGNOSIS

- Iliotibial band friction syndrome may cause painful snapping on the lateral side of the knee.
- Patellofemoral pain syndrome commonly presents with popping around or under the patella.

MAKING THE DIAGNOSIS

- Radiographs typically reveal a widened lateral joint space, squaring of the lateral femoral condyle, and cupping of the lateral tibial spine.
- Magnetic resonance imaging confirms the diagnosis with a block-shaped meniscus at least 5 mm thick on at least 3 contiguous slices (Figure 31-8).

TREATMENT

- An asymptomatic discoid meniscus requires no treatment.
- Those with recurrent swelling, catching, or locking require surgical treatment.
  — Unstable (type 3) menisci usually require complete meniscectomy.
  — Types 1 and 2 require partial meniscectomy or saucerization to create a more normally shaped meniscus.
- Tears in otherwise stable discoid menisci may be repaired, saucerized, debrided, or resected, depending on the type of tear.

EXPECTED OUTCOMES/PROGNOSIS

- Poor long-term outcomes with increased risk for early osteoarthritis are more likely for menisci that require significant debridement or resection.

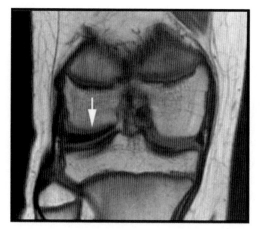

Figure 31-8. Discoid meniscus. T1-weighted magnetic resonance imaging scan showing a discoid lateral meniscus. Note that the lateral meniscus measures more than 12 mm wide (arrow) and is larger than the medial mensicus. Reproduced with permission from Johnson TR, Steinbach LS (eds): *Essentials of Musculoskeletal Imaging.* Rosemont, IL: American Academy of Orthopaedic Surgeons; 2004.

WHEN TO REFER

- To a pediatric orthopaedic surgeon
  — Patients with recurrent swelling, catching, or locking should be made non-weight bearing until evaluated by an orthopaedic surgeon.

RELEVANT *ICD-9-CM* CODES

- **717.5** Discoid meniscus
- **836.1** Meniscus tear, lateral
- **836.2** Meniscus tear, medial

Osteochondritis Dissecans

INTRODUCTION/ETIOLOGY/EPIDEMIOLOGY

- Avascular necrosis of the subchondral bone that can progress to fissuring of the overlying cartilage and separation of the osteochondral fragment from surrounding bone
- Affects children between 9 and 18 years of age.
- More common in boys
- The most commonly affected joint is the knee (medial more than the lateral femoral condyle) followed by the ankle (talus) and the elbow (capitellum). Rarely, the shoulder, hip, wrist, and hand may be affected.
- Etiology is not completely understood but is probably repetitive microtrauma to an incompletely vascularized area of developing bone. It may be familial.

SIGNS AND SYMPTOMS

- There may not be a history of trauma.
- The most common presenting symptom is joint pain followed by swelling and limited motion.
- Catching and locking may occur if the fragment displaces.
- Physical examination findings are usually nonspecific and include effusion, altered gait, and muscle atrophy.
- There may be tenderness at the medial femoral condyle.

DIFFERENTIAL DIAGNOSIS

- Other causes of a painful, swollen knee with nonspecific physical examination findings include patellofemoral pain, juvenile arthritis, infection, and tumor. Imaging studies or laboratory tests can differentiate these from OCD.

MAKING THE DIAGNOSIS

- Radiographs reveal the lesion if it is large and progressive.
  — Notch (tunnel) view of the knee is the most sensitive view (Figure 31-9).
  — Lesions in the posterior aspect of the femoral condyle may represent irregular ossification rather than OCD.
- Magnetic resonance imaging confirms the diagnosis of OCD when radiographs are negative and determines the stage of the lesion (Table 31-3).
- Bone scans are sometimes used to determine the lesion's healing potential.

TREATMENT

- *Grade I and II injuries*
  — Avoidance of high-impact exercise (running and jumping) until pain is resolved and the lesion shows healing on imaging studies
  — A knee immobilizer or crutches may be required until ambulation is pain-free.
  — Low-impact activities such as walking, swimming, and bicycling are allowed if not painful.
  — A rehabilitation program of strengthening and range of motion exercises will address any muscle atrophy and may promote cartilage healing.

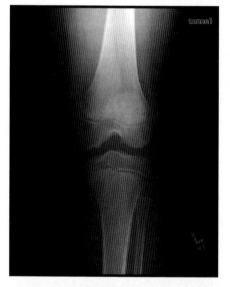

Figure 31-9. Notch (tunnel) view of knee demonstrates osteochondritis dissecans of medial femoral condyle. From Metzl JD. *Sports Medicine in the Pediatric Office.* Elk Grove Village, IL: American Academy of Pediatrics; 2008.

Table 31-3. Berndt and Harty Classification of Osteochondritis Dissecans Lesions

Stage	Description
I	Small area of subchondral compression
II	Partially detached fragment
III	Completely detached fragment remaining in the crater
IV	Fragment loose in the joint

- *Grade III and IV injuries*
  — These require surgical fixation or removal of the unstable fragment and drilling of the underlying bone to stimulate bleeding and healing with fibrous tissue.

EXPECTED OUTCOMES/PROGNOSIS

- In patients with open physes, up to 81% of grade I and II lesions will heal with nonoperative treatment.
  — Smaller lesions may heal in 3 months; larger lesions usually take 6 to 12 months.
- Skeletally mature patients are less likely to heal grade I and II lesions with nonoperative treatment.
- Grade III and IV lesions treated with surgical fixation have good functional outcomes.
- Osteoarthritis in adulthood is a common sequela and more likely with large lesions, grade III and IV lesions, and those in weight-bearing areas of the joint.

WHEN TO REFER

- To a pediatric orthopaedic surgeon
  — Grade III and IV lesions
  — Any grade lesion in a skeletally mature patient
  — Patients with catching or locking
  — Grade I and II lesions that progress or have unresolved symptoms after nonoperative treatment

RELEVANT *ICD-9-CM* CODE

- **732.7   OCD**

Bibliography

Accousti WK, Willis RB. Tibial eminence fractures. *Orthop Clin North Am.* 2003;34:365–375

Aichroth PM, Patel DV, Zorrilla P. The natural history and treatment of rupture of the anterior cruciate ligament in children and adolescents. A prospective review. *J Bone Joint Surg Br.* 2002;84:38–41

American Academy of Family Physicians, American Academy of Pediatrics, American College of Sports Medicine, American Medical Society for Sports Medicine, American Orthopaedic Society for Sports Medicine, American Osteopathic Academy of Sports Medicine. *Preparticipation Physical Evaluation.* 3rd ed. New York, NY: McGraw-Hill; 2005:31–32

American Academy of Pediatrics Committee on Adolescence, American College of Obstetricians and Gynecologists Committee on Adolescent Health Care. Menstruation in girls and adolescents: using the menstrual cycle as a vital sign. *Pediatrics.* 2006;118:2245–2250

American Academy of Pediatrics Committee on Sports Medicine and Fitness. Climatic heat stress and the exercising child and adolescent. *Pediatrics.* 2000;106:158–159

American Academy of Pediatrics Committee on Sports Medicine and Fitness. Protective eyewear for young athletes. *Pediatrics.* 2004;113:619–622

An YH, Friedman RJ. Multidirectional instability of the glenohumeral joint. *Orthop Clin North Am.* 2000; 31:275–285

Andrish JT. Anterior cruciate ligament injuries in the skeletally immature patient. *Am J Orthop.* 2001;30:103–110

Arendt E, Dick R. Knee injury patterns among men and women in collegiate basketball and soccer. NCAA data and review of literature. *Am J Sports Med.* 1995;23:694–701

Arendt EA, Bershadsky B, Agel J. Periodicity of noncontact anterior cruciate ligament injuries during the menstrual cycle. *J Gend Specif Med.* 2002;5:19–26

Arnoczky SP, Warren RF. Microvasculature of the human meniscus. *Am J Sports Med.* 1982;10:90–95

Aronowitz ER, Ganley TJ, Goode JR, Gregg JR, Meyer JS. Anterior cruciate ligament reconstruction in adolescents with open physes. *Am J Sports Med.* 2000;28:168–175

Atkin DM, Fithian DC, Marangi KS, Stone ML, Dobson BE, Mendelsohn C. Characteristics of patients with acute lateral patellar dislocation and their recovery within the first 6 months of injury. *Am J Sports Med.* 2000;28:472–479

Beasley L, Faryniarz DA, Hannafin JA. Multidirectional instability of the shoulder in the female athlete. *Clin Sports Med.* 2000;19:331–349

Berndt AL, Harty M. Transchondral fractures (osteochondritis dissecans) of the talus. *J Bone Joint Surg Am.* 1959;41-A:988–1020

Boden BP, Dean GS, Feagin JA Jr, Garrett WE Jr. Mechanisms of anterior cruciate ligament injury. *Orthopedics.* 2000;23:573–578

Buch KA, Campbell J. Acute onset meralgia paraesthetica after fracture of the anterior superior iliac spine. *Injury.* 1993;24:569–570

Carek PJ, Futrell M, Hueston WJ. The preparticipation physical examination history: who has the correct answers? *Clin J Sport Med.* 1999;9:124–128

Castro FP Jr. Stingers, cervical cord neurapraxia, and stenosis. *Clin Sports Med.* 2003;22:483–492

Chappell JD, Yu B, Kirkendall DT, Garrett WE. A comparison of knee kinetics between male and female recreational athletes in stop-jump tasks. *Am J Sport Med.* 2002;30:261–267

Cherf J, Paulos LE. Bracing for patellar instability. *Clin Sports Med.* 1990;9:813–821

Cleeman E, Flatow EL. Shoulder dislocations in the young patient. *Orthop Clin North Am.* 2000;31:217–229

Cofield RH, Bryan RS. Acute dislocation of the patella: results of conservative treatment. *J Trauma.* 1977;17:526–531

Cohen DA, Nsuami M, Martin DH, Farley TA. Repeated school-based screening for sexually transmitted diseases: a feasible strategy for reaching adolescents. *Pediatrics.* 1999;104:1281–1285

Collins M, Giola G. Acute concussion evaluation. Available at: http://www.cdc.gov/TraumaticbrainInjury/pdf/ACE-a.pdf. Accessed February 11, 2010

Corrado D, Basso C, Pavei A, Michieli P, Schiavon M, Thiene G. Trends in sudden cardiovascular death in young competitive athletes after implementation of a preparticipation screening program. *JAMA.* 2006;296:1593–1601

Deie M, Sakamaki Y, Sumen Y, Urabe Y, Ikuta Y. Anterior knee laxity in young women varies with their menstrual cycle. *Int Orthop.* 2002;26:154–156

DeMaio M, McHale K. Anterior cruciate ligament injuries in female athletes. In: Garrick JG, ed. *Orthopaedic Knowledge Update: Sports Medicine 3.* 3rd ed. Rosemont, IL: American Academy of Orthopaedic Surgeons; 2004:403–410

Dickhaut SC, DeLee JC. The discoid lateral-meniscus syndrome. *J Bone Joint Surg Am.* 1982;64:1068–1073

Dorizas JA, Stanitski CL. Anterior cruciate ligament injury in the skeletally immature. *Orthop Clin North Am.* 2003;34:355–363

Dragoo JL, Lee RS, Benhaim P, Finerman GA, Hame SL. Relaxin receptors in the human female anterior cruciate ligament. *Am J Sports Med.* 2003;31:577–584

Dubow JS, Kelly JP. Epilepsy in sports and recreation. *Sports Med.* 2003;33:499–516

DuRant RH, Seymore C, Linder CW, Jay S. The preparticipation examination of athletes. Comparison of single and multiple examiners. *Am J Dis Child.* 1985;139:657–661

Edwards MR, Terry J, Gibbs J, Bridle S. Proximal anterior cruciate ligament avulsion fracture in a skeletally immature athlete: a case report and method of physeal sparing repair. *Knee Surg Sports Traumatol Arthrosc.* 2007;15:150–152

Emery CA, Meeuwisse WH, Hartmann SE. Evaluation of risk factors for injury in adolescent soccer: implementation and validation of an injury surveillance system. *Am J Sports Med.* 2005;33:1882–1891

Emery KH. Imaging of sports injuries of the upper extremity in children. *Clin Sports Med.* 2006;25:543–568

Fernbach SK, Wilkinson RH. Avulsion injuries of the pelvis and proximal femur. *AJR Am J Roentgenol.* 1981;137:581–584

Field M, Collins MW, Lovell MR, Maroon J. Does age play a role in recovery from sports-related concussion? A comparison of high school and collegiate athletes. *J Pediatr.* 2003;142:546–553

Fithian DC, Paxton EW, Stone ML, et al. Epidemiology and natural history of acute patellar dislocation. *Am J Sports Med.* 2004;32:1114–1121

Ford KR, Myer GD, Toms HE, Hewett TE. Gender differences in the kinematics of unanticipated cutting in young athletes. *Med Sci Sports Exerc.* 2005;37:124–129

Fountain NB, May AC. Epilepsy and athletics. *Clin Sports Med.* 2003;22;605–616

Goldberg B, Saraniti A, Witman P, Gavin M, Nicholas JA. Pre-participation sports assessment—an objective evaluation. *Pediatrics.* 1980;66:736–745

Griffin LY, Agel J, Albohm MJ, et al. Noncontact anterior cruciate ligament injuries: risk factors and prevention strategies. *J Am Acad Orthop Surg.* 2000;8:141–150

Guskiewicz KM, Weaver NL, Padua DA, Garrett WE Jr. Epidemiology of concussion in collegiate and high school football players. *Am J Sports Med.* 2000;28:643–650

Hawkins RJ, Bell RH, Anisette G. Acute patellar dislocations. The natural history. *Am J Sports Med.* 1986;14:117–120

Heidt RS, Sweeterman LM, Carlonas RL, Traub JA, Tekulve FX. Avoidance of soccer injuries with preseason conditioning. *Am J Sports Med.* 2000;28:659–662

Hewett TE, Lindenfeld TN, Riccobene JV, Noyes FR. The effect of neuromuscular training on the incidence of knee injury in female athletes. A prospective study. *Am J Sports Med.* 1999;27:699–706

Hewett TE, Myer GD, Ford KR. Anterior cruciate ligament injuries in female athletes: part 1, mechanisms and risk factors. *Am J Sports Med.* 2006;34:299–311

Hewett TE, Myer GD, Ford KR. Decrease in neuromuscular control about the knee with maturation in female athletes. *J Bone Joint Surg Am.* 2004;86-A:1601–1608

Hewett TE, Myer GD, Ford KR, et al. Biomechanical measures of neuromuscular control and valgus loading of the knee predict anterior cruciate ligament injury risk in female athletes: a prospective study. *Am J Sport Med.* 2005;33:492–501

Hovelius L, Olofsson A, Sandstrom B, et al. Nonoperative treatment of primary anterior shoulder dislocation in patients forty years of age and younger. A prospective twenty-five-year follow up. *J Bone Joint Surg Am.* 2008;90:945–952

Hurwitz KM, Argyros GJ, Roach JM, Eliasson AH, Phillips YY. Interpretation of eucapnic voluntary hyperventilation in the diagnosis of asthma. *Chest.* 1995;108:1240–1245

Jarvinen M, Lehto M, Sorvari T, et al. Effect of some anti-inflammatory agents on the healing of ruptured muscle: an experimental study in rats. *J Sports Traumatol Relat Res.* 1992;14:19–28

Kark JA, Posey DM, Schumacher HR, Ruehle CJ. Sickle-cell trait as a risk factor for sudden death in physical training. *N Engl J Med.* 1987;317:781–787

Kazakova SV, Hageman JC, Matava M, et al. A clone of methicillin-resistant *Staphylococcus aureus* among professional football players. *N Engl J Med.* 2005;352:468–475

Kelly JP, Rosenberg JH. The development of guidelines for the management of concussion in sports. *J Head Trauma Rehabil.* 1998;13:53–65

Kerkhoffs GM, Rowe BH, Assendelft WJ, Kelly KD, Struijs PA, van Dijk CN. Immobilisation for acute ankle sprain. A systematic review. *Arch Orthop Trauma Surg.* 2001;121:462–471

King SJ, Carty HM, Brady O. Magnetic resonance imaging of knee injuries in children. *Pediatr Radiol.* 1996; 26:287–290

Kirkwood MW, Yeates KO, Wilson PE. Pediatric sport-related concussion: a review of the clinical management of an oft-neglected population. *Pediatrics.* 2006;117:1359–1371

Kowatari K, Nakashima K, Ono A, Yoshihara M, Amano M, Toh S. Leovofloxacin-induced bilateral Achilles tendon rupture: a case report and review of the literature. *J Orthop Sci.* 2004;9:186–190

Kuhn JE. Treating the initial anterior shoulder dislocation—an evidence-based approach. *Sports Med Arthrosc.* 2006;14:192–198

Kujala UM, Orava S, Karpakka J, Leppavuori J, Mattila K. Ischial tuberosity apophysitis and avulsion among athletes. *Int J Sports Med.* 1997;18:149–155

LaBella C. Common acute sports-related lower extremity injuries in children and adolescents. *Clin Pediatr Emerg Med.* 2007:31–42

LaBella C. Overuse injuries unique to young athletes. *The Child's Doctor Journal of Children's Memorial Hospital, Chicago.* 2005;22:2–6

LaBella C. Patellofermoral pain syndrome: evaluation and treatment. *Prim Care Clin Office Pract.* 2004; 31:977–1003

Lephart SM, Ferris CM, Riemann BL, Myers JB, Fu FH. Gender differences in strength and lower extremity kinematics during landing. *Clin Orthop Relat Res.* 2002;401:162–169

Lo IK, Bell DM, Fowler PJ. Anterior cruciate ligament injuries in the skeletally immature patient. *Instr Course Lect.* 1998;47:351–359

MacKnight JM. Infectious mononucleosis: ensuring a safe return to sport. *Phys Sportsmed.* 2002;30:27–41

MacNab I. Recurrent dislocation of the patella. *J Bone Joint Surg Am.* 1952;34A:957–967

Malinzak RA, Colby SM, Kirkendall DT, Yu B, Garrett WE. A comparison of knee joint motion patterns between men and women in selected athletic tasks. *Clin Biomech (Bristol, Avon).* 2001;16:438–445

Mandelbaum BR, Silvers HJ, Watanabe DS, et al. Effectiveness of a neuromuscular and proprioceptive training program in preventing anterior cruciate ligament injuries in female athletes: 2-year follow-up. *Am J Sport Med.* 2005;33:1003–1010

Mannix ET, Roberts M, Fagin DP, Reid B, Farber MO. Prevalence of airways hyperresponsiveness in members of an exercise training facility. *J Asthma.* 2003;40:349–355

Maron BJ. Hypertrophic cardiomyopathy in childhood. *Pediatr Clin North Am.* 2004;51:1305–1346

Maron BJ, Thompson PD, Puffer JC, et al. Cardiovascular preparticipation screening of competitive athletes. A statement for health professionals from the Sudden Death Committee (clinical cardiology) and Congenital Cardiac Defects Committee (cardiovascular disease in the young), American Heart Association. *Circulation.* 1996;94:850–856

Maron BJ, Zipes DP. Introduction: eligibility recommendations for competitive athletes with cardiovascular abnormalities—general considerations. *J Am Coll Cardiol.* 2005;45:1318–1321

Martin TJ, American Academy of Pediatrics Committee on Sports Medicine and Fitness. Knee brace use in the young athlete. *Pediatrics.* 2001;108:503–507

McCrory P, Johnston K, Meeuwisse W, et al. Summary and agreement statement of the 2nd International Conference on Concussion in Sports, Prague 2004. *Br J Sports Med.* 2005;39:196–204

McLean SG, Lipfert SW, van den Bogert AJ. Effect of gender and defensive opponent on the biomechanics of sidestep cutting. *Med Sci Sports Exerc.* 2004;36:1008–1016

McNair PJ, Marshall RN, Matheson JA. Important features associated with acute anterior cruciate ligament injury. *N Z Med J.* 1990;103:537–539

Messina DF, Farney WC, DeLee JC. The incidence of injury in Texas high school basketball. A prospective study among male and female athletes. *Am J Sports Med.* 1999;27:294–299

Metzmaker JN, Pappas AM. Avulsion fractures of the pelvis. *Am J Sports Med.* 1985;13:349–358

Meyers MH, McKeever FM. Fracture of the intercondylar eminence of the tibia. *J Bone Joint Surg Am.* 1959; 41-A:209–222

Micheli LJ, Metzl JD, Di Canzio J, Zurakowski D. Anterior cruciate ligament reconstructive surgery in adolescent soccer and basketball players. *Clin J Sports Med.* 1999;9:138–141

Mickleborough TD, Lindley MR, Turner LA. Comparative effects of a high-intensity warm-up and salbutamol on the bronchoconstrictor response to exercise in asthmatic athletes. *Int J Sports Med.* 2007;28:456–462

Mishra DK, Friden J, Schmitz MC, Lieber RL. Anti-inflammatory medication after muscle injury. A treatment resulting in short-term improvement but subsequent loss of muscle function. *J Bone Joint Surg Am.* 1995;77: 1510–1519

Moeller JL. Pelvic and hip apophyseal avulsion injuries in young athletes. *Curr Sports Med Rep.* 2003;2:110–115

Mounsey JP, Ferguson JD. The assessment and management of arrhythmias and syncope in the athlete. *Clin Sports Med.* 2003;22:67–79

Myklebust G, Engebretsen L, Braekken IH, Skjolberg A, Olsen OE, Bahr R. Prevention of anterior cruciate ligament injuries in female team handball players: a prospective intervention study over three seasons. *Clin J Sport Med.* 2003;13:71–78

Napier SM, Baker RS, Sanford DG, Easterbrook M. Eye injuries in athletics and recreation. *Surv Ophthalmol.* 1996;41:229–244

National High Blood Pressure Education Program Working Group on High Blood Pressure in Children and Adolescents. The fourth report on the diagnosis, evaluation, and treatment of high blood pressure in children and adolescents. *Pediatrics.* 2004;114:555–576

Neer CS. Involuntary inferior and multidirectional instability of the shoulder: etiology, recognition, and treatment. *Instr Course Lect.* 1985;34:232–238

Nietosvaara Y, Aalto K, Kallio PE. Acute patellar dislocation in children: incidence and associated osteochondral fractures. *J Pediatr Orthop.* 1994;14:513–515

Nomura E, Inoue M, Kurimura M. Chondral and osteochondral injuries associated with acute patellar dislocation. *Arthroscopy.* 2003;19:717–721

Olsen O, Myklebust G, Engebretsen L, Holme I, Bahr R. Exercises to prevent lower limb injuries in youth sports: cluster randomized controlled trial. *BMJ.* 2005;330:449

Paluska SA. An overview of hip injuries in running. *Sports Med.* 2005;35:991–1014

Powell JW, Barber-Foss KD. Injury patterns in selected high school sports: a review of the 1995-1997 seasons. *J Athl Train.* 1999;34:277–284

Rice SG, American Academy of Pediatrics Council on Sports Medicine and Fitness. Medical conditions affecting sports participation. *Pediatrics.* 2008;121:841–848

Rizzo M, Holler SB, Bassett FH 3rd. Comparison of males' and females' ratios of anterior-cruciate-ligament width to femoral-intercondylar-notch width: a cadaveric study. *Am J Orthop.* 2001;30:660–664

Rossi F, Dragoni S. Acute avulsion fractures of the pelvis in adolescent competitive athletes: prevalence, location and sports distribution of 203 cases collected. *Skeletal Radiol.* 2001;30:127–131

Rowe CR. Prognosis in dislocations of the shoulder. *J Bone Joint Surg Am.* 1956;38-A:957–977

Rundell KW, Jenkinson DM. Exercise-induced bronchospasm in the elite athlete. *Sports Med.* 2002;32:583–600

Scholten RJ, Opstelten W, van der Plas CG, Bijl D, Deville WL, Bouter LM. Accuracy of physical diagnostic tests for assessing ruptures of the anterior cruciate ligament: a meta-analysis. *J Fam Pract.* 2003;52:689–694

Shea KG, Pfeiffer R, Wang JH, Curtin M, Apel PJ. Anterior cruciate ligament injury in pediatric and adolescent soccer players: an analysis of insurance data. *J Pediatr Orthop.* 2004;24:623–628

Shelbourne KD, Davis TJ, Klootwyk TE. The relationship between intercondylar notch width of the femur and the incidence of anterior cruciate ligament tears. A prospective study. *Am J Sports Med.* 1998;26:402–408

Silvers HJ, Giza ER, Mandelbaum BR. Anterior cruciate ligament tear prevention in the female athlete. *Curr Sports Med Rep.* 2005;4:341–343

Smith J, Laskowski ER. The preparticipation physical examination: Mayo Clinic experience with 2,739 examinations. *Mayo Clinic Proc.* 1998;73:419–429

Stanitski CL. Correlation of arthroscopic and clinical examinations with magnetic resonance imaging findings of injured knees in children and adolescents. *Am J Sports Med.* 1998;26:2–6

Stanitski CL, Harvell JC, Fu F. Observations on acute knee hemarthrosis in children and adolescents. *J Pediatr Orthop.* 1993;13:506–510

Stanitski CL, Paletta GA Jr. Articular cartilage injury with acute patellar dislocation in adolescents. Arthroscopic and radiographic correlation. *Am J Sports Med.* 1998;26:52–55

Sundar M, Carty H. Avulsion fractures of the pelvis in children: a report of 32 fractures and their outcome. *Skeletal Radiol.* 1994;23:85–90

Sundgot-Borgen J, Torstveit MK. Prevalence of eating disorders in elite athletes is higher than in the general population. *Clin J Sport Med.* 2004;14:25–32

Swirtun LR, Jansson A, Renstrom P. The effects of a functional knee brace during early treatment of patients with a nonoperated acute anterior cruciate ligament tear: a prospective randomized study. *Clin J Sport Med.* 2005;15:299–304

Thanikachalam M, Petros JG, O'Donnell S. Avulsion fracture of the anterior superior iliac spine presenting as acute-onset meralgia paresthetica. *Ann Emerg Med.* 1995;26:515–517

Tolo V. Fractures and dislocations about the knee. In: Green NE, Swiontkowski MF, eds. *Skeletal Trauma in Children.* Philadelphia, PA: WB Saunders; 1998:444–447

Treloar AE, Boynton RE, Behn BG, Brown BW. Variation of the human menstrual cycle through reproductive life. *Int J Fertil.* 1967;12:77–126

Waninger KN, Harcke HT. Determination of safe return to play for athletes recovering from infectious mononucleosis: a review of the literature. *Clin J Sport Med.* 2005;15:410–416

Washington ER 3rd, Root L, Liener UC. Discoid lateral meniscus in children. Long-term follow-up after excision. *J Bone Joint Surg Am.* 1995;77:1357–1361

Watanabe M, Takeda S, Kieuchi H. *Atlas of Arthroscopy.* 3rd ed. Tokyo, Japan: Igaku-Shoin; 1979

Weiler JM, Layton T, Hunt M. Asthma in United States Olympic athletes who participated in the 1996 Summer Games. *J Allergy Clin Immunol.* 1998;102:722–726

Wessel LM, Scholz S, Rusch M, et al. Hemarthrosis after trauma to the pediatric knee joint: what is the value of magnetic resonance imaging in the diagnostic algorithm? *J Pediatr Orthop.* 2001;21:338–342

Willis RB, Blokker C, Stoll TM, Paterson DC, Galpin RD. Long-term follow-up of anterior tibial eminence fractures. *J Pediatr Orthop.* 1993;13:361–364

Winkler AR, Barnes JC, Ogden JA. Break dance hip: chronic avulsion of the anterior superior iliac spine. *Pediatr Radiol.* 1987;17:501–502

Wojtys EM, Ashton-Miller JA, Huston LJ. A gender-related difference in the contribution of the knee musculature to sagittal-plane shear stiffness in subjects with similar knee laxity. *J Bone Joint Surg Am.* 2002;84-A:10–16

Wojtys EM, Huston LJ, Boynton MD, Spindler KP, Lindenfeld TN. The effect of the menstrual cycle on anterior cruciate ligament injuries in women as determined by hormone levels. *Am J Sports Med.* 2002;30:182–188

Zobel MS, Borrello JA, Siegel MJ, Stewart NR. Pediatric knee MR imaging: pattern of injuries in the immature skeleton. *Radiology.* 1994;190:397–401

Part 12: Common Fractures and Physeal Injuries

CHAPTER 32

Imaging Fractures

Pediatric Trauma in the United States

- Leading cause of death and disability in children
- Annually accounts for 11 million hospitalizations, 100,000 permanent disabilities, and 15,000 deaths.
- Pediatric trauma rate in the United States is one of the highest in the world and is related to a mechanized society and urban violence.
- Direct costs of childhood injury exceed 8 billion dollars per year.
- Many areas of the United States have regionalized trauma care.
- Studies have suggested that mortality may increase when patients are treated by surgeons who see fewer than 35 seriously injured patients per year.
- Several studies have demonstrated lower severity-adjusted mortality and better functional outcomes at discharge for those treated at pediatric trauma centers.
- Presence of an in-house pediatric surgeon improves survival rates from trauma.
- In a recent study, musculoskeletal injuries constituted the predominant category of pediatric trauma, representing up to 50% of emergency department consultations.
- Treatment of musculoskeletal trauma is the most likely cause for hospital admission and surgical intervention among children sustaining pediatric trauma.
- *Radiographs* are the imaging study of choice for pediatric fractures and should be performed first and before advanced imaging study.
- Long bone injuries: obtain at least 2 views taken at 90 degrees to each other and include the joint above and below the site of pain to evaluate for any associated fractures or dislocations (Table 32-1).
- Include clinical information on the requisition such as the age of the patient, location of pain, and mechanism of injury to assist the radiologist in interpretation.
- Variants of normal anatomy are common. Keats and Anderson's *Atlas of Normal Roentgen Variants That May Simulate Disease* can help differentiate an injury from one of these variants.
- Imaging the opposite extremity is helpful for comparing physeal appearance or differentiating an accessory ossification center from a fracture or an avulsion.

Table 32-1. Common Radiographic Series to Evaluate Fractures

Area	Series
Cervical spine	AP/lateral/obliques/flexion and extension
Thoracic spine	AP/lateral
Lumbar spine	AP/lateral/spot L5-S1/obliques
Sacrum	AP/lateral
Pelvis	AP/obliques
Shoulder	AP with internal and external rotation, axillary, Y view
Elbow	AP/lateral/obliques
Wrist	PA/lateral/scaphoid/carpal tunnel view
Hand	AP/lateral/oblique
Finger	AP/lateral/oblique
Hip	AP/frog lateral
Femur	AP/lateral
Knee	AP/lateral/sunrise/obliques
Tibia/Fibula	AP/lateral
Ankle	AP/lateral/oblique
Foot	AP/lateral/mortise
Toes	AP/lateral/oblique

AP, anteroposterior; PA, posteroanterior.

- Some fractures (eg, scaphoid, toddler, stress) are not visible on radiographs.
  - If a fracture is suspected and radiographs are normal, the patient can be treated as if there is a fracture and radiographs repeated in 1 to 2 weeks when a fracture line or periosteal reaction may become visible.
  - If an immediate answer is needed, *magnetic resonance imaging* is very sensitive and can rule out a fracture.
- *Computed tomography* is more sensitive than radiographs for detecting fractures or hematoma in cases of spinal or pelvic trauma.

CHAPTER 33

Fracture Types

Plastic Deformation

- Instead of breaking, an immature bone can bend or bow (Figure 33-1).
- Occurs in response to a longitudinally applied force but has also been described after a transverse blow.
- Most commonly occurs in the ulna or fibula.
- Remodeling potential is good in children younger than 6 years.
- A deformity of more than 10 degrees in a child older than 6 years should be corrected.

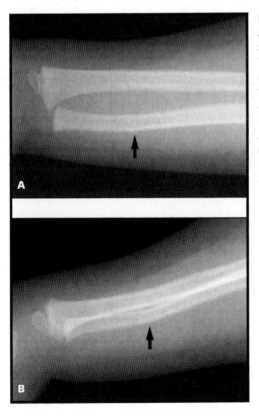

Figure 33-1. A, Plastic deformation. Anteroposterior view of the distal forearm shows mild ulnar apex angular deformity. The arrow indicates plastic deformation of the distal ulna. B, Lateral view of the distal forearm shows a volar apex angular deformity of the ulna (arrow). Reproduced with permission from Johnson TR, Steinbach LS (eds): *Essentials of Musculoskeletal Imaging.* Rosemont, IL: American Academy of Orthopaedic Surgeons; 2004.

Buckle or Torus Fractures

- Occur at the diaphyseal-metaphyseal junction, when more dense diaphyseal bone compresses the metaphysis (Figure 33-2).
- Most common fracture type in children
- Often subtle radiographically
- Frequently present without swelling, loss of motion, or much pain

Greenstick Fractures

- Occur in the diaphysis when the cortex on the tension side fails and breaks but the fracture does not propagate through to the opposite cortex (Figure 33-3; see also Figure 36-10).
- Reduction may be difficult and sometimes the fracture must be completed to achieve

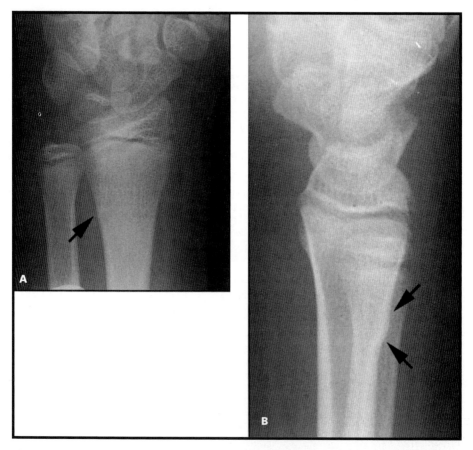

Figure 33-2. Torus fracture. A, Anteroposterior view of distal forearm and wrist shows a torus fracture. The arrow points to buckling of the distal radius in the metaphyseal region. B, Lateral view. Arrows indicate buckling of the distal radius on the metaphseal region, consistent with a torus fracture. Reproduced with permission from Johnson TR, Steinbach LS (eds): *Essentials of Musculoskeletal Imaging.* Rosemont, IL: American Academy of Orthopaedic Surgeons; 2004.

Fracture type	Characteristics	
Transverse	Fracture line perpendicular to the shaft of the bone	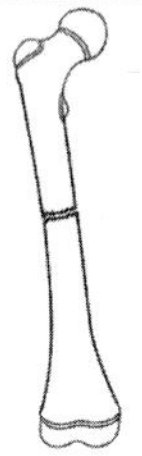
Oblique	Angulated fracture line	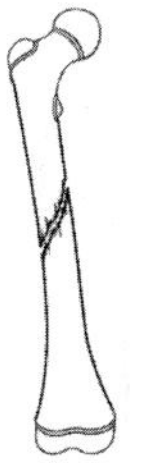
Spiral	A multiplanar and complex fracture line	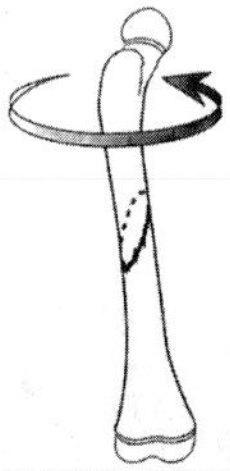
Torus	An incomplete buckle fracture	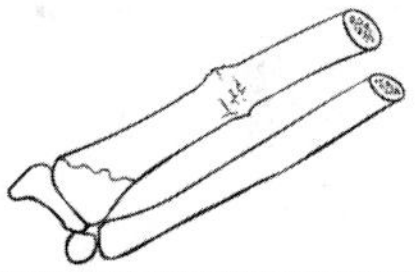
Greenstick	An incomplete fracture with angular deformity	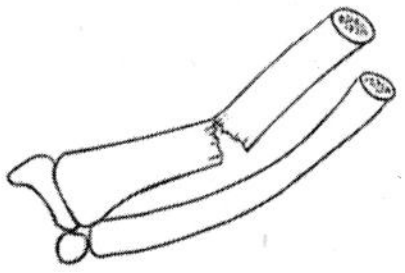

Figure 33-3. Fracture types of long bones in children. Reproduced with permission from Johnson TR, Steinbach LS (eds): *Essentials of Musculoskeletal Imaging.* Rosemont, IL: American Academy of Orthopaedic Surgeons; 2004.

proper anatomic alignment.

Spiral Fractures

• Caused by a rotational force
• Inflicted trauma must be considered.

Oblique Fractures

• Occur diagonally at the diaphysis.
• Usually associated with periosteal disruption
• Because of the slope and loss of periosteum, these fractures are often difficult to keep in proper alignment even after appropriate reduction and immobilization.

Transverse Fractures

• Occur at a right angle to the cortex usually near the bone mid-shaft.
• After closed reduction, can usually be held in position with immobilization.

Physeal Fractures

• Common because the cartilage plate is weaker than the bone and therefore much more susceptible to injury

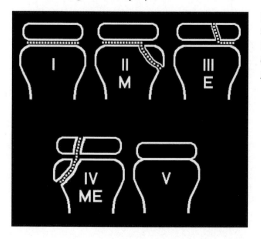

Figure 33-4. Salter-Harris classification system for epiphyseal fractures. From Metzl JD. *Sports Medicine in the Pediatric Office.* Elk Grove Village, IL: American Academy of Pediatrics; 2008.

• Most commonly classified using the Salter-Harris method (Figure 33-4).
• See Chapter 35 for a detailed discussion of diagnosis and treatment.

CHAPTER 34

Stages of Fracture Healing

Inflammatory Phase

- This occurs during approximately the first 10 days after the injury (Figure 34-1a).
- Hematoma forms around and within the broken bone.
- Platelets, inflammatory cells, and chemical mediators released as a result of the hematoma stimulate vascularization and recruit osteoblasts.
- Initially blood vessels on either side of the fracture are disrupted. This results in sclerosis of the fracture margins and resorption of the bony matrix within the fracture site, which causes the fracture to appear more visible on plain radiographs. Physicians should anticipate this and reassure parents this is a normal phase of fracture healing, even though the radiograph may look worse.
- The hematoma is subsequently replaced with an interwoven collagen mesh, which will serve as the scaffolding for new bone formation.

Reparative Phase

- This usually occurs between 10 and 14 days after the injury (Figure 34-1b).
- Enhanced vascularization and the differentiation of mesenchymal cells into cartilage, bone, or fibrous precursors.
- As osteoblasts are recruited, bone mineralization occurs and the healing callus becomes visible on radiographs.
- The reparative phase ends with clinical union, which is when the radiograph demonstrates visible callus filling in the fracture site and it is no longer painful to manipulation. At this point the fracture is stable in that no further displacement (without trauma) is expected, but the callus is still relatively weak, structurally disorganized, and not functionally ready for the typical stresses placed on bone.

Remodeling Phase

- Lengthiest phase of fracture healing; can continue for years (Figure 34-1c).
- Healing bone gradually returns to its pre-injury shape and strength.

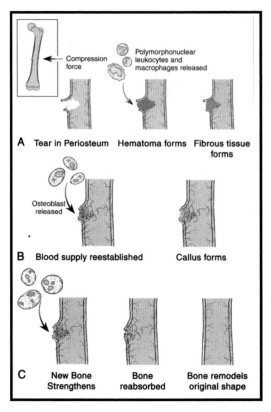

Figure 34-1. Phases of secondary fracture healing. A, Early inflammatory phase. B, Callus formation. C, New bone formation, with remodeling of bone to original shape. Reproduced with permission from Sullivan JA, Anderson SJ (eds). *Care of the Young Athlete.* Rosemont, IL: American Academy of Orthopaedic Surgeons; 2000.

- Osteoblasts respond to external stress placed on the bone, intrinsic muscle action, and movement of the adjacent articulation by filling in the bony matrix appropriately. This is why early mobilization is recommended (once clinical union is present) for optimal fracture healing.
- Osteoclasts initiate bony resorption to remove any excess bone that is formed.
- During this phase if the child falls without a protective splint or cast, the bone may be reinjured.

Healing Fractures

- Fractures heal more rapidly in children because of the following factors:
  — Skeletally immature bone is inherently more biologically active than adult bone.
  — Children have a more rapid and pronounced inflammatory response.
  — Children have a thicker, stronger, more anatomically distinct periosteum.
    ▪ Acts as a restraint for displacement, which allows the bony bridge to form more rapidly and efficiently.
    ▪ Contains the hematoma so the biologically active cells and chemical mediators can work locally at the fracture site.
    ▪ Has osteogenic potential and can augment bone formation taking place in the hematoma.

Fracture Remodeling Principles

- Amount of potential remodeling depends on age, fracture type, and anatomic location.
  - *Age*
    - In patients younger than 5 years, 20 to 30 degrees of angulation in a long bone fracture is acceptable; in an adolescent with 1 to 2 years of growth potential, less than 5 to 10 degrees of angulation is acceptable. Adults require near-perfect alignment from the start of treatment to maximize cosmetic and functional outcome (Figure 34-2).
    - Patients with wide-open physes, pre-menarchal females, and males without secondary sex characteristics have more remodeling potential than older adolescents.
    - Children remodel varus or valgus angulation better than older adolescents and adults.
    - Children younger than 10 years usually remodel well if there is at least 50% apposition.

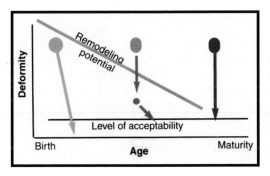

Figure 34-2. Age-determined changes affecting reduction. As age increases, the potential for remodeling declines (green line). For a given angulation, age determines the required degree of reduction. In infancy, (green arrow), reduction is not necessary because remodeling is rapid and complete. The same angulation in a child (blue arrows) requires partial reduction, with remodeling connecting the remaining deformity. Adolescents (red arrow) require anatomic reduction. From Staheli LT. *Practice of Pediatric Orthopedics.* Philadelphia, PA: Lippincott Williams & Wilkins; 2001. Used by permission.

  - *Fracture type*
    - Low-energy Salter-Harris type I and II injuries generally remodel well.
    - Injuries involving the articular surface (Salter-Harris types III and IV) will not remodel well if there is significant displacement, and early arthritis is a potential complication. A step off at the articular surface greater than 2 mm on computed tomography scan requires surgical fixation.
    - Diaphyseal fractures have less remodeling potential than metaphyseal fractures.
    - Plastic deformation does not remodel well in patients older than 6 years.
    - Remodeling potential is greater if the deformity is in the plane of motion of the adjacent joint.

- Rotational deformities do not remodel.
— *Anatomic location*
  - Clavicle and proximal humerus fractures have great remodeling potential.
  - Toddler fractures (spiral fractures of the tibia in children younger than 5 years) have good remodeling potential.
  - *The distal radius can remodel angulation of up to 30 degrees in young children* (Figure 34-3).
  - The elbow has poor remodeling potential, especially for supracondylar and lateral epicondyle fractures, which often require operative management for optimal results.
  - Forearm shaft fractures also have limited remodeling potential.
    - ◆ Dorsal/volar angulation remodels better than radial/ulnar angulation because of the stress applied to the bone with normal motion.
    - ◆ Angulation in both planes usually requires operative management.
- Longitudinal bone growth may be stimulated after a fracture, especially in the tibia or femur, such that the bone grows longer than would have occurred without injury; therefore, some overlap of fracture fragments is often desirable to balance this excess growth.

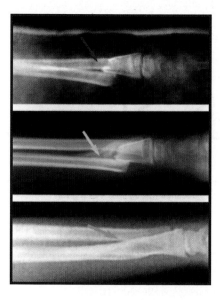

Figure 34-3. Remodeling of distal radius. Fracture fragments were in bayonette apposition (red arrow). Three months later remodeling was in progress (yellow arrow). At 2 years (orange arrow) remodeling was nearly complete. From Staheli LT. *Practice of Pediatric Orthopedics.* Philadelphia, PA: Lippincott Williams & Wilkins; 2001. Used by permission.

CHAPTER 35

Physeal Fractures

Introduction/Etiology/Epidemiology

- Physes are organized into zones of function, with cartilage cells growing continually on the epiphyseal side and bony replacement occurring on the metaphyseal side at the end of a long bone.
- These zones persist until skeletal maturity when the cartilage of the physis has been completely replaced by bone.
- While the physes are open, it is more common for a child to sustain a fracture or an injury through the relatively weaker physis than to sustain a ligamentous injury (sprain) or dislocation of a joint.
- Salter-Harris classification of physeal fractures is the standard terminology to describe and categorize injuries involving the growth plate (see Figure 33-4).
  — Describes the plane or trajectory of the fracture through the physeal plate.
  — Has implications for treatment and prognosis of potential growth arrest.
  — Salter-Harris type I fracture
    ▪ Traverses across the physis without entering the epiphysis or metaphysis.
    ▪ Eight-point-five percent of physeal fractures
    ▪ Common in infants and younger children
  — Salter-Harris type II fracture
    ▪ Extends across the physis for a variable distance and then exits into the metaphysis.
    ▪ Most common type representing 73% of physeal fractures
    ▪ Usually occurs in children older than 10 years.
  — Salter-Harris type III and IV fractures
    ▪ Extend into the articular surface.
    ▪ Six-point-five percent (type III) and 12% (type IV) of physeal fractures
    ▪ Because accuracy of reduction is necessary for subsequent physeal function, it is important that anatomic reduction is achieved.
  — Salter-Harris type V fracture
    ▪ Crush injury to the physis
    ▪ Rare
    ▪ High risk of physeal growth arrest is expected.
- Physeal fractures are common and account for 18% to 30% of all fractures in children.

- Distal radius physeal fractures comprise between 25% and 30% of physeal fractures, followed by the distal tibia, distal fibula, distal humerus, distal ulna, proximal humerus, and distal femur.
- Physeal fractures are more likely to occur around the most rapidly growing physes and during times of most rapid growth.
- Physeal injuries occur over the entire span of childhood years, increasing in occurrence with increasing age.
- Highest incidence is in the preadolescent period, with girls peaking at 11 years of age and boys peaking at 12 to 14 years of age.
- The risk of physeal fractures in boys extends longer, consistent with their slower development and later skeletal maturation.
- Fractures through the physis occur during infancy as birth-related trauma or as a result of abusive trauma or child abuse.
  — Almost always physeal separations (Salter-Harris type I)
  — Overall, these are rare injuries, with the most common occurring in the distal humerus and distal femur.
  — Occasionally, proximal femur physeal separation may be seen.
  — Can be challenging to differentiate from a developmentally dislocated hip or a septic arthritis of the hip.

Signs and Symptoms

- History of trauma or overuse
- Point tenderness at physis
- Pain with attempted active or passive range of motion of the affected joint
- Depending on the severity of the injury, there may be swelling, ecchymosis, and deformity of the limb.
- Infants and younger children will not be able to describe what is hurting them and may only be able to protect the affected limb, limiting use and mobility (pseudoparalysis).

Differential Diagnosis

- A displaced physeal fracture is likely to be obvious on radiographic examination.
- It may be difficult to differentiate a nondisplaced physeal fracture from a soft tissue injury or a sprain.
  — If the point of maximal tenderness is over a growth plate and the radiographs are normal, the patient is treated as if he or she has a Salter-Harris type I fracture.
- Infection, metabolic disorders, and neoplasm, as well as normal variants in growth patterns, may have radiographic similarities to physeal fractures or injuries.

Making the Diagnosis

- *Radiographs* should include oblique views if no obvious fracture is present on the anteroposterior and lateral images.
  - Some physeal fractures can be difficult to visualize with radiographs because the potentially displaced segment is cartilaginous and radiolucent.
  - Salter-Harris type I fractures commonly have normal radiographs.
- *Computed tomography* scan may be helpful for evaluating type III and IV fractures that have extension into the articular surface, to assess the magnitude of articular displacement.
- *Magnetic resonance imaging* may help to differentiate bony versus soft tissue injury and may identify a subtle, non-displaced injury

Treatment

- Displaced fractures require urgent referral to an orthopaedic surgeon. If a closed manipulation is required, it must be performed acutely.
- Non-displaced fractures should be splinted and the patient made non-weight bearing or placed in a sling until reevaluation by a pediatric orthopaedic specialist or pediatric sports medicine physician within 10 to 14 days.
- A non-displaced physeal fracture may not be apparent on the initial radiographs, despite symptoms and clinical findings that suggest a fracture.
  - In such cases, splinting of the limb and non-weight bearing for protection and pain control is recommended.
  - The patient should be reevaluated by a pediatric orthopaedic specialist or pediatric sports medicine physician within 10 to 14 days
  - Repeat radiographs in 10 to 14 days may reveal evidence of bony healing, with the appearance of periosteal new bone verifying the diagnosis.
- Fracture management depends on the severity of the injury, location of the injury, and age of the patient.
  - Depending on the age of the child, significant potential remodeling may occur and thus, a less than anatomic reduction may be acceptable.
  - As a child gets closer to skeletal maturity, remodeling is less reliable and criteria for acceptable alignment are more strict.
  - Surgical intervention is required for treatment of open fractures or for a fracture that cannot be adequately reduced by closed means.
  - Open reduction is commonly required for type III and IV fractures to ensure anatomic reduction of joint surface and physis.

Expected Outcomes/Prognosis

- Physeal fractures heal much more quickly than diaphyseal fractures.
- Most physeal injuries heal without complication.
- Incidence of *physeal arrest* after physeal fracture is low, ranging from 1% to 6.5%.
  — Manifests by formation of a bony bridge across some, or all, of the cartilage of the growth plate. This is referred to as a bony bar (Figure 35-1).
  — Cessation of normal growth from the involved physis leads to development of a progressive angular deformity or a limb-length discrepancy.
  — Premature cessation of growth depends on several factors including the location of the fracture, the bone involved, the extent of injury to the physis, and the amount of remaining growth.
  — Physeal arrest is most common with fractures of the distal femur, distal tibia, and proximal tibia.
  — Partial growth arrest secondary to bony bar formation is most common with type IV fractures.
- Continued monitoring over 12 to 24 months is required.
- Harris growth arrest lines may be seen during follow-up and may be helpful in early identification of a problem with physeal function (Figure 35-2).
- Complete premature physeal closure cannot be repaired. If the child has considerable growth remaining, a treatment intervention would be required to prevent a significant limb-length discrepancy.
  — Treatment might include a closure of the contralateral limb physis (epiphysiodesis) or a limb-lengthening procedure.
  — For partial premature physeal closure, a physeal bar resection
  — A realignment osteotomy to improve angular deformity may be required (combined with an epiphysiodesis procedure to address potential limb-length discrepancy.)

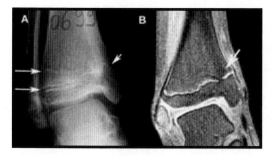

Figure 35-1. A, Radiograph. B, Magnetic resonance imaging. Demonstrate physeal arrest with bar formation and growth abnormality (arrow). Courtesy of Kristina Kjeldsberg, MD.

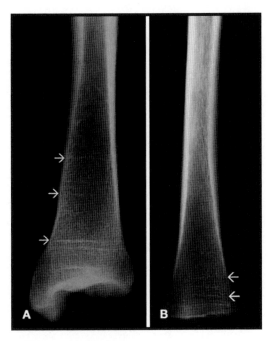

Figure 35-2. Harris growth arrest lines (arrows). Available at: www.proteinpower.com/drmike/ wp-content/uploads/2009/04/ harris-lines-blog.jpg.

When to Refer

- See "Treatment" on page 361.

Relevant *International Classification of Diseases, Ninth Revision, Clinical Modification* Codes

- **813.42** Fracture, distal radius
- **824.8** Fracture, distal tibia
- **824.8** Fracture, distal fibula
- **812.49** Fracture, distal humerus
- **813.43** Fracture, distal ulna
- **812.09** Fracture, proximal humerus
- **821.29** Fracture, distal femur

CHAPTER 36

Common Fractures of the Upper and Lower Extremities

Fractures About the Elbow

GENERAL INFORMATION

- The most common severe low-energy injuries in children
- Most pediatric elbow fractures are sustained by a fall on an outstretched hand (commonly abbreviated as FOOSH).
- Because most pediatric elbow fractures result from a fall, physical abuse is an unlikely mechanism unless the child is non-ambulatory or there are other indications of non-accidental trauma.
- Referral to an orthopaedic specialist is recommended (Box 36-1).

Box 36-1. Reasons to Refer Swollen Elbows to an Orthopaedic Specialist

While not all pediatric elbow injuries are severe, many have the potential for adverse outcomes; therefore, every elbow fracture should be referred to a pediatric orthopaedic surgeon.

Because of the difficulty of pediatric elbow injury differential diagnosis, every child with a swollen elbow after trauma should be referred to a pediatric orthopaedic surgeon.

Supracondylar Elbow Fracture (Supracondylar Fracture of the Humerus)

INTRODUCTION/ETIOLOGY/EPIDEMIOLOGY

- Fracture of the distal humerus
- The most common and most dangerous pediatric elbow fracture
- Typically caused by a fall on an outstretched hand

- The average age is between 4 and 8 years, but may occur between walking age and 12 years of age. The reason for this age distribution is the frequency of falling in addition to the development of the distal humerus and elbow joint.
  - During early childhood, the supracondylar region of the elbow is composed of a small amount of relatively soft bone with a large hole in it—the olecranon fossa.
  - The olecranon fossa accommodates the proximal end of the ulna, the olecranon, when the elbow is extended.
  - Normal childhood ligamentous laxity allows the elbow to *hyperextend*. Hence, when the child falls on an outstretched hand, the elbow hyperextends and drives the olecranon into the olecranon fossa, fracturing the humerus just above the medial and lateral elbow condyles proximal to the elbow joint; hence the term *supracondylar* fracture of the humerus.

SIGNS AND SYMPTOMS

- The mechanism is usually a fall on an outstretched hand (FOOSH).
- Often parents may incorrectly infer and state that the child "fell on his elbow." This is true only in the very rare *flexion type* of supracondylar fracture.
- Sometimes, with mild fractures in toddlers, there is no history other than "She just doesn't want to use her arm," and presentation for medical care may be delayed. This is not an indication of abuse or neglect.
- The fracture is far more likely to have serious neurovascular complications if the child fell from a height, such as a tree, window, or bars, compared with a slip and fall on level ground.
- Tips for evaluating elbow fractures are shown in Box 36-2.

Box 36-2. Tips for Evaluating Fractures About the Elbow

Evaluate shoulder, wrist, and hand for associated injuries.
- Concomitant injuries include scuffing of the hand, distal radius and ulna fractures, and proximal humerus or clavicle fractures.
- In the rare flexion-type supracondylar fracture, there may be scraping or bruising over the posterior olecranon (point of the elbow).

Evaluate neurovascular status of the hand including color, temperature, pulse, capillary refill in the digits, strength, and sensation. Compare with uninjured side.
- For the *radial nerve,* check sensation in the dorsal first web space and ability to actively extend the thumb.
- For the *median nerve,* check sensation on the palmar surface of the index finger and active thumb interphalangeal joint flexion.
- For the *ulnar nerve,* check sensation in the palmar tip of the little finger and active abduction of the little finger.
  - Ability to form a circle with thumb and index finger (the O sign) indicates intact median and ulnar nerve function (Figure 36-1).
  - In severe fractures, there is often immediate bruising and dimpling of the skin in the antecubital fossa where the sharp spike of bone of the proximal fracture fragment impales the deep dermis. The spike may completely penetrate the anterior skin resulting in an open fracture.

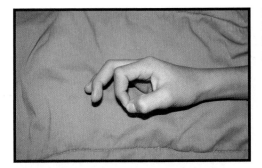

Figure 36-1. Clinical examination indicating the O sign. The anterior interosseous nerve (branch of the median nerve) is intact.

- Physical examination findings depend on severity and displacement of the fracture.
  — Type 1 fractures: minimal swelling and mild loss of elbow motion
  — Type 2 fractures: moderate swelling, loss of motion and deformity
  — Type 3 fractures: severe pain, rapid swelling, ecchymosis, and deformity
    - Nerve injuries are common, but fortunately nearly all are neurapraxias (stretch injuries) and resolve spontaneously over several days to months.
    - Vascular injuries are less common but can be devastating, resulting in Volkmann ischemic contracture (Figure 36-2). The brachial artery lies directly anterior to the elbow in the antecubital fossa and can be damaged by stretching or direct impalement by a spike of bone.

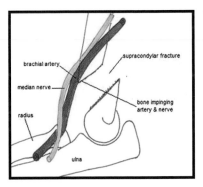

Figure 36-2. Volkman ischemic fracture is caused by damage to the brachial artery.

MAKING THE DIAGNOSIS

- Diagnosis is made on anteroposterior (AP) and lateral radiographs of the elbow (Figure 36-3).
- If the elbow is minimally swollen and gentle positioning is comfortably allowed, an oblique view is also obtained, which is best for evaluating for subtle lateral condyle, olecranon, or radial head fracture.
- Supracondylar fractures are classified as closed versus open and displaced versus non-displaced using the Gartland classification (Box 36-3).

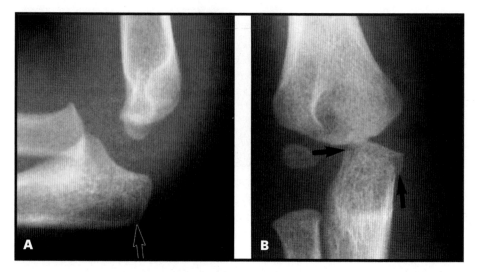

Figure 36-3. A, Lateral view of the elbow shows the fracture line beginning at the posterior tip of the olecranon (arrow). B, Anteroposterior view of the elbow shows mild medial displacement of the proximal metaphyseal region of the olecranon (arrows). Reproduced with permission from Johnson TR, Steinbach LS (eds): *Essentials of Musculoskeletal Imaging.* Rosemont, IL: American Academy of Orthopaedic Surgeons; 2004.

Box 36-3. Modified Gartland Classification of Pediatric Supracondylar Fractures

Type 1	Fracture is undisplaced or minimally displaced.
Type 2	Obvious fracture line with displacement, cortex still intact.
Type 3	Fracture is displaced with no cortical contact.

TREATMENT

- Type 1 fractures are treated in a long arm cast for about 3 weeks.
  — Recovery is rapid and full.
  — Therapy is not required.
- Type 2 fractures are treated by closed reduction (manipulation) and percutaneous pinning.
  — Reduction is required to prevent cubitus varus (gunstock) deformity (see Figure 4-21). While this deformity causes little or no dysfunction or pain, parents are most unhappy.
  — Pinning is a more secure method of maintaining reduction and is safer than casting.
- Type 3 fractures require surgical repair with closed reduction and percutaneous pinning, using fluoroscopy under general anesthesia (Figure 36-4).
  — Several recent studies have shown that these fractures may be safely observed in the hospital overnight, allowing for fasting and daytime surgery under better operating conditions.
  — There is no incision unless the reduction is difficult or there is a vascular problem.
  — Open fractures are surgically debrided.

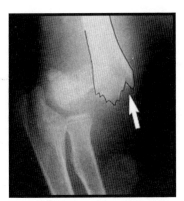

Figure 36-4. Radiograph of a displaced supracondylar fracture (humerus is outlined). Reproduced with permission from Sullivan JA, Anderson SJ (eds). *Care of the Young Athlete*. Rosemont, IL: American Academy of Orthopaedic Surgeons; 2000.

— Fasciotomies are performed if there was any significant period of ischemia.
— The immediate postoperative period may be the most dangerous time for ischemia. Tight bandages, true casts, and hyperflexion of the elbow must be avoided during this period.
— Even with meticulous care, an initially silent intimal tear may later thrombose and obstruct arterial supply to the forearm. Microvascular surgery may be required to repair or vein graft a brachial artery injury.
— After surgery, the elbow is immobilized for about 3 weeks, followed by removal of the pins in the office without the need for anesthesia.
— Normal range of motion and full activities are restored by 3 months in most cases.

EXPECTED OUTCOMES/PROGNOSIS

• Results are favorable for all fracture types when adequate reduction is achieved.
• Little if any remodeling can be expected about a child's distal humerus fracture. Therefore, any deformity noted shortly after fracture healing is likely permanent.
• Unreduced type 3 fractures invariably lead to cubitus varus. This deformity will not remodel and requires osteotomy for correction.

WHEN TO REFER

• All supracondylar fractures should be referred to a pediatric orthopaedic surgeon.
• The urgency of orthopaedic evaluation will depend on the severity of the fracture, the comfort of the child, and whether there are associated soft tissue injuries.
— A pulseless extremity or open fracture are orthopaedic emergencies that warrant immediate surgical attention.
— A non-displaced fracture that is already several days old can be splinted and seen by an orthopaedist nonurgently.

RELEVANT *INTERNATIONAL CLASSIFICATION OF DISEASES, NINTH REVISION, CLINICAL MODIFICATION (ICD-9-CM)* CODES

• **812.41**   Supracondylar fracture of humerus, closed
• **812.51**   Supracondylar fracture of humerus, open

LATERAL CONDYLE ELBOW FRACTURE

Introduction/Etiology/Epidemiology

- Fractures of varying portions of the lateral half of the distal humerus (Figure 36-5).
- Twenty percent of pediatric elbow fractures
- Two generally accepted mechanisms
  — The fracture is avulsed off the distal humerus by a bending varus force as the child falls onto an outstretched hand.
  — The radial head knocks off the lateral condyle when an axial force is applied to a partially flexed elbow.
- The large portion of cartilage and small sliver of attached bone makes lateral condyle fractures difficult to diagnose and heal. Cartilage is radiographically invisible and does not easily heal to adjacent cartilage even if rigidly fixed.

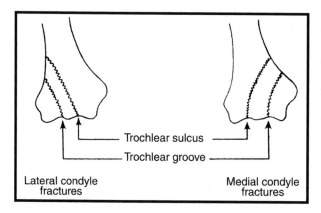

Figure 36-5. Typical fracture patterns of lateral and medial condyles of distal humerus in children. From Milch H. Fractures and fracture-dislocations of the humeral condyles. *J Trauma.* 1964;3:592–607. Reprinted by permission of Wolters Kluwer Health.

Signs and Symptoms

- Non-displaced fractures present with minimal lateral soft tissue swelling and tenderness and no deformity.
- Grossly displaced and rotated fracture fragments present with severe swelling and bruising.
- Rarely associated with nerve and vascular problems because the elbow soft tissue envelope is mostly intact.
- Radial nerve injuries and compartment syndromes can occur, so careful evaluation is always required (see Box 36-2).

Making the Diagnosis

- In an older child with a grossly displaced fracture, *AP and lateral radiographs of the elbow* will reveal the fracture.
- In a young child with a minimally displaced fracture, the only radiographic indication may be a *fat pad sign*, also known as a sail sign. These lucencies are caused by the normal periarticular fat pads being displaced by an acute effusion of the elbow joint. A fat pad sign following trauma, despite the absence of a clear fracture line, indicates a probable fracture.

- An *oblique elbow view* is obtained when AP and lateral views do not show a fracture but there is clinical suspicion or a fat pad sign.

Treatment

- Non-displaced fractures are casted for several weeks with the elbow at 90 degrees and the forearm supinated to decrease distraction at the fracture site.
- Minimally displaced fractures may be casted or percutaneously pinned.
- Displaced fractures (greater than 2 mm displacement) require open reduction and internal fixation with pinning.

Expected Outcomes/Prognosis

- With proper treatment, results are generally favorable.
- Adequate reduction is essential, as nonunions have been reported even with minimally displaced fractures.
- Because of their frequent subtle clinical and radiographic presentation, lateral condyle fractures may be misdiagnosed as contusions, sprains, or pulled elbows, or undertreated with a splint or cast when surgery is indicated. These may present years later with progressive elbow deformity, limitation of motion, and tardy ulnar nerve palsy.
  — Tardy ulnar nerve palsy is due to tension and tethering of the nerve in the cubital tunnel caused by the deformity.
  — Not all require surgery. Factors to consider are age of the child, stable versus progressive deformity, limitations of motion, pain, athletic or occupational pursuits, and tardy ulnar nerve palsy.
  — Elbow deformity surgery is challenging and may involve osteotomy of the humerus, nerve transfer, and grafting or fixation of the nonunion site.

When to Refer

- All lateral condyle fractures should be referred to a pediatric orthopaedic surgeon.

Relevant ICD-9-CM Codes

- **812.42**   Lateral condyle elbow fracture, closed
- **812.52**   Lateral condyle elbow fracture, open

MEDIAL EPICONDYLE ELBOW FRACTURE

Introduction/Etiology/Epidemiology

- Avulsion of the medial epicondyle from the remainder of the distal humerus, through the medial apophyseal growth plate
- Five percent to 10% of all pediatric elbow fractures
- Most common between 9 and 14 years of age
- More common in males
- Up to 50% are associated elbow dislocation.

- Common mechanisms
  - Fall onto outstretched hand with valgus stress applied to the elbow
  - Sudden, forceful contraction of the flexor or pronator muscle group that originates from the medial epicondyle
  - Chronic forms of this fracture occur with repetitive stress from pitching, as seen in Little League elbow (see Chapter 29).
  - Acute-on-chronic fractures may also occur.

Signs and Symptoms

- Swelling, bruising, tenderness of the medial elbow, and limited elbow motion
- The ulnar nerve, because of its proximity to the medial epicondyle, may be injured, causing pain paresthesias or numbness along the medial forearm into the fourth and fifth fingers.
- If elbow motion is greatly limited, entrapment of the medial epicondyle within the elbow joint must be considered.
- If the elbow is dislocated, there will be an obvious deformity.
- If there was a transient subluxation or dislocation with spontaneous relocation, there will be considerable swelling of the entire elbow and laxity with valgus elbow stress testing, indicating additional injury to capsular and ligamentous structures.

Making the Diagnosis

- Diagnosis is made on *AP and lateral radiographs of the elbow.*
  - In non-displaced fractures, the AP film will show some mild medial soft tissue swelling and slight widening of the medial apophyseal growth plate when compared with the uninjured elbow.
  - In displaced fractures, there is more soft tissue swelling and the fragment is clearly displaced medially and distally (Figure 36-6).
  - If the fragment is not clearly seen, consider intra-articular entrapment.

Treatment

- Treatment is somewhat controversial and depends on degree of displacement, associated elbow instability, intended sports participation, and handedness.
- Most are treated nonoperatively, with less than 3 weeks of immobilization in a long-arm cast or splint followed by 4 to 6 weeks of physical therapy for motion and strengthening.
- Indications for surgical fixation
  - Displacement more than 10 mm
  - Fracture fragment entrapped within joint
  - Ulnar neuropathy
  - Valgus instability
- Displaced fractures (greater than 5 mm) in the throwing arm of athletes or in gymnasts are more likely to undergo internal fixation with a screw.

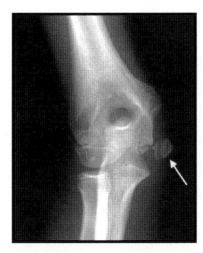

Figure 36-6. Radiograph demonstrating a displaced fracture of the medial epicondyle (arrow). Reproduced with permission from Griffin LY (ed): *Essentials of Musculoskeletal Care,* 3rd edition. Rosemont, IL: American Academy of Orthopaedic Surgeons; 2005.

Expected Outcomes/Prognosis

- Non-displaced fractures have excellent outcomes with good elbow function and little elbow instability.
- Displaced fractures treated nonoperatively also have good outcomes despite healing via fibrous union.
- Outcome after surgical fixation is generally good but depends on the accuracy of the reduction and stability of the fixation. Potential long-term complications include chronic pain, instability, loss of motion, or ulnar neuropathy.

When to Refer

- Refer to a pediatric orthopaedist
  — Displaced fractures
  — Intra-articular entrapment
  — Associated instability
  — Ulnar nerve involvement

Relevant ICD-9-CM Code

- **812.43**   Medial epicondyle elbow fracture, closed

Distal Radius Fractures

- Most common childhood fractures
- Fall on an outstretched hand is most common mechanism but can also occur with direct blow or fall on a flexed wrist.
- Commonly accompanied by fractures of the distal ulna
- The newly formed metaphyseal bone of the distal radius and ulna is soft and easily broken.
- Fractures may range from tiny buckle (torus) fractures of the distal radius to completely displaced and angulated fractures of the distal radius and ulna.

- Because of the mild signs and symptoms, many children with minimal fractures will present for medical care late or not at all.

Distal Radius Fractures: Physical Examination Pearls

- **Evaluate wrist range of motion in pronation and supination, as well as flexion extension and radial and ulnar deviation.**
- **Begin by palpating distal to the injured part, then working toward it.**
- **Examine the elbow carefully, especially if the distal radius fracture is deformed and distracting.**
- **Palpate the scaphoid in the anatomic snuff box, the dorsal space between the extensor pollicis brevis and longus (Figure 36-7).**
- **Palpate the distal radius to determine whether tenderness is localized over the growth plate.**

Distal Radius Fractures: Radiographic Pearl

If a fracture involves bone proximal to the metaphysis, or if there is forearm pain, 2 views of the entire forearm including the elbow and wrist should be obtained.

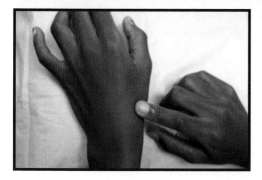

Figure 36-7. Anatomic snuff box.

Buckle (Torus) Fractures

INTRODUCTION/ETIOLOGY/EPIDEMIOLOGY

- Impaction injuries of a single cortex
- If there is even the slightest fracture in the opposite cortex, it is not a buckle fracture.

SIGNS AND SYMPTOMS

- Children often present several days after the event with a guilt-ridden parent stating, "We thought it was only a sprain."
- There is no bruising or deformity and little or no swelling.
- Wrist motion may be complete or partly limited because of pain.

MAKING THE DIAGNOSIS

- *Radiographs (AP and lateral views)* of the wrist are sufficient to make the diagnosis (Figure 36-8).

TREATMENT

- Evidence indicates that buckle fractures have been overtreated in the past.
- There is growing literature addressing treatment with a simple splint that may be gradually removed and non-sport activities resumed at the patient and family's discretion (Figure 36-9).
- Healing is reliable, so follow-up radiographs are unnecessary.
- Average splinting time is 2 to 4 weeks.
- If the child wishes to play sports at anytime up to 6 weeks after the fracture, a cast or splint can be used to protect the extremity from further injury.
- The major concern with returning to play in a cast or splint is protecting *other* players from impact by the hard cast. Most soccer leagues allow players to participate if their casts are over-wrapped with a soft material.

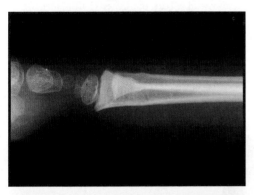

Figure 36-8. Typical buckle (torus) fracture of the distal radius. Note that only one cortex is fractured.

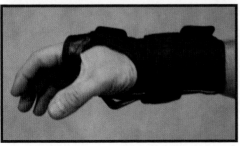

Figure 36-9. Commercial wrist splint for immobilization of buckle fracture.

WHEN TO REFER

- Most buckle fractures can be treated by the child's pediatrician or primary care physician.
- Refer to a pediatric orthopaedic specialist if symptoms persist after 3 to 4 weeks of immobilization.

EXPECTED OUTCOMES/PROGNOSIS

- Prognosis is excellent for complete healing without complications.

RELEVANT *ICD-9-CM* CODE

- **813.45**   Torus fracture of distal radius

Greenstick Fractures

INTRODUCTION/ETIOLOGY/EPIDEMIOLOGY

- Complete fracture through the bone with varying degrees of angulation
- A minimal greenstick fracture of the distal radius, usually at the metaphyseal and diaphyseal junction, has also been called a slipper fracture because of its propensity to angulate (slip) if treated with the same benign neglect as with a buckle fracture.

SIGNS AND SYMPTOMS

- Mild to moderate pain, little swelling, no bruising, and a deformity
  — The child's thick layer of periosteum, like the flexible bark of a green (living) tree branch, explains these findings—the periosteum limits motion and thus pain at the fracture site, and contains any bleeding, thus limiting swelling and bruising.

MAKING THE DIAGNOSIS

- *Radiographs (AP and lateral views)* of the wrist are sufficient to make the diagnosis (Figure 36-10).

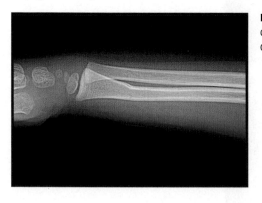

Figure 36-10. Radiograph of the wrist demonstrating greenstick fracture of distal radius.

TREATMENT

- Most are treated by closed reduction (manipulation) and casting.
- Follow-up radiographs in the cast are necessary to detect loss of reduction.
- Repeat manipulation is sometimes required.
- Duration of cast immobilization is 4 weeks; this is sometimes followed by a week of splinting.

WHEN TO REFER

- Refer all greenstick distal radius fractures immediately to a pediatric orthopaedic specialist for reduction.

EXPECTED OUTCOMES/PROGNOSIS

- Some re-angulation may occur during the healing process, but fortunately most angulated fractures of the distal radius will eventually remodel.
- In a child with 5 years of growth remaining, angulation of up to 30 degrees has the potential to remodel acceptably. Remodeling potential decreases by 5 degrees for every remaining year of growth less than 5 years.

RELEVANT *ICD-9-CM* CODE

- **813.40**   Distal radius fracture, closed

Displaced Fractures of the Distal Radius

INTRODUCTION/ETIOLOGY/EPIDEMIOLOGY

- If sufficient energy is imparted to the palm in a fall, the distal radius, with or without the distal ulna, can be broken off, with various degrees of displacement.
- In high-energy falls, such as out of a tree, the fracture may be open.

SIGNS AND SYMPTOMS

- Acute pain and deformity
- Limited ability to move wrist or fingers or rotate forearm
- Acute swelling and compression of the median nerve causes pain and numbness in the median dermatome (palm and palmar surfaces of thumb, index, and middle fingers).
- Bleeding and swelling may cause a *compartment syndrome* of the volar forearm, clinically manifested by severe pain refractory to normal measures of splinting and opioid adminis-tration, inability to wiggle the fingers, and severe pain with passive finger stretch (Chapter 39). This is an acute surgical emergency requiring fasciotomy.

- Open fractures are usually obvious, but sometimes the only indication may be a tiny puncture wound on the volar surface of the forearm, where the proximal fracture fragment transiently exited the skin at the time of injury.
  — It is critical to recognize an open fracture because of the potential for contamination of the bone and fracture hematoma, leading to infection and possible devastating consequences if not urgently surgically debrided, and treated with antibiotics and tetanus prophylaxis as indicated.

MAKING THE DIAGNOSIS

- *Radiographs (AP and lateral views)* of the wrist are sufficient to make the diagnosis.

TREATMENT

- Most can be treated by closed reduction.
- Rarely, open reduction is required to achieve satisfactory alignment, such as for a displaced overriding fracture of the distal radius with an intact ulna—the reduction is more difficult than if both bones are fractured.
- Following manipulation, the reduction is held with a cast or percutaneous pin.

WHEN TO REFER

- Refer all displaced distal radius fractures immediately to a pediatric orthopaedic specialist for reduction.

EXPECTED OUTCOMES/PROGNOSIS

- With prompt and proper treatment, most displaced distal radius fractures have an excellent long-term prognosis.
  — Residual angulation is the most common complication.
  — There may also be some loss of forearm rotation.
  — Less common complications include median nerve injury and compartment syndrome.

Articular Fractures

- **Fractures extending to the joint surface of the distal radius are much less common in children than in adults because the softer metaphyseal bone and epiphyseal plate have a protective effect by failing first with axial force.**
- **When fractures of the articular surface do occur in children, they are far less likely to be comminuted than in the more brittle bone of an adult.**
- **The goal of treatment is anatomic reduction.**

RELEVANT *ICD-9-CM* CODES

- **813.40**   Distal radius fracture, closed
- **813.44**   Distal radius and ulna fracture, closed
- **813.50**   Distal radius fracture, open
- **813.54**   Distal radius and ulna fracture, open

Scaphoid Fractures

INTRODUCTION/ETIOLOGY/EPIDEMIOLOGY

- Scaphoid is the most commonly fractured carpal bone in children and adults.
- Rare in young children but incidence rises with age, peaking at 15 years of age.
- Fall on an outstretched hand is most common mechanism, often while engaged in sports.
- Often associated with other injuries (eg, lunate or distal radius fractures)

SIGNS AND SYMPTOMS

- May present late (days to years) because it was thought to be a sprain due to minimal swelling and lack of deformity.
- Tenderness in the anatomic snuff box, the dorsal space between the extensor pollicis longus and brevis
- There may be tenderness and swelling on the palmar surface of the scaphoid.
- Bruising and deformity are not typically seen.
- Wrist motion and grip strength are limited by pain.

MAKING THE DIAGNOSIS

- Diagnosis is made on *radiographs—3 views (AP, lateral, oblique) of the wrist* are typically sufficient.
  - If a scaphoid fracture is suspected and 3 views of the wrist are negative, an additional oblique or scaphoid view (AP view with wrist in ulnar deviation) is ordered (Figure 36-11).
  - In younger children, more of the scaphoid is cartilage, making it less likely that a fracture will be seen. A radiographic clue is displacement of the periarticular wrist fat pad (wrist fat pad sign).
- If a scaphoid fracture is clinically suspected but radiographs are negative, a thumb spica cast is applied and films are repeated out of the cast 2 to 3 weeks later. *Magnetic resonance imaging* is ordered if an immediate determination is needed (Figure 36-12).

TREATMENT

- Non-displaced fractures are immobilized for 6 weeks in a thumb spica cast.
- Non-displaced fractures that are identified late (more than 10 days) may require up to 10 weeks of immobilization.

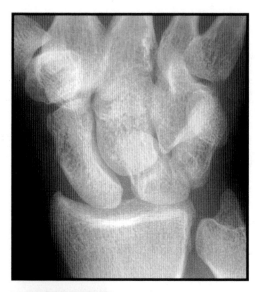

Figure 36-11. Anteroposterior radiograph of wrist demonstrating scaphoid fracture. From Metzl JD. *Sports Medicine in the Pediatric Office.* Elk Grove Village, IL: American Academy of Pediatrics; 2008.

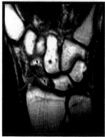

Figure 36-12. Magnetic resonance imaging (MRI) of wrist demonstrating scaphoid fracture. It is important to note that most cases of scaphoid fracture will not show on initial radiograph series. Diagnosis is made by history and physical examination. MRI can be used to confirm presence of a scaphoid fracture. From Metzl JD. *Sports Medicine in the Pediatric Office.* Elk Grove Village, IL: American Academy of Pediatrics; 2008.

- Displaced fractures undergo surgical open reduction and internal fixation because of the risk of nonunion and avascular necrosis.
- Because of the importance and fragility of the scaphoid and the possibility of long-term disability, orthopaedists are more reluctant to allow sports participation by children casted for scaphoid fractures than for greenstick or buckle fractures.

WHEN TO REFER

- Refer all scaphoid fractures to a pediatric orthopaedic specialist.

EXPECTED OUTCOMES/PROGNOSIS

- The scaphoid is particularly prone to nonunion and avascular necrosis because of its fragile blood supply.

RELEVANT *ICD-9-CM* CODE

- **814.01**   Scaphoid fracture

Common Fractures of the Lower Extremity

FEMORAL SHAFT FRACTURES

Introduction/Etiology/Epidemiology

- Account for 1.4% to 1.7% of pediatric fractures.
- Incidence is highest between 2 and 3 years of age and in mid-adolescence.
- Incidence is 2.6 times higher in boys than in girls.
- Most common mechanism in early childhood is a fall.
- Most common mechanisms in adolescents are sports and motor vehicle accidents.
- In infants, most femoral shaft fractures are caused by nonaccidental trauma.
- Pathologic fractures, while rare, can occur with osteogenesis imperfecta, tumor, or osteopenia.

Signs and Symptoms

- Thigh pain, swelling, and inability to bear weight after acute trauma
- Can be associated with significant bleeding within the thigh, although unlike in adults, the need for blood replacement is rare.

Making the Diagnosis

- Anteroposterior and lateral radiographs of the femur that include the hip and knee joints are sufficient (Figure 36-13).

Treatment

- Treatment depends on age and size of the patient.
  - *Infants* are treated with a single leg spica cast or Pavlik harness for 4 weeks. Up to 45 degrees of angulation is acceptable, given the capacity for remodeling.
  - *Children up to 6 years of age* are most commonly treated with intraoperative closed reduction and spica casting for 6 weeks.
  - *Children between 6 and 10 years of age* can be treated in a variety of ways, including immobilization in spica cast for 8 weeks, although current preferred method is flexible intramedullary nail fixation.
  - *Larger patients* and those in their *postadolescent years*
    - Because of greater risk for angulation or loss of fracture position with the flexible nail, rigid intramedullary rod fixation is sometimes used. Insertion of these rods carries a risk of avascular necrosis. Alternative methods of treatment include sub-muscular plating and external fixation.

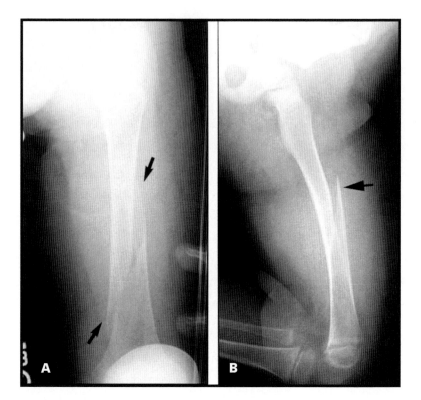

Figure 36-13. A, Fracture of the femoral shaft—anteroposterior (AP) view. AP view of the femur in a young (aged 2 to 4 years) child shows a spiral fracture of the distal third of the femur with mild lateral displacement (arrows). B, Fracture of the femoral shaft—lateral view. Lateral view of the femur in the same patient shown in A shows a spiral fracture of the distal third of the femur with mild anterior displacement (arrow). Reproduced with permission from Johnson TR, Steinbach LS (eds): *Essentials of Musculoskeletal Imaging.* Rosemont, IL: American Academy of Orthopaedic Surgeons; 2004.

Expected Outcomes/Prognosis

- Most femoral shaft fractures heal well without complications or long-term disability.
- Potential complications include angular and rotational deformities, nonunion (rare), infection, muscle weakness, and leg-length discrepancy (most common).
  - In children between 2 and 10 years of age, leg-length discrepancy most commonly results from overgrowth of the injured side caused by growth acceleration.
  - Patients older than 10 years are more likely to have shortening of the injured side.
  - Patients with leg-length discrepancy less than 2 cm generally notice no alteration in their stride or knee mechanics.

When to Refer

- Promptly refer all femur fractures to an orthopaedic surgeon.

Relevant ICD-9-CM *Codes*

- **821.01**   Fracture, femur, closed
- **821.11**   Fracture, femur, open

DISTAL FEMORAL PHYSEAL FRACTURES

Introduction/Etiology/Epidemiology

- Account for approximately 5% of all physeal fractures.
- Usually result from high-energy trauma to a hyperextended knee, leading to anterior displacement of the epiphysis.
- Most are Salter-Harris type I or II.
- Associated with a high potential for growth problems.

Signs and Symptoms

- Knee pain, swelling, limited range of motion, and inability to bear weight
- Tenderness over distal femoral growth plate
- Careful neurovascular examination is performed to rule out injury to the popliteal artery or sciatic nerve.

Making the Diagnosis

- Anteroposterior and lateral radiographs of the knee are usually sufficient.
- A notch or tunnel view may necessary to identify Salter-Harris III fractures.

Treatment

- Anatomic reduction is required for Salter-Harris type II, III, and IV fractures because even a small amount of physeal displacement can result in formation of an osseous bar, increasing the risk for limb-length discrepancy or angular deformity.
- Closed reduction may be possible for non-displaced and minimally displaced fractures, although screw or pin fixation is advised for most of these unstable injuries.

Expected Outcomes/Prognosis

- Approximately 50% develop leg-length discrepancy or angular deformity caused by formation of osseous bars that bridge the physis.
- Loss of joint motion is a less common complication.

When to Refer

- Promptly refer all distal femoral physeal fractures to an orthopaedic surgeon.

Relevant ICD-9-CM *Code*

- **821.22**   Fracture, femur, distal physis

PROXIMAL TIBIAL PHYSEAL FRACTURES

Introduction/Etiology/Epidemiology

- Rare but have a high rate of complication.
- Usually result from a direct blow to the lateral aspect of the knee.

Signs and Symptoms

- Knee pain, swelling, and inability to bear weight after acute trauma
- Tenderness over proximal tibial growth plate
- Careful neurovascular examination is performed to rule out injury to the popliteal artery or sciatic nerve.

Making the Diagnosis

- Anteroposterior and lateral radiographs of the knee are sufficient.

Treatment

- Non-displaced fractures are usually treated in a long leg cast with the knee flexed approximately 15 degrees.
- Displaced fractures must be treated with great care because the patient is at high risk for vascular injury and compartment syndrome.

Expected Outcomes/Prognosis

- These patients must be followed for several years because they are at high risk for angular deformity or leg-length discrepancy.

When to Refer

- Promptly refer all proximal tibial physeal fractures to an orthopaedic surgeon.

Relevant ICD-9-CM Code

- **823.00**   Fracture, tibia, proximal physis

TIBIAL TUBERCLE AVULSION FRACTURES

Introduction/Etiology/Epidemiology

- Avulsion of the tibial tubercle apophysis caused by sudden forceful contraction of the quadriceps
- Account for less than 3% of physeal injuries.
- Most common during adolescence (14–16 years of age)
- Usually occur during sports or activities with repetitive jumping and contraction of the quadriceps (eg, basketball, volleyball).
- Osgood-Schlatter disease is a risk factor.

Signs and Symptoms

- Acute onset of painful pop in the knee during jumping or landing
- Difficulty bearing weight
- Swelling and tenderness over tibial tubercle
- Unable to perform a straight leg raise

Making the Diagnosis

- Anteroposterior and lateral radiographs of the knee are sufficient.
  — Distinguish from Osgood-Schlatter disease in which there is pain at the tibial tubercle and sometimes mild fragmentation of the apophysis on radiographs, but no fracture.
- Watson-Jones classification system
  — Type I: fracture through the small distal portion of the tibial tuberosity
  — Type II: fracture line divides the tuberosity from the proximal tibial plateau.
  — Type III: fracture line extends from the tibial tuberosity through the primary ossification center into the joint.

Treatment

- Types I and II
  — Long leg cast immobilization with knee in extension for 4 to 6 weeks
  — Physical therapy is often necessary following immobilization.
  — Return to play is allowed when range of motion, strength, and flexibility are normal and pain is resolved.
  — Significantly displaced fractures may require surgical fixation.
- Type III—surgical fixation

Expected Outcomes/Prognosis

- With proper treatment, prognosis is excellent for complete healing and return to previous level of activity.
- Growth disturbance does not occur.

When to Refer

- Non-displaced type I fractures may be managed by primary care physicians who are comfortable with casting.
- Promptly refer to an orthopaedic surgeon
  — Significantly displaced fractures
  — Type III fractures

Relevant ICD-9-CM Code

- **823.00** Avulsion fracture, tibial tubercle

TIBIAL SHAFT FRACTURES

Introduction/Etiology/Epidemiology

- Fractures of the tibia midshaft account for 39% of tibial fractures.
- Most are spiral fractures because of rotation of body weight around the planted foot.
- Isolated, transverse fractures are usually from a high-energy direct blow.

Signs and Symptoms

- Pain, tenderness, and swelling over fracture site
- Difficulty bearing weight

Making the Diagnosis

- Radiographs (AP, lateral) of the tibia that include the knee and ankle joints are sufficient for diagnosis.
- Fracture is nondisplaced if
  — Less than 5 mm displacement in AP and mediolateral directions
  — Less than 15 degrees angulation in AP plane
  — Less than 5 degrees angulation in mediolateral plane
  — Less than 10 degrees of rotation

Treatment

- Non-displaced fractures
  — Closed reduction followed by non-weight bearing, long leg cast with knee in 30 degrees of flexion
  — When radiographs demonstrate sufficient callous, long leg weight-bearing cast may be used until healing is compete (usually 6–10 weeks).
- Displaced fractures
- Require operative management followed by casting for 6 to 8 weeks.

Expected Outcomes/Prognosis

- Patients can resume previous level of activity when clinical and radiographic healing is complete and strength and joint range of motion are normal.
- Physical therapy may be required to regain knee range of motion, muscle strength, flexibility, and function.
- Potential complications include compartment syndrome, nonunion (no signs of radiographic healing by 12 weeks), malunion (varus angulation greater than 15 degrees does not remodel well), and postoperative infection.

When to Refer

- Non-displaced fractures may be managed by primary care physicians who are comfortable with casting.
- Promptly refer to an orthopaedic surgeon
  — All displaced fractures
  — Tibia/fibula fractures

Relevant ICD-9-CM Code

- **823.20**   Tibia shaft fracture

TODDLER FRACTURE

Introduction/Etiology/Epidemiology

- An oblique fracture of the distal tibial shaft with no injury to the fibula
- Usually occur between 9 months and 6 years of age.
- Occur with minimal trauma, usually during a trip and fall while running or playing.

Signs and Symptoms

- Pain
- Refusal to walk or bear weight.
- Tenderness over mid-lower tibia
- No swelling, bruising, or deformity

Making the Diagnosis

- Radiographs (AP, lateral) of the tibia may show the faint oblique fracture line through the distal metaphysis (Figure 36-14), but often appear normal.
  — Oblique views may help delineate the fracture.
- When suspicion is high and radiographs are negative, a *bone scan* can be performed to make the diagnosis, or radiographs can be repeated in 7 to 10 days when fracture line or periosteal reaction may be present.

Treatment

- Immobilization in long leg walking cast for 2 to 3 weeks.
- If fracture presents late (2 or more weeks after injury), casting is not necessary unless symptoms are significant.

Expected Outcomes/Prognosis

- Heals completely within 6 to 8 weeks.

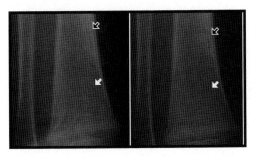

Figure 36-14. Toddler fracture: radiographs of the tibia may show the faint oblique fracture line through the distal metaphysis; radiograph may not show the fracture and seem normal. Courtesy of Loren Yamamoto, MD.

When to Refer

- Toddler fractures may be managed by primary care physicians who are comfortable with casting.
- Refer to an orthopaedic surgeon for casting as necessary.

Relevant ICD-9-CM Code

- **823.20**   Toddler fracture

SALTER-HARRIS TYPE I DISTAL FIBULA FRACTURES

Introduction/Etiology/Epidemiology

- In the skeletally immature athlete, the most common acute injury of the foot and ankle is a Salter-Harris type I fracture of the distal fibula.
- Mechanism is same as for an ankle sprain—acute inversion to the ankle, usually during sports.
- Because the distal fibular physis is weaker than the surrounding ligaments, children are more likely to have a physeal fracture than a ligament sprain after an ankle inversion injury.

Signs and Symptoms

- Lateral ankle pain after an inversion injury
- Painful weight bearing
- Sometimes there is mild swelling.
- Tenderness directly over the distal fibular physis (1 cm above the tip of the fibula)

Differential Diagnosis

- Distinguish from an ankle sprain, which will be associated with tenderness more distally over the ligaments that attach the fibula to the talus.

Making the Diagnosis

- Diagnosis is based on history, physical examination, and radiographs (AP, lateral, and mortise views of the ankle).
- Radiographs may show soft tissue swelling adjacent to the physis or slight widening of the physis, but frequently are normal.
- *Regardless of radiographic findings, any skeletally immature athlete with tenderness at the distal fibula after an inversion injury to the ankle is treated for a Salter-Harris type I fracture of distal fibula.*

Treatment

- Treatment is largely symptomatic and consists of casting or immobilization in a walker boot or air stirrup for 3 to 4 weeks, whichever allows pain-free weight bearing. Otherwise, crutches are required until weight bearing is pain-free.
- Reevaluation should occur in 2 to 3 weeks.
- Athletes can return to play when there is no longer any tenderness at the physis and weight bearing is pain-free, which typically takes about 3 to 4 weeks.

- Rehabilitation is rarely necessary.
- Displaced fractures require reduction and sometimes surgical fixation.

Expected Outcomes/Prognosis

- Prognosis is excellent for compete healing and full return to previous level of activity.
- Growth disturbance occurs in less than 1% and does not affect function.

When to Refer

- Salter-Harris type I injuries may be treated by the primary care physician.
- Refer displaced fractures to a pediatric orthopaedic surgeon.

Relevant ICD-9-CM Code

- **823.81**   Distal fibula fracture

TRANSITIONAL ANKLE FRACTURES (JUVENILE TILLAUX, TRIPLANE)

Introduction/Etiology/Epidemiology

- Occur during early adolescence (12–15 years of age) when the physis is in the process of closing, termed the *transition* period near cessation of skeletal growth.
- The asymmetrical closure of the distal tibial physis (from posteromedial to anterolateral) produces distinct fracture patterns.
- *Tillaux fractures*
  — On external rotation of the ankle, the anterior tibiofibular ligament avulses a small portion of the distal lateral tibial epiphysis, involving the articular surface (Figure 36-15).
  — Common mechanisms include sliding in baseball or softball and skateboard falls.
  — More common in girls
- *Triplane fracture*
  — More severe than Tillaux fracture, resulting from a higher energy trauma
  — Most common mechanism is external rotation (eversion) of a planted foot.
  — Fracture lines propagate in 3 planes of the distal tibial growth plate—axial, sagittal, and frontal (Figure 36-16).
  — Can be 2 or 3 part, depending on degree of physeal closure.
  — Commonly associated with fibular fracture
  — More common in boys

Signs and Symptoms

- Pain, swelling, bruising, and inability to bear weight
- Tenderness at anterior ankle
- Palpate the proximal fibula to evaluate for Maisonneuve fracture.

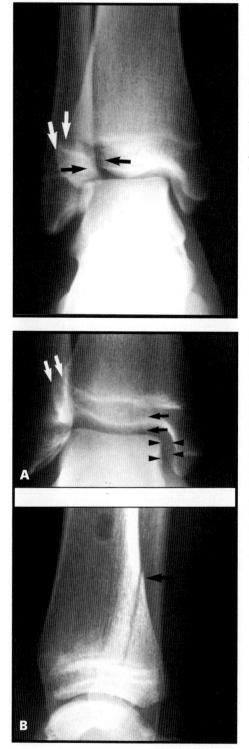

Figure 36-15. Juvenile Tillaux fracture, anteroposterior view of the ankle shows a small anterolateral epiphyseal fragment that is displaced toward the fibula and away from the remaining portion of the epiphysis (black arrows). The white arrows show a subtle displacement of the epiphyseal fragment in relationship to the metaphysis. Reproduced with permission from Johnson TR, Steinbach LS (eds): *Essentials of Musculoskeletal Imaging.* Rosemont, IL: American Academy of Orthopaedic Surgeons; 2004.

Figure 36-16. Triplane fracture. A, Anteroposterior view of the ankle shows a fracture through the anterior portion of the epiphysis (black arrows). The white arrows indicate subtle lateral displacement of the epiphysis, causing widening of the medial ankle mortise (arrowheads). B, Lateral view of ankle shows a posterior metaphyseal fragment (arrow) extending from the physis to the posterior cortex of the tibia. Reproduced with permission from Johnson TR, Steinbach LS (eds): *Essentials of Musculoskeletal Imaging.* Rosemont, IL: American Academy of Orthopaedic Surgeons; 2004.

Making the Diagnosis

- Diagnosis can usually be made on radiographs.
  — Anteroposterior, lateral, and mortise views of ankle are usually sufficient.
  — Oblique view may help identify triplane fracture.
  — Two views of the fibula are performed if there is any fibular tenderness.
- Computed tomography scan is often used to define the propagation of the fracture and amount of intra-articular displacement. Three-dimensional reconstructions are also helpful.

Treatment

- Tillaux fractures
  — Most are nondisplaced so can be treated in non–weight-bearing short leg cast for 4 to 6 weeks.
  — Physical therapy after cast is removed to regain motion and strength
  — For displaced fractures, treatment is similar to that for triplane fractures.
- Triplane fractures
  — For displacement less than 2 mm, closed reduction may be attempted and is successful in 30% to 50% of cases.
  — Displacement of more than 2 mm requires open reduction and internal fixation.
  — After adequate reduction, patients are non-weight bearing in long leg cast for 4 to 6 weeks, followed by limited weight bearing in short leg cast for 4 more weeks.
  — Physical therapy after cast is removed to regain motion and strength
  — After surgery, patients are non-weight bearing in long leg cast for 4 to 6 weeks.

Expected Outcomes/Prognosis

- Prognosis is good for return to previous activity level.
- Complications are uncommon.
- Patients are at risk for early arthritis when reduction is inadequate.

When to Refer

- Promptly refer all transitional fractures to a pediatric orthopaedic surgeon.

Relevant ICD-9-CM Code

- **824.8**   Closed ankle fracture

FRACTURES OF BASE OF THE FIFTH METATARSAL

Introduction/Etiology/Epidemiology

- The 2 most common types of fifth metatarsal fractures in children and adolescents are tuberosity fractures and apophyseal avulsion fractures.
- Caused by the same mechanism that causes an ankle sprain—excessive inversion on a plantar flexed ankle.

Signs and Symptoms

- Sudden, painful pop or snap at lateral foot during inversion injury
- Difficulty bearing weight
- Tenderness, swelling, and bruising along the lateral aspect of the foot

Making the Diagnosis

- Radiographs (AP, lateral, and oblique views of the foot) are sufficient for diagnosis.
- *Tuberosity fracture:* transverse fracture through the tuberosity oriented perpendicular to the long axis of the metatarsal (Figure 29-10b)
  — Differentiate from the normal apophysis, a fleck of bone parallel to the long axis of the fifth metatarsal, visible in girls 9 to 11 years of age and in boys 11 to 14 years of age. The normal apophysis is distinguished from an acute fracture by its lack of tenderness and longitudinal orientation on radiographs.
- *Apophyseal avulsion fracture:* widening or separation of the apophysis
  — Comparison views of the opposite foot can confirm this diagnosis.
  — Tenderness at the apophysis without a history of acute trauma suggests *Iselin disease,* a traction apophysitis of the fifth metatarsal tuberosity (see Chapter 29).

Treatment

- Weight bearing as tolerated in a short leg walking cast, cast shoe, or walking boot
- Return to sports is possible when there is no tenderness at the fracture site and weight bearing is pain-free, which usually occurs at 3 to 4 weeks.
- Rehabilitation is rarely necessary.
- Tuberosity fractures with more than 2 mm of displacement may require surgical fixation for optimal healing.

Expected Outcomes/Prognosis

- Prognosis is excellent for complete healing and return to previous activity level.

When to Refer

- Most of these fractures can be treated by the primary care physician.
- Refer significantly displaced fractures to a pediatric orthopaedic surgeon.

Relevant ICD-9-CM Code

- **825.25**   Closed fracture of metatarsal

CHAPTER 37

Casting and Splinting

Introduction

- Acute management of musculoskeletal injuries often involves splinting or casting for comfort, maintaining alignment, or protection for return to play.
- Appropriate management varies widely by type and location of injury. Refer to appropriate chapters for more detail on injury-specific treatments.
- General guidelines
  — Unstable fractures require secure immobilization. Displaced fractures are usually unstable.
    ▪ Immobilize a joint above and below the site of injury to maintain alignment.
  — Stable fractures, such as buckle fractures (see Figure 36-8) and radiographically healing fractures (Figure 37-1), require less immobilization.
    ▪ Span the injury to adequately stabilize and provide protection, including the nearest joint.
  — Joint injuries are immobilized to the body part above and below.

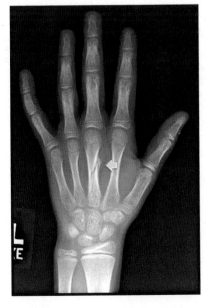

Figure 37-1. Healing fracture with callus formation that will prevent future displacement if there is no reinjury.

Fracture Reduction

* Adequate anesthesia facilitates quick and effective reduction of displaced fractures.
  — Regional blocks or hematoma blocks with local anesthesia (eg, lidocaine) are often effective for phalangeal, metacarpal, and distal radial fractures in older children. Administration should not exceed 4.5 mg/kg lidocaine.
  — Conscious sedation, or even general anesthesia, may be used in younger children, for lower extremity fractures, or for those failing to reduce on initial attempts.

Purpose of Immobilization

* Splint (non-circumferential)
  — May be modified as needed to immobilize and stabilize an acute fracture or soft tissue injury (Table 37-1).
  — At the time of injury
    ▪ Provides stability, limits motion, and offers pain relief until the time of definitive treatment or recovery.
    ▪ Provides protection, but allows for swelling and removal for neurovascular checks.
  — For stable fractures
    ▪ Permits removal for rehabilitation during or prior to return to activities.
* Cast (circumferential)
  — More securely limits motion and prevents easy removal.
  — For potentially unstable fractures, a well-molded, custom-fit cast maintains reduction and decreases the risk for complications.
  — For stable fractures, cast affords protection during return to high-risk athletic activities.

Table 37-1. Stabilization of Fractures and Injuries Based on Location

Location	Preferred Method of Stabilization
Distal interphalangeal joint	Stack splint
Fifth metacarpal fracture	Boxer splint
Thumb ulnar collateral	Gamekeeper splint
Scaphoid	Thumb spica splint
Wrist	Colles splint
Shoulder	Shoulder immobilizer, shoulder stabilizer
Clavicle	Figure-of-eight brace or sling
Cervical spine	C-collar
Hip	Hip abduction brace
Knee	Knee extension brace, hinged knee brace, patellar stabilizing brace
Ankle	Cast boot, stirrup brace, lace-up/figure-of-eight brace
Foot	Post-op shoe

Choice of Immobilization Materials

- Premade splints
  - *Aluminum and foam constructs*
    - Most commonly used to immobilize fingers.
    - Bend to the desired position and are secured with tape or elastic bandage.
  - *Injury-specific prefabricated splints* exist for almost any location and type of injury.
    - Models may include soft (eg, elastic, neoprene, nylon), semirigid (metal stays within a soft body), rigid (eg, plastic, metal), pneumatic, or even dynamic material.
    - Many have built-in hinges that allow movement in some planes.
    - Provide protection for soft tissue injuries or stabilized fractures where low but not negligible risk for reinjury exists, although use for acute management of stable fractures is growing (Table 37-2).
- Plaster—it still works!
  - Easily moldable in any plane and over any prominence
  - May be used for a cast or splint.
  - Preferred for initial management after fracture reduction
- Fiberglass
  - Durable, water-tolerant material. Lighter than plaster.
  - Used for casting non-displaced and stable fractures, although some institutions use it for nearly all fractures.
  - Material of choice for athletes who return to play with a healing but stable fracture
- "Soft" fiberglass
  - Incompletely sets, creating a semirigid cast that allows for some motion and may be removed by the patient when treatment is complete.
  - Appropriate for most buckle fractures.
- Fiberglass encased in synthetic padding
  - Molds in multiple planes for a closer fit.
  - Used to temporarily stabilize a fracture until definitive treatment
  - Products come in precut lengths or may be cut to length from a roll, dipped in (or run under) water (wringing or blotting out the excess), molded to a padded extremity, and secured with an elastic bandage as the product hardens (Figure 37-2a–d).

Table 37-2. Types of Splint Constructs

Splint Type	Use
Volar slab	Distal radius, carpal (except scaphoid)
Ulnar gutter	Fourth or fifth metacarpal or phalangeal
Radial gutter	Scaphoid, gamekeeper thumb
Coaptation	Humerus
Sugar tong	Forearm, lower leg
Posterior	Leg, elbow

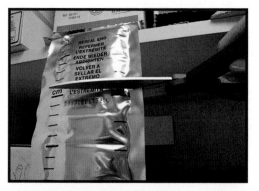

Figure 37-2a. Encased fiberglass is cut to desired length.

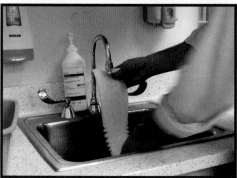

Figure 37-2b. Exposure to water accelerates hardening; excess water should be wrung out.

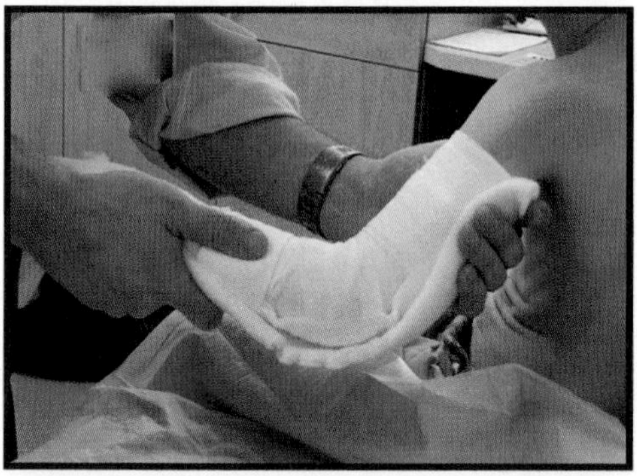

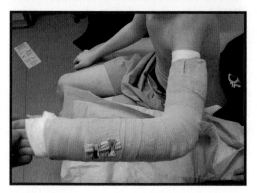

Figure 37-2c. Molding of the splint in the desired position over a padded extremity.

Figure 37-2d. Splint is secured with an elastic bandage.

Application of Plaster or Fiberglass

- Safe and effective application of casts and splints requires experience and should be approached with caution to avoid complications.
- Casting should be performed by providers who have had supervised training in proper application.
- Padding
  — Placed over the skin to protect from irritation during wear and injury during removal.
  — Cotton rolls
    ▪ Preferred for initial treatment
    ▪ Accommodates mild to moderate swelling.
    ▪ Conforms to prominences and is easily removed.
    ▪ After the cast or splint sets, the cotton must remain dry.
  — Synthetic (polypropylene)
    ▪ Repels water, so may allow for getting the cast wet, although some patients may still experience skin problems.
    ▪ More restrictive, so use with caution if continued swelling is a concern.
    ▪ Polypropylene requires a synthetic stockinette to prevent skin reaction.
    ▪ Place protective strips between polypropylene and fiberglass for additional protection during removal.
  — Start distally, wrapping circumferentially and overlapping 50% with each turn while moving proximally.
  — If there is concern for excessive swelling, padding is applied longitudinally.
  — Avoid wrinkles in the lining that may create pressure sites.
  — Four layers suffice in most cases and reduce the risk of burns during removal. A well-padded cast or splint is not the goal—excess padding prevents close molding and allows for increased motion and shear forces that may lead to loss of alignment.
- Splints
  — Apply padding as appropriate (Figure 37-3a).
  — Unwind the roll of plaster or fiberglass and fold over repeatedly at the desired length to create a stack 6 to 10 layers thick, depending on the site to be immobilized and the age of the patient (Figure 37-3b).

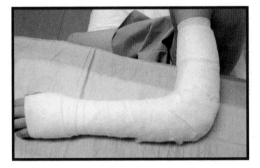

Figure 37-3a. Padding: use 2 to 3 layers of webroll; 3 to 4 over bony prominences.

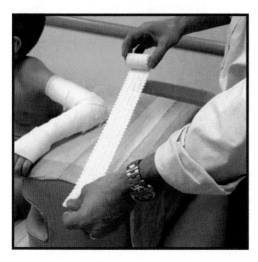

Figure 37-3b. Plaster is creased and folded on itself.

— Do not double the plaster. Excess thickness (more than 12 layers) may lead to burns.
— Dip the stack in water (at manufacturer's recommended temperature), gently remove excess water (Figure 37-3c), then apply to the site and mold in place (Figure 37-3d).
— Secure the splint with an elastic bandage (Figure 37-3e).
• Casts
  — Apply stockinette as appropriate for a clean edge (Figure 37-4a).
  — Place the extremity in the position required to maintain reduction or alignment, or in a neutral position to prevent contractures (see additional chapters for injury-specific recommendations).
  — Apply padding as appropriate (Figure 37-4b).
  — If casting over an ankle, knee, or elbow, first make a splint consisting of 4 to 6 layers to place over the convexity of the joint (Figure 37-4c). To make a cast strong enough using only circumferential wraps results in a cast 3 times thicker in the concavity as in the convexity.
  — Dip the roll of wrap in water (at the manufacturer's suggested temperature), leaving the tail free.
  — Start distally, unwinding the roll as the site is wrapped without stretching. During curing the weave will contract and constrict.
  — Overlap each wrap 50%, avoiding prominent folds or creases (Figure 37-4d). Plaster may need to be folded and tucked (Figure 37-4e).
  — For fiberglass, the wrap may be cut to smoothly wrap the layers. Smooth each circumferential wrap into the prior one to incorporate the layers.
  — After one layer has been placed, position the splint, then wrap back down the extremity to incorporate.
  — Apply additional layers (2–4) as necessary to strengthen the cast.
  — Mold the cast around prominences and as necessary to maintain fracture alignment.

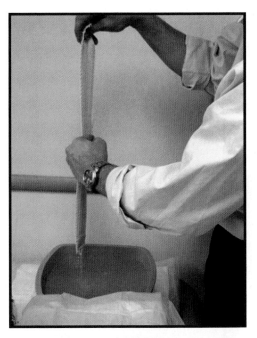

Figure 37-3c. Excess water is removed after dripping.

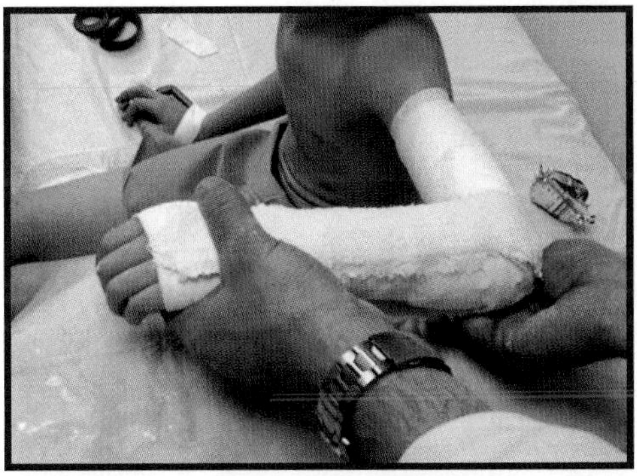

Figure 37-3d. The splint is applied to the extremity and molded.

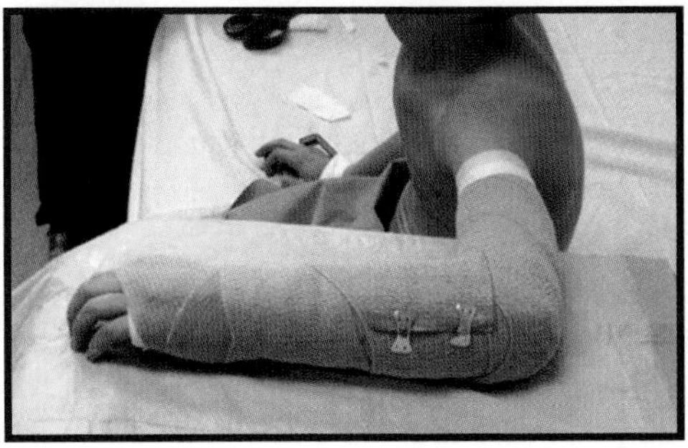

Figure 37-3e. An elastic bandage holds the splint in place.

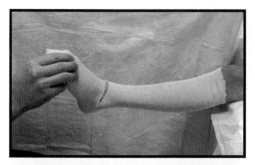

Figure 37-4a. Lower extremity stockinette is applied over the skin.

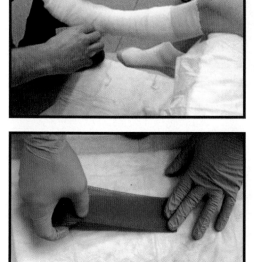

Figure 37-4b. Padding is applied.

Figure 37-4c. A splint is preconstructed for use behind the heel.

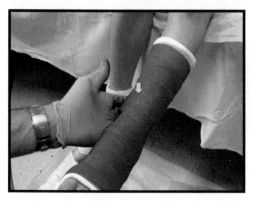

Figure 37-4d. The fiberglass cast is molded to avoid prominent folds and creases.

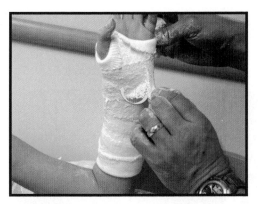

Figure 37-4e. As plaster is wrapped, prominent edges should be folded and tucked.

— Casts may be cut longitudinally (univalve for plaster or bivalve for fiberglass) after hardening if there is concern for additional soft tissue swelling.
  ▪ Over-wrap the cast with an elastic bandage to hold the halves together.
  ▪ Once the swelling resolves, over-wrap the cast with fiberglass for a longer lasting construct.

Continued Fracture Care

- Elevate the injured extremity above the level of the heart as much as possible for 3 to 4 days to minimize swelling.
- Prevent exposure of casts and splints to water.
- Treat pain with acetaminophen or narcotic analgesics. Because fracture healing requires inflammation, avoid nonsteroidal anti-inflammatory medications because they may delay bone healing.
- Modify activity as appropriate for fracture type and location (eg, non-weight bearing for lower extremity fractures, limited use for upper extremity fractures).
- Follow-up
  — Unstable fractures are reevaluated in 1 week with radiographs to assess alignment. Radiographs in the cast are usually acceptable, except for elbows.
  — Stable fractures are reevaluated as necessary to remove cast or splint and provide instruction on appropriate return to play (3–6 weeks).

Duration of Wear

- Decisions about initiation of and transition between casting and splinting should be based on clinical and radiographic findings, risk for complications from casting, and risk for reinjury.
- Refer to appropriate chapters for injury-specific guidelines.
- For stable fractures, splint until re-fracture risk is minimized, usually 3 to 6 weeks (Figure 37-5).

- For unstable fractures, casting precedes splinting until the reparative phase of bone healing is well established whereby the fracture stabilizes and bridging callus develops, typically 4 to 8 weeks in children (see Chapter 33) (Figure 37-6).
- Casting may continue longer for protection during high-risk sports.

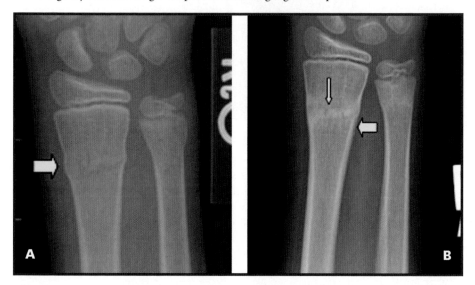

Figure 37-5. A, Buckle fracture in a 13-year-old child, day of injury. B, After 4 weeks, periosteal reaction (large arrow) and sclerosis (small arrow) at the fracture site are present.

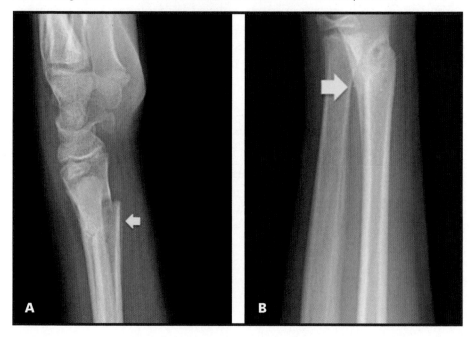

Figure 37-6. A, A transverse fracture after 4 weeks demonstrates periosteal reaction. B, Callus is evident at 6 weeks.

Complications

- Burns from plaster or fiberglass application (rare)
  — As moldable constructs harden, an exothermic reaction occurs.
    - Thicker constructs generate more heat.
    - Hot water adds to the heat generation and may burn the skin, so water temperature should not exceed manufacturer suggestions.
- Water exposure
  — Plaster breaks down and loses its integrity when wet. Cotton padding remains wet once exposed to water. In both circumstances, the cast should be replaced promptly.
  — Synthetic padding does not absorb water or will dry out over a number of hours, allowing some flexibility in water exposure. Repeated exposure to water is not advised because many children may still develop skin problems (Figure 37-7).
- Skin breakdown (Avoid it!)
  — Do not change the position of an extremity once plaster or fiberglass has been applied. This creates folds that will erode through the skin (Figure 37-8).

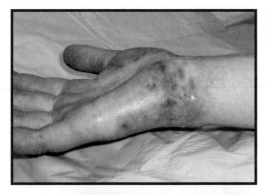

Figure 37-7. Skin reaction following prolonged exposure to water in a "waterproof" cast.

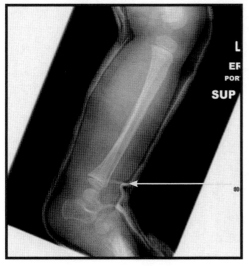

Figure 37-8. Folds (arrow) in the concavity of a cast were generated by placing the cast while the foot was in equinus, then dorsiflexing the foot into the desired position afterwards.

— Poorly molded casts that allow excess motion may lead to skin irritation and break-down, as well as loss of fracture alignment.

— Children often place objects in their cast that can lead to pressure sores if not promptly removed.

• Neurovascular compromise

— A tight or malpositioned cast poses a risk for neurovascular impingement or even compartment syndrome. Examine the patient before and after application and instruct on proper monitoring at home.

• Foreign bodies

— Children often place objects in their cast and deny doing so (Figure 37-9). Pain from a cast always requires investigation.

• Proper removal

— A cast saw may cause abrasions or burns. Blades become hot during removal, especially when cutting through thick casts. Intermittent pauses allow it to cool.

— The saw blade should not be drawn across the cast, but rather only pressed through the cast to prevent cutting the skin.

— Use of plastic guards or placement of protective strips under the cast reduce injury risk (Figure 37-10).

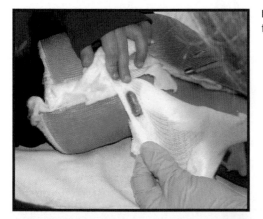

Figure 37-9. Foreign body (capsule) was found in this cast on removal.

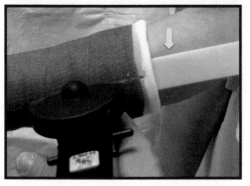

Figure 37-10. A cutting guard provides additional protection against injury to the underlying skin during removal.

- Prolonged immobilization
  — Immobilization results in joint and tendon contractures, muscle atrophy, and loss of proprioception. Many children improve on their own, but some require formal rehabilitation.

Return to Play Guidelines

- The safety of returning to sport with a cast or splint depends on
  — Degree of fracture healing
  — Risk of reinjury
  — Ability to adequately protect the injury with a splint or cast
  — Whether the sport's rules or officials permit play with casts or splints
- If return to play in a splint or cast is allowed, the cast or splint is covered with bubbled plastic wrap or foam padding to decrease the risk of injury to other players.
  — Splints may need to be secured to the injured extremity with cloth tape to prevent shifting during activity.
  — Athletes are instructed to adjust and retighten splints periodically because they often loosen during activity.
- If bracing or casting of the injury is not feasible or not allowed for return to play, athletes should attain radiographic healing and the return of functional motion and strength before resuming high-risk activities.

CHAPTER 38

Occult Fractures

Introduction/Etiology/Epidemiology

- Occult fractures are difficult-to-diagnose fractures in a child with extremity pain, disuse, and a history of trauma.
- A child's skeleton is composed of varying amounts of cartilage depending on age. Radiographs are often not definitive in ruling out a fracture.
- Physical examination becomes important in this clinical setting.
- The foot is a common site of missed fractures, with fractures of the calcaneus, cuboid, and first metatarsal being most prevalent.

Signs and Symptoms

- History of trauma
- Extremity pain
- Disuse
- Swelling is sometimes present.

Differential Diagnosis

- Sprain
- Contusion

Making the Diagnosis

- Diagnosis is made on radiographs but may not be confirmed until fracture healing has become evident (10–14 days).
  — Include oblique views if no obvious fracture is present on the anteroposterior and lateral images.
  — When the point of maximal tenderness cannot be identified (eg, the preschool-aged child who cannot verbalize the site of pain or is crying throughout the examination), the entire extremity is imaged.
  — If the point of maximal tenderness is over a growth plate and the radiographs are normal, the diagnosis is a Salter-Harris type I fracture.
  — Children's fractures are sometimes seen only on one view.

— Children have multiple *apophyses* in varying locations that can be confused with fracture fragments.
  ▪ Apophyses have smooth rounded borders, unlike the irregular, jagged edges of fracture fragments.
  ▪ Comparison views of the contralateral extremity may help to distinguish a normal apophysis from a fracture.
— *Occult fractures are frequently suspected in the elbow.*
  ▪ When bony injury is not evident, evaluate the soft tissues, particularly the anterior and posterior fat pads.
  ▪ Swelling within the elbow joint elevates the fat pads from the bone, making them apparent on a lateral radiograph of the elbow.
  ▪ The posterior fat pad is larger than the anterior fat pad and its elevation is much more sensitive for fracture of the distal humerus, proximal radius, or olecranon.

Treatment

- Immobilize the affected extremity, make non-weight bearing, and refer to an orthopaedic surgeon or pediatric sports medicine physician for reevaluation in 10 to 14 days.
  — Children can be immobilized for short periods without risk of stiffness or limitation in motion.
- Reevaluation includes clinical and radiographic examinations.
  — Persistent bony tenderness over the affected area supports the diagnosis of a fracture.
  — Repeat radiographs of the affected area may show signs of bony healing, most likely periosteal reaction (see Figure 29-11).
  — A bone scan or magnetic resonance imaging is helpful if a fracture is clinically suspected yet follow-up radiographs appear normal.

Expected Outcomes/Prognosis

- Depends on the specific injury.
- Majority heal completely with appropriate treatment.

When to Refer

- Children with suspected fractures should be immobilized and referred to an orthopaedic surgeon or a pediatric sports medicine physician for reevaluation in 10 to 14 days.

CHAPTER 39

Compartment Syndrome

Introduction/Etiology/Epidemiology

- Increased pressure within a myofascial compartment
- Can lead to compromised blood flow to muscle and nerves with resultant tissue damage.
- May be acute or chronic.
- *Acute compartment syndrome*
  - Typically secondary to trauma, often with an underlying fracture, crush injury, or contusion
  - May also be associated with reperfusion after ischemia and circumferential burns.
  - Most common locations include lower leg, forearm, thigh, and upper arm.
  - Most common clinical scenario is a tibia fracture and resultant compartment syndrome of the leg.
- *Chronic compartment syndrome*
  - Often called chronic exertional compartment syndrome
  - Symptoms occur with exercise and resolve with rest.
  - Usually involves the anterior and lateral compartments of the lower leg.

Signs and Symptoms

- Acute compartment syndrome—the 5 *Ps*
  - *Pain* out of proportion to clinical setting and with passive range of motion of adjacent joints
  - *Paresthesias* in the area supplied by the affected nerve
  - *Pallor*
  - *Paralysis*
  - *Pulselessness*
  - Involved compartments are tense to palpation.
- Chronic compartment syndrome
  - Patients complain of pain, aching, or throbbing of the affected compartment triggered by activity and relieved with rest.
  - Physical examination is most often normal.

Differential Diagnosis

- Acute compartment syndrome
  — Arterial occlusion
  — Neurapraxia
  — Cellulitis
  — Deep vein thrombosis
- Chronic compartment syndrome
  — Medial tibial stress syndrome (shin splints)
  — Stress fracture
  — Nerve entrapment
  — Popliteal artery entrapment

Making the Diagnosis

- Acute compartment syndrome
  — In an awake, alert patient the diagnosis is clinical based on appropriate clinical history and physical examination findings.
  — In comatose or equivocal cases the compartment pressures can be measured using a Stryker compartment pressure monitor or an arterial line setup.
  — Resting compartment pressures under 30 mm Hg are considered abnormal.
- Chronic compartment syndrome
  — Diagnosed by measuring compartment pressures at rest and 1 and 5 minutes after exercise.
  — Resting pressures greater than 15 mm Hg, 1-minute postexercise greater than 30 mm Hg, and 5-minute postexercise greater than 20 mm Hg are all considered abnormal.
- *There are currently no radiographic studies available to diagnose acute or chronic compartment syndrome.*

Treatment

- Acute compartment syndrome requires immediate orthopaedic consultation and emergent fasciotomies of the affected compartments.
- Chronic compartment syndrome may respond to nonoperative treatment with activity modification, nonsteroidal anti-inflammatory drugs, lower extremity stretching, soft tissue massage, and orthotics. Nonoperative care is often unsuccessful, and surgical fasciotomy is recommended for these cases.

Expected Outcomes/Prognosis

- Failure to perform emergent fasciotomies for acute compartment syndrome leads to irreversible nerve and muscle damage and poor outcomes.
- Surgical treatment for chronic compartment syndrome has a success rate of greater than 90% with most patients being able to return to their activities.

When to Refer

- Acute compartment syndrome requires emergent referral to an orthopaedic surgeon.
- Chronic compartment syndrome
  — A pediatric sports medicine physician can assist with making the diagnosis and managing nonoperative treatment.
  — If nonoperative treatment fails, refer to an orthopaedic surgeon.

Resource for Physicians and Families

- http://orthoinfo.aaos.org/topic.cfm?topic=a00204

Relevant *International Classification of Diseases, Ninth Revision, Clinical Modification* Codes

- **729.7** Non-traumatic (chronic) compartment syndrome
- **958.9** Traumatic (acute) compartment syndrome

CHAPTER 40

Child Abuse

Introduction/Etiology/Epidemiology

- The spectrum of child maltreatment includes neglect, psychological abuse, sexual abuse, and physical abuse (sometimes called non-accidental trauma).
- For 2006, the US Department of Health and Human Services reported 906,000 confirmed cases of child maltreatment and at least 1,500 confirmed deaths.
- Infants and children with physical or mental disabilities are at higher risk for abuse.
- In more than 80% of cases a parent is the abuser.
- Risk factors for child abuse are listed in Box 40-1.

Signs and Symptoms

- Caregiver provides an explanation for an injury that does not match the mechanism causing the injury.
- Caregiver provides no explanation for an injury that could only occur with a caregiver's knowledge of the event. For example, caregivers have no explanation for a 3-month-old child's humerus fracture.
- Child is too young or developmentally incapable of causing the injury described; for example, a 4-month-old with a toddler fracture.
- *Soft tissue injuries* are the most common physical findings in the abused child. Consider abuse if
  — Bruises, ecchymoses, and other soft tissue injuries are on cheeks, ears, neck, back, buttocks, chest, abdomen, or genitourinary area, or over other non-bony areas.
  — Child is not yet cruising.
  — Bruise has a pattern of an object or an instrument; for example, loop marks.
  — Child has multiple bruises (more than 4) and bruises in clusters.

Clinical Pearl

Soft tissue injuries in a nonambulatory child should raise suspicion for abuse. "Those who don't cruise rarely bruise."

Box 40-1. Factors That Place Children at Risk for Child Abuse

Domestic violence

Maternal depression

Parental alcohol abuse

Parental drug use

Premature birth

Parents' unrealistic expectations of a child

Parents' negative perception of a child.

* *Fractures* can be caused by child abuse or result from an accident. Fractures that commonly occur as a result of an accident can also be caused by child abuse, making the determination of causation sometimes difficult.
  — Consider abuse if
  * History provided is inconsistent with the mechanisms required to cause the particular type of fracture.
  * Child has multiple fractures or fractures in different stages of healing.
  * Child has other evidence of abuse, for example, bruises, head trauma, or neglect.
  — *Fractures with a high specificity for child abuse*
  * Rib fractures
  * Classic metaphyseal fractures (Figure 40-1).
  * Scapular fractures
  * Spinous process fractures
  * Sternal fractures
  — *Long bone fractures* are another common finding in non-accidental trauma.
  * Diaphysis of the femur, humerus, and tibia are the most frequent sites of injury.
  * Transverse fractures are more commonly associated with child abuse than spiral fractures.
  * A single, isolated fracture is more common than multiple fractures.
  * Long bone fracture mechanisms
    * *Transverse* fractures are caused by application of compressive and tensile loads perpendicular to the bone (ie, bending). A high-impact force applied to a single location can cause a transverse fracture.
    * *Spiral* fractures are caused by torsional loading of the bone (ie, twisting) (Figure 40-2).
    * *Buckle* or *torus* fractures are caused by compressive or axial loading of the bone.
    * *Oblique* fractures are caused by a combination of torsion and bending of the bone.

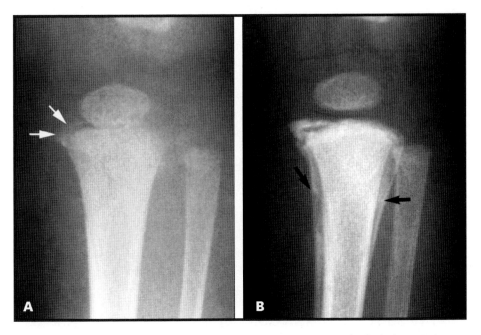

Figure 40-1. A, Child abuse (corner fracture of the tibia)—anteroposterior (AP) view. AP view of the proximal tibia in a 3-month-old infant shows a metaphyseal fracture (corner fracture) and evidence of periosteal separation between the physis and metaphysis (arrows), most likely secondary to a forceful downward pulling on the extremity. B, Child abuse (new bone formation in the tibia)—AP view. AP view of the same child shown in A approximately 1 month later shows new periosteal bone formation along the medial and lateral cortices (arrows). Note that the first signs of new periosteal bone can occur as early as 7 to 10 days after the injury. Reproduced with permission from Johnson TR, Steinbach LS (eds): *Essentials of Musculoskeletal Imaging.* Rosemont, IL: American Academy of Orthopaedic Surgeons; 2004.

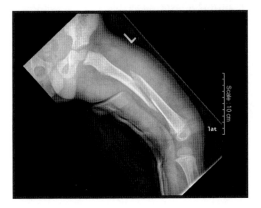

Figure 40-2. Spiral femur fracture.

Making the Diagnosis

- A high index of suspicion for inflicted trauma must be maintained when evaluating any child with a fracture or other musculoskeletal injury.
- Take a *detailed history* of the event causing the fracture.
  — Specific details about the patient's position just prior to and immediately following the injury event may provide information about the mechanism.
  — If a history of trauma is described, determine if it is a plausible cause for the injuries sustained by the child.
  — Suspect abuse if the parent or caregiver provides no explanation for an injury, gives inconsistent or conflicting histories, or blames a nonverbal or developmentally immature child.
- Conduct a thorough *physical examination* checking the skin carefully for bruises and other evidence of abuse.
- Obtain appropriate *radiographs* to evaluate for other fractures.
  — The "babygram" is inadequate for identifying subtle fractures in infants.
  — The American Academy of Pediatrics suggests that a *skeletal survey* be completed on all children younger than 2 years (Table 40-1).
  — A skeletal survey for patients between 2 and 5 years of age should be determined on an individual basis; for example, if the child has bony deformities, limited use of an extremity, or pain on palpation, or is disabled or non-ambulatory.
  — Skeletal survey in patients older than 5 years has not been proven to be beneficial.
  — Radiographic dating of fractures has been proven to be imprecise but can grossly differentiate between fresh and older fractures.
  — Repeating the skeletal survey 10 to 14 days after the patient's initial evaluation may identify fractures not seen previously, confirm the previously diagnosed fractures, and assess fracture healing.
- *Head computed tomography* is indicated to evaluate for intracranial injury in the following cases:
  — Any child younger than 1 year for whom abuse is suspected (eg, multiple fractures, soft tissue injuries)
  — Any child older than 1 year with signs and symptoms of head trauma (eg, vomiting, change in mental status)
- Many hospitals have multidisciplinary child abuse teams including child abuse pediatricians who can assist the general practitioner in evaluating for possible abuse.

Differential Diagnosis

- For fractures
  — Accidental trauma
  — Osteogenesis imperfecta (OI)
    - Osteogenesis imperfecta is much less common than child abuse.
    - Suspect OI if family history of multiple fractures or early onset hearing loss, or child has blue sclera or osteopenic bones on skeletal survey.

Table 40-1. Radiographs Included in a Skeletal Survey

Appendicular Skeleton
Humeri (AP)
Forearms (AP)
Hands (PA)
Femurs (AP)
Lower legs (AP)
Feet (PA or AP)
Axial Skeleton
Thorax (AP and lateral), to include ribs, thoracic, and upper lumbar spine Consider oblique radiographs of the chest.
Pelvis (AP; including mid and lower lumbar spine)
Lumbar spine (lateral)
Cervical spine (lateral)
Skull (frontal and lateral)

AP, anteroposterior; PA, posteroanterior.

— Rickets
  - Bones have characteristic radiologic appearance.
  - Premature neonates may have osteopenia but are also more vulnerable to be abused.

Treatment

- Treatment for specific fractures is covered in other sections.
- Reporting suspected cases of child abuse is as important to the child's welfare as treating the injuries.
- Health care professionals are required by state law to report all suspected cases of child abuse to state child protection authorities.
- The Child Abuse Prevention and Treatment Act "provides protection from criminal and civil liability to health care professionals who report suspected cases of child abuse in good faith."
- Physicians who have reported suspected child abuse in good faith have never been successfully sued for malpractice.

Expected Outcomes/Prognosis

- Without appropriate intervention, children who are victims of abuse are likely to experience repeated episodes of abuse.
- Twenty percent of fatalities related to child abuse had contact with the health care community for nonroutine care within a month of their deaths.

Prevention

- Identify families at risk to abuse their child (Box 40-1).
- Make appropriate referrals that will provide the family with resources and appropriate intervention.
  — Learn about your local resources for alcohol and drug treatment programs, parenting classes, and parenting support groups.
  — If domestic violence is suspected
    - The National Domestic Violence Hotline
      ◆ www.ndvh.org
      ◆ 800/799-SAFE (7233)
  — If postpartum depression is suspected
    - Postpartum Support International (www.postpartum.net)

When to Refer

- All suspected cases of child abuse should be reported to state authorities. Hospital-based child abuse teams can assist with this process.
- Fractures should be referred to an orthopaedist for management as indicated in other sections.

Resources for Physicians and Families

- Hospital-based child abuse multidisciplinary teams
- Prevent Child Abuse America (www.preventchildabuse.org)
- Parents Anonymous (www.parentsanonymous.org)
- Home visitation programs such as Nurse-Family Partnership (www.nursefamilypartnership.org) and Healthy Families America (www.healthyfamiliesamerica.org)
- Early childhood programs
- Childhelp
  — www.childhelpusa.org/gethelp/local-phone-numbers
  — 800/4-A-CHILD directs people to their local agency to make a report.

Relevant *International Classification of Diseases, Ninth Revision, Clinical Modification* Codes

- **995.51**   Child abuse, psychological/emotional
- **995.52**   Child abuse, neglect (nutritional)
- **995.53**   Child abuse, sexual
- **995.54**   Child abuse, physical
- **995.55**   Shaken baby syndrome

Bibliography

Aitken ME, Jaffe KM, DiScala C, Rivera FP. Functional outcome in children with multiple trauma without significant head injury. *Arch Phys Med Rehabil.* 1999;80:889–895

American Academy of Pediatrics Section on Radiology. Diagnostic imaging of child abuse. *Pediatrics.* 2000;105:1345–1348

Barsness KA, Cha ES, Bensard DD, et al. The positive predictive value of rib fractures as an indicator of nonaccidental trauma in children. *J Trauma.* 2003;54:1107–1110

Beaty JH, Kasser JR. *Rockwood and Wilkins' Fractures in Children.* 6th ed. Philadelphia, PA: Lippincott Williams and Wilkins; 2005

Bond SJ, Gotschall CS, Eichelberger MR. Predictors of abdominal injury in children with pelvic fracture. *J Trauma.* 1991;31:1169–1173

Bouche RT. Chronic compartment syndrome of the leg. *J Am Podiatr Med Assoc.* 1990;80:633–648

Canale ST. Physeal injuries. In: Green NE, Swiontkowski MF, eds. *Skeletal Trauma in Children.* 2nd ed. Philadelphia, PA: WB Saunders; 1998

Close BJ, Strouse PJ. MR of physeal fractures of the adolescent knee. *Pediatr Radiol.* 2000;30:756–762

Cooper A, Barlow B, DiScala C, String D, Ray K, Mottley L. Efficacy of pediatric trauma care: results of a population-based study. *J Pediatr Surg.* 1993;28:299–305

Cooper A, Hannan EL, Bessey PQ, Farrell LS, Cayten CG, Mottley L. An examination of the volume-mortality relationship for New York State trauma centers. *J Trauma.* 2000;48:16–24

Daltroy LH, Liang MH, Fossel AH, Goldberg MJ. The POSNA pediatric musculoskeletal functional health questionnaire: report on reliability, validity, and sensitivity to change. Pediatric Outcomes Instrument Development Group. Pediatric Orthopaedic Society of North America. *J Pediatr Orthop.* 1998;18:561–571

Delee JC, Drez D Jr, Miller MD. *Delee and Drez's Orthopaedic Sports Medicine.* 3rd ed. Philadelphia, PA: WB Saunders; 2009

Detmer DE, Sharpe K, Sufit RL, Girdley FM. Chronic compartment syndrome: diagnosis, management, and outcomes. *Am J Sports Med.* 1985;13:162–170

Doolin EJ, Browne AM, DiScala C. Pediatric trauma center criteria: an outcomes analysis. *J Pediatr Surg.* 1999; 34:885–890

Edwards P, Myerson M. Exertional compartment syndrome of the leg: steps for expedient return to activity. *Phys Sports Med.* 1996;24:31–37

Guillamondegui OD, Mahboubi S, Stafford PW, Nance ML. The utility of the pelvic radiograph in the assessment of pediatric pelvic fractures. *J Trauma.* 2003;55:236–240

Halanski M, Noonan KJ. Cast and splint immobilization: complications. *J Am Acad Orthop Surg.* 2008;16:30–40

Halanski MA, Halanski AD, Oza A, Vanderby R, Munoz A, Noonan KJ. Thermal injury with contemporary cast-application techniques and methods to circumvent morbidity. *J Bone Joint Surg Am.* 2007;89:2369–2377

Heinrich SD. Proximal femur fractures: hip dislocations. In: MacEwen GD, Kasser JR, Heinrich SD, eds. *Pediatric Fractures—A Practical Approach to Assessment and Treatment.* Philadelphia, PA: Lippincott Williams and Wilkins; 1993

Howard JL, Mohtadi NG, Wiley JP. Evaluation of outcomes in patients following surgical treatment of chronic exertional compartment syndrome in the leg. *Clin J Sports Med.* 2000;10:176–184

Johnstone EW, Foster BK. The biologic aspects of children's fractures. In: Beaty JH, Kasser JR, eds. *Rockwood and Wilkins' Fractures in Children.* 5th ed. Philadelphia, PA: Lippincott Williams and Wilkins; 2001

Keenan HT, Runyan DK, Marshall SW, Nocera MA, Merten DF. A population-based comparison of clinical and outcome characteristics of young children with serious inflicted and noninflicted traumatic brain injury. *Pediatrics.* 2004;114:633–639

King J, Diefendorf D, Apthorp J, Negrete VF, Carlson M. Analysis of 429 fractures in 189 battered children. *J Pediatr Orthop.* 1988;8:585–589

King WK, Kiesel EL, Simon HK. Child abuse fatalities: are we missing opportunities for intervention? *Pediatr Emerg Care.* 2006;22:211–214

Kleinman PK. *Diagnostic Imaging of Child Abuse.* 2nd ed. St. Louis, MO: Mosby; 1998

Krauss BS, Harakal T, Fleisher GR. General trauma in a pediatric emergency department: spectrum and consultation patterns. *Pediatr Emerg Care.* 1993;9:134–138

Loder RT, Bookout C. Fracture patterns in battered children. *J Orthop Trauma.* 1991;5:428–433

Maguire S, Mann MK, Sibert J, Kemp A. Are there patterns of bruising in childhood which are diagnostic or suggestive of abuse? A systematic review. *Arch Dis Child.* 2005;90:182–186

Mann DC, Rajmaira S. Distribution of physeal and nonphyseal fractures in 2,650 long-bone fractures in children aged 0-16 years. *J Pediatr Orthop.* 1990;10:713–716

Mars M, Hadley GP. Raised intracompartmental pressures and compartment syndrome. *Injury.* 1998;29:403–411

Martens MA, Backaert M, Vermaut G, Mulier JC. Chronic leg pain in athletes due to a recurrent compartment syndrome. *Am J Sports Med.* 1984;12:148–151

Matsen FA, Winquist RA, Krugmire RB. Diagnosis and management of compartment syndromes. *J Bone Joint Surg Am.* 1980;62:286–291

McMahon P, Grossman W, Gaffney M, Stanitski C. Soft-tissue injury as an indication of child abuse. *J Bone Joint Surg Am.* 1995;77:1179–1183

Mizuta T, Benson WM, Foster BK, Paterson DC, Morris LL. Statistical analysis of the incidence of physeal fractures. *J Pediatr Orthop.* 1987;7:518–523

Mubarak SJ, Owen CA, Hargens AR, Garetto LP, Akeson WH. Acute compartment syndromes: diagnosis and treatment with the aid of the wick catheter. *J Bone Joint Surg Am.* 1978;60:1091–1095

Nakayama DK, Copes WS, Sacco W. Differences in trauma care among pediatric and nonpediatric trauma centers. *J Pediatr Surg.* 1992;27:427–431

Naranja RJ Jr, Gregg JR, Dormans JP, Drummond DS, Davidson RS, Hahn M. Pediatric fracture without radiographic abnormality. Description and significance. *Clin Orthop Relat Res.* 1997;342:141–146

Pedowitz RA, Hargens AR, Mubarak SJ, Gershuni DH. Modified criteria for the objective diagnosis of chronic compartment syndrome of the leg. *Am J Sports Med.* 1990;18:35–40

Peterson HA, Madhok R, Benson JT, Ilstrup DM, Melton LJ. Physeal fractures: part I. Epidemiology in Olmstead County, Minnesota, 1979-1988. *J Pediatr Orthop.* 1994;14:423–430

Pierce MC, Bertocci G. Fractures resulting from inflicted trauma: assessing injury and history compatibility. *Clin Ped Emerg Med.* 2006;7:143–148

Pierce MC, Bertocci GE, Vogeley E, Moreland MS. Evaluating long bone fractures in children: a biomechanical approach with illustrative cases. *Child Abuse Negl.* 2004;28:505–524

Plint AC, Perry JJ, Correll R, Gaboury I, Lawton L. A randomized, controlled trial of removable splinting versus casting for wrist buckle fractures in children. *Pediatrics.* 2006;117:691–697

Pollack MM, Alexander SR, Clarke N, Ruttimann UE, Tesselaar HM, Bachulis AC. Improved outcomes from tertiary center pediatric intensive care: a statewide comparison of tertiary and nontertiary care facilities. *Crit Care Med.* 1991;19:150–159

Prosser I, Maguire S, Harrison SK, Mann M, Sibert JR, Kemp AM. How old is this fracture? Radiologic dating of fractures in children: a systematic review. *AJR Am J Roentgenol.* 2005;184:1282–1286

Rorabeck CH, Fowler PJ, Nott L. The results of fasciotomy in the management of chronic exertional compartment syndrome. *Am J Sports Med.* 1988;16:224–227

Salter RB, Harris WR. Injuries involving the epiphyseal plate. *J Bone Joint Surg Am.* 1963;45:587–622

Shuler FD, Grisafi FN. Cast-saw burns: evaluation of skin, cast, and blade temperatures generated during cast removal. *J Bone Joint Surg Am.* 2008;90:2626–2630

Silfverskiold JP. Splinting tips. *Postgrad Med.* 1989;86:185–188

Slongo TF. The choice of treatment according to the type and location of the fracture and the age of the child. *Injury.* 2005;36(Suppl 1):A12–A19

Sugar NF, Taylor JA, Feldman KW. Bruises in infants and toddlers: those who don't cruise rarely bruise. Puget Sound Pediatric Research Network. *Arch Pediatr Adolesc Med.* 1999;153:399–403

Vitale MG, Vitale MA, Lehmann CL, et al. Towards a national pediatric musculoskeletal trauma outcomes registry: the Pediatric Orthopaedic Trauma Outcomes Research Group (POTORG) experience. *J Pediatr Orthop.* 2006;26:151–156

Vuolteenaho K, Moilanen T, Moilanen E. Non-steroidal anti-inflammatory drugs, cyclooxygenase-2 and the bone healing process. *Basic Clin Pharmacol Toxicol.* 2008;102:10–14

West S, Andrews J, Bebbington A, Ennis O, Alderman P. Buckle fractures of the distal radius are safely treated in a soft bandage: a randomized prospective trial of bandage versus plaster cast. *J Pediatr Orthop.* 2005;25:322–325

Part 13: Foot and Ankle

TOPICS COVERED

CHAPTER 41

General Considerations

Physical Examination

- The most helpful part of the examination is palpation with a single finger or thumb to identify the anatomic structure that is tender (point of maximal tenderness) (Figure 41-1)

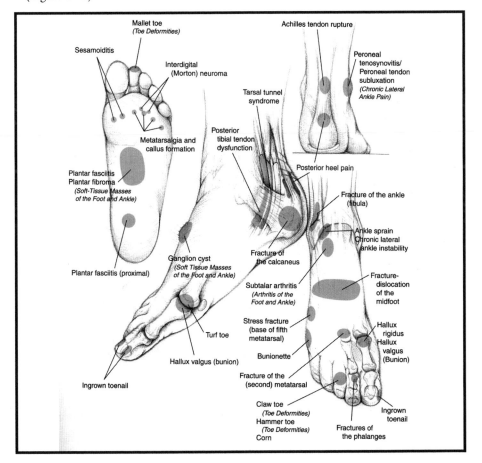

Figure 41-1. Pain diagram of foot and ankle. Reproduced with permission from Griffin LY (ed): *Essentials of Musculoskeletal Care,* 3rd edition. Rosemont, IL: American Academy of Orthopaedic Surgeons; 2005.

- Tenderness along the anterior joint line may indicate an intra-articular process.
- Swelling that is diffuse or circumferential around the ankle suggests an ankle joint effusion, a sign of intra-articular pathology.

Accessory Centers of Ossification

- Common around the foot and ankle
- Most eventually fuse with the parent bone.
- Some persist as separate ossicles attached to parent bone by cartilage or fibrous tissue.
- May be confused with fractures.
- Can become symptomatic if fibrocartilaginous connection is strained or disrupted from direct or repetitive trauma.
  — Most frequently occurs at navicular or lateral malleolus (Figure 41-2).
  — Treat symptomatically with relative rest and shoe wear modifications.
  — Shoe inserts with arch support may be helpful to unload an irritated accessory navicular.

Footwear Assessment

- *Evaluate general wear and condition.* Particularly in athletic footwear, the midsole is the weakest link and tends to break down after about 300 to 400 miles of wear. This leads to a significant loss of support and cushioning and may occur while the upper and outer soles still appear to be in good condition.
- *Identify pressure points that may correlate with symptoms.* This can be particularly problematic over the first metatarsophalangeal joint in patients with bunions, or over the metatarsal heads in patients with forefoot complaints.
- *Evaluate suitability of shoe for foot type.* Planus feet are often more comfortable in shoes that provide some medial arch support. Cavus feet tend to be more rigid and will often benefit from shoes that provide adequate cushioning and shock absorption.

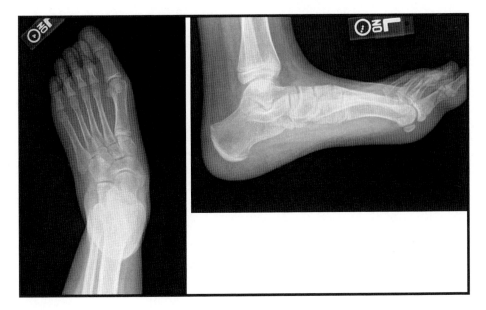

Figure 41-2. Accessory navicular bone.

CHAPTER 42

Clubfoot

Introduction/Etiology/Epidemiology

- *Congenital talipes equinovarus,* clubfoot, is a complex *severe* foot deformity, characterized by hindfoot (heel) varus and equinus, smaller calf muscles, and forefoot cavus and adductus (Figure 42-1a, b).
    — Pathologically, the ligaments of the posterior aspect of the ankle and of the medial and plantar aspects of the foot are shortened and thickened.
    — Gastrocnemius, tibialis posterior, and toe flexors are shortened and are smaller in size.
    — Connective tissue rich in collagen tends to spread into the Achilles tendon and deep fascia.
- Clubfoot may occur in the normal child (idiopathic) or as part of a disorder such as myelomeningocele, arthrogryposis, and others (Box 42-1).

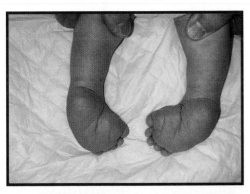

Figure 42-1a. Posterior view of moderate infant clubfoot deformity demonstrating heel varus, equinus, and forefoot cavus.

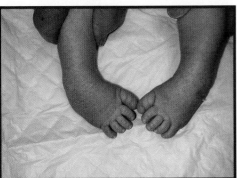

Figure 42-1b. Anterior view of moderate bilateral infant clubfoot deformity demonstrating forefoot adduction.

Box 42-1. Syndromes and Disorders Associated With Clubfoot

Arthrogryposis

Meningocele

Amniotic band syndrome

Proximal femoral focal deficiency

Freeman-Sheldon syndrome

Larson syndrome

Diastrophic dwarfism

- Idiopathic clubfoot incidence varies from 0.3 to 8 per 1,000 live births.
- Males are more commonly affected than females (2:1).
- Approximately 50% of cases are bilateral.
- Present at birth (congenital). Not a malformation, but a developmental disorder.
  — A normally developing foot becomes a clubfoot during the second trimester of pregnancy. Clubfoot is rarely detected by ultrasonography before the 14th to 16th week of gestation.
- The etiology and pathogenesis of clubfoot remains unknown.
- Clubfoot clusters in some families and affects family members across generations, suggesting a genetic role.
  — The occurrence rate is 17 times higher for first-degree relatives compared with the general population.
  — Mode of inheritance does not follow a distinctive pattern, but several studies support a single, major genetic factor.

Signs and Symptoms

- Forefoot cavus and adductus (Figure 42-1a, b)
- Heel varus and equinus (Figure 42-1a, b)
- Smaller calf muscles

Differential Diagnosis

- In some cases, the deformity is positional due to intrauterine "packing."
- Metatarsus adductus (see Chapter 44)
- Calcaneovalgus deformity (see Chapter 47)
  — Hyperdorsiflexion of the foot, often with the dorsum of the forefoot resting on the anterior surface of the lower leg
  — Resolves spontaneously without treatment.
- Congenital vertical talus (very rare) (Figure 42-2)
  — Commonly associated with neuromuscular and genetic disorders including trisomy 13-15 and trisomy 18.
  — Involvement is bilateral in 50% of cases.
- Clubfoot may also be associated with a number of syndromes and disorders (Box 42-1).

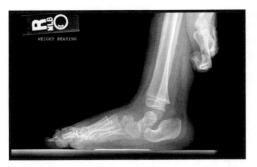

Figure 42-2. Congenital vertical talus.

Making the Diagnosis

- Diagnosis is usually made at birth by identifying the abnormality on physical examination.
- In many cases, the diagnosis is made by prenatal ultrasound.

Treatment

- *Standards of care for clubfoot*
  — The *Ponseti method* has become the worldwide gold standard for the treatment of clubfoot.
    - Very safe, efficient, economical, easy to teach, and radically decreases the need for extensive corrective surgeries.
    - Effective even in the most challenging and severe cases that include neglected clubfeet up to 10 to 12 years of age.
    - Technique involves gentle manipulation and well-molded plaster casts.
      - Casting begins within a few days of life.
      - Manipulation of the foot is performed before each cast change, every 5 to 7 days (Figure 42-3).
      - A series of 5 to 8 toe-to-groin plaster casts should be sufficient to obtain the maximum correction possible (Figure 42-4).
      - A simple percutaneous tenotomy of the Achilles tendon facilitates the final correction of the deformity.
      - After full correction has been obtained, a brace is worn during sleeping hours until the age of 4 years to prevent relapses (Figure 42-5).

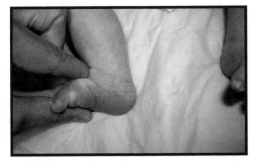

Figure 42-3. Stretching is part of the serial casting program.

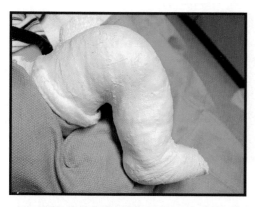

Figure 42-4. Long leg cast for clubfoot deformity, part of a serial casting program.

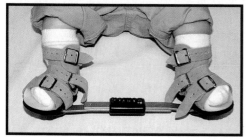

Figure 42-5. Bracing for clubfoot abnormality after serial casting.

Expected Outcomes/Prognosis

- The Ponseti method results in early and full correction of all components of the deformity.
- The more muscle atrophy and stiffness, the more resistance to correction and the higher the possibilities for a relapse if the brace is not used appropriately.
- In general, clubfoot associated with a syndrome is more resistant to treatment but may still have good outcomes with conservative management.
- Long-term results at an average of 34 years (range 25–45 years)
  — Seventy-eight percent of the feet had excellent or good scores (using pain and functional limitation as outcome criteria), compared with 85% in a control population of normal feet (not a statistically significant difference) (Figure 42-6).

Prevention

- While there is no known prevention for clubfoot, prenatal screening is available that allows for provision of anticipatory guidance and counseling to families.

When to Refer

- At the time of diagnosis, referral should be made to a pediatric orthopaedic specialist.

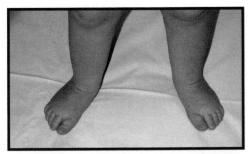

Figure 42-6. Feet after serial casting program for clubfoot deformity.

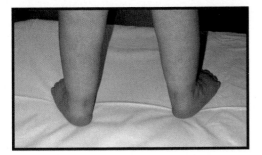

Relevant *International Classification of Diseases, Ninth Revision, Clinical Modification* Codes

- **754.51** Talipes equinovarus (clubfoot)
- **754.59** Talipes calcaneovarus
- **754.61** Congenital vertical talus
- **754.53** Metatarsus adductus

CHAPTER 43

Flatfoot

Introduction/Etiology/Epidemiology

- Common condition
- Loss of the medial longitudinal arch of the foot
- Flatfeet in children are a common concern among parents.
- High incidence of physiologic (flexible) flatfoot in children younger than 2 years because of
  — Increased ligamentous laxity
  — Medial fat pad normally present at birth
- Rapid development of the medial longitudinal arch occurs during normal growth from 2 to 6 years of age due to atrophy of the medial fat pad and decline in ligamentous laxity.
- Rigid flatfeet may be associated with an underlying etiology such as tarsal coalition or congenital vertical talus.

Signs and Symptoms

- Medial arch of the foot is collapsed with weight bearing.
- Physiologic (flexible) flatfoot
  — Medial arch is reconstituted when non-weight bearing or with toe walking (see Figure 4-37).
  — Typically asymptomatic
- Nonphysiologic (rigid) flatfoot
  — Medial arch is not reconstituted when non-weight bearing or with toe walking.
  — Passive subtalar motion is limited.
  — Patients often complain of activity-related pain around the midfoot or hindfoot.
- Limited ankle dorsiflexion caused by tight Achilles tendon can also pull the hindfoot into valgus and lead to a flatfoot deformity.
  — Evaluate ankle dorsiflexion with the hindfoot in slight eversion to avoid dorsiflexing through the midfoot.
  — Patients should be able to dorsiflex the ankle at least 10 degrees beyond neutral while the knee is extended (see Figure 4-4).

Differential Diagnosis

- Accessory navicular (see Figure 41-2)
  — Will usually present with a painful and tender medial prominence.
- Achilles contracture
- Congenital vertical talus
  — Rocker bottom foot
- Tarsal coalition

Making the Diagnosis

- Most flatfeet are flexible and can be confirmed on physical examination by good tibiotalar and subtalar motion and reconstitution of the medial arch with toe rise or non-weight bearing.
- Radiographs for painless flatfeet are rarely indicated.
- Obtain weight-bearing anteroposterior and lateral radiographs to evaluate rigid or painful flatfeet.
  — Bones of the foot not well ossified until 5 years of age
  — To evaluate for congenital vertical talus, lateral radiographs of the foot in maximum dorsiflexion and maximum plantarflexion should be obtained (see Figure 42-2).
  — In adolescents, oblique views of the foot may help identify a tarsal coalition.
- Computed tomography scan or magnetic resonance imaging may be used to identify an occult coalition or determine the extent of a coalition (Figure 43-1).

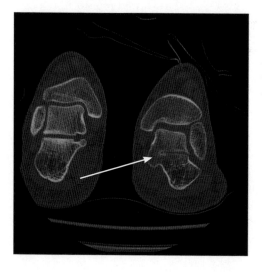

Figure 43-1. Talo-calcaneal coalition: Coronal computed tomography scan image of bilateral feet. The foot on the left demonstrated a rigid flatfoot, with loss of motion of the subtalar joint and subtaler coalition (arrow).

Treatment

- *Asymptomatic flexible flatfeet require no specific treatment.*
- Rigid flatfeet are more likely to become symptomatic without treatment.
- Nonoperative treatment
  — Orthotics or casting can be used to selectively off-load symptomatic portions of the foot.
  — Soft-shoe inserts can be used to pad around a symptomatic accessory navicular.
  — Stretching exercises for the heel cord are beneficial when the flatfoot is associated with an Achilles contracture.
- Surgery
  — May be considered for significant symptoms unresponsive to nonoperative treatment or for rigid flatfeet.
  — Procedures to lengthen the Achilles tendon or remove an accessory navicular may be beneficial in some patients.
  — Excision of symptomatic tarsal coalitions also provides good results.
  — Congenital vertical talus requires casting followed by surgery to reduce the talonavicular joint.

Expected Outcomes/Prognosis

- Flexible flatfeet rarely become symptomatic and can be managed conservatively with excellent long-term prognosis.
- Rigid flatfeet typically result in hindfoot or midfoot pain during adolescence and usually require surgical treatment to address the underlying etiology.

When to Refer

- Adolescents with flexible flatfeet that have not responded to orthotics and activity modification should be referred to a sports medicine physician or orthopaedist.
- Any rigid flatfoot should be referred to a pediatric orthopaedic surgeon.

Resource for Physicians and Families

- http://orthoinfo.aaos.org/topic.cfm?topic=a00046

Relevant *International Classification of Diseases, Ninth Revision, Clinical Modification* Codes

- **734**   Flexible flatfoot
- **754.61**   Rigid flatfoot
- **755.67**   Accessory navicular
- **755.67**   Tarsal coalition
- **754.61**   Congenital vertical talus
- **727.81**   Achilles contracture

CHAPTER 44

Metatarsus Adductus

Introduction/Etiology/Epidemiology

- Metatarsus adductus (MTA) is a common foot deformity.
- The forefoot deviates medially with respect to the hindfoot, giving the foot a bean-shaped appearance such that the lateral aspect of the foot is convex.
- Incidence is 1 per 1,000 live births.
- Some authors have postulated a relationship between MTA and hip dysplasia because of in utero positioning and molding. The incidence of hip dysplasia in children with MTA ranges from 1% to 13% in some series (Jacobs, Kumar), while others have found no correlation between the 2 disorders (Betz).

Signs and Symptoms

- One or both feet curve medially (see Figure 22-4).
- The forefoot is flexible and can easily be positioned into normal alignment with the hindfoot.

Differential Diagnosis

- Metatarsus varus
- A "searching" or "seeking" great toe
  — The tendency for the foot to deviate medially may not be noticed at birth. When the child stands and walks, the great toe abductor muscles pull the forefoot medially due to a primitive grasping reflex.
  — Not true with MTA.
- Clubfoot
  — The most important distinction between MTA and clubfoot is that the ankle and hindfoot in MTA are flexible.
  — Although the infant may hold the foot in an equinovarus position, the MTA foot can be easily manipulated into a normal foot posture.

Making the Diagnosis

- Metatarsus adductus is a clinical diagnosis.
- Radiographs of the feet are not necessary to diagnose or assess results of treatment.
- Routine pelvic radiographs in children with foot deformities are not recommended unless there are other risk factors or physical findings suggestive of hip dysplasia.

Treatment

- No treatment is necessary in most.
- Metatarsus adductus feet will develop normally and fit into regular shoes.
- Manipulations for MTA have not been proven to improve the long-term function of the foot.
- The patient can be fitted with straight or reverse last shoes, or instructed to wear his or her usual shoes on opposite feet.
  — The shoes are worn full-time until the child can stand, and then only while sleeping until a normal foot position is maintained.

Expected Outcomes/Prognosis

- Prognosis is excellent for normal function and shoe wear throughout life.

When to Refer

- If the deformity is no longer flexible, refer to a pediatric orthopaedic surgeon.

Relevant *International Classification of Diseases, Ninth Revision, Clinical Modification* Code

- **754.53**   MTA

CHAPTER 45

Metatarsus Varus

Introduction/Etiology/Epidemiology
- Uncommon, rigid deformity of the forefoot
- The forefoot deviates medially with respect to the hindfoot, giving the foot a bean-shaped appearance such that the lateral aspect of the foot is convex.

Signs and Symptoms
- One or both feet curve medially.
- Feet have a deep medial crease and are stiff, so that the forefoot is difficult to manipulate into normal alignment with the hindfoot.

Differential Diagnosis
- Metatarsus adductus (MTA)
- A "searching" or "seeking" great toe
  — The tendency for the foot to deviate medially may not be noticed at birth. When the child stands and walks, the great toe abductor muscles pull the forefoot medially due to a transient, primitive grasping reflex.
  — Not true in MTA
- Clubfoot
  — The most important distinction between metatarsus varus and clubfoot is that the ankle and hindfoot in metatarsus varus are flexible.
  — Although the infant may hold the foot in an equinovarus position, the foot can be easily manipulated into a normal foot posture.

Making the Diagnosis
- Radiographs or other imaging of the feet are not necessary.

Treatment
- Gentle manipulation, followed by casting of the feet to stretch the medial structures
- Casts are changed each week until the foot is flexible. Best results occur in patients younger than 8 months.

Expected Outcomes/Prognosis

- Prognosis is excellent for normal function and shoe wear throughout life.
- Rarely, surgical treatment is necessary if casting is ineffective. The most common surgical procedures for metatarsus varus include abductor hallucis recession, medial release of the soft tissues and midfoot joints, and metatarsal osteotomies or osteotomy of the medial cuneiform and cuboid, after age 4 years.

When to Refer

- Patients with metatarsus varus should be referred to an orthopaedic surgeon before 8 months of age for serial casting.

Relevant *International Classification of Diseases, Ninth Revision, Clinical Modification* Code

- **754.53**   Metatarsus varus

CHAPTER 46

Pes Cavus and Cavovarus

Introduction/Etiology/Epidemiology

- Pes cavus is a high-arched foot.
- Pes cavovarus is a high-arched foot with plantarflexed first ray, forefoot pronation or adduction, and a variable degree of hindfoot varus.
- The high arch is caused by tight plantar fascia and variable weakness of the foot intrinsic muscles, peroneals, or anterior tibialis.
- Usually presents in children older than 3 years.
- *May be idiopathic, but a neurogenic cause is eventually identified in up to 66% of patients with pes cavus or pes cavovarus.* Neurologic etiologies include central nervous system abnormalities, spinal abnormalities, peripheral neuropathies, and isolated nerve injury (Box 46-1).

Signs and Symptoms

- High arches, tall midfoot (Figure 46-1)
- Flexibility of the deformity is determined by inverting and everting the hindfoot. Early in the pathogenesis of pes cavus, the hindfoot varus may be flexible, but as the deformity progresses, the hindfoot varus becomes more rigid.
- Toe walking with inability to lower heels
- Pain or calluses under metatarsal heads
- Recurrent ankle sprains
  - When the foot is in the weight-bearing position, it functions as a tripod with weight evenly distributed between the heel and the first and fifth metatarsal heads. In pes cavovarus, the first ray is plantarflexed, so the heel must tilt into varus to maintain the tripod. This tendency to tilt into varus makes walking on uneven terrain difficult. The ankle and hindfoot may roll inward, causing a lateral ankle sprain.
- Parents will note that the feet are not growing. The length of the foot may appear short, but the height of the foot may be increasing because of worsening cavus.
- There may be signs and symptoms or family history of neuromuscular disease.

Box 46-1. Etiology of Pes Cavus and Cavovarus

Neurologic—No. 1 Cause; Estimated at About 66%

- Charcot-Marie-Tooth disease
- Friedreich ataxia
- Roussy-Levy syndrome
- Poliomyelitis
- Cerebral palsy
- Dejerine-Sottas hypertrophic interstitial neuritis

Congenital

- Spina bifida
- Talipes equinovarus
- Myelodysplasia
- Clubfoot

Iatrogenic

- Post surgery or trauma
  - —Peroneal nerve injury
  - —Weak anterior muscles
  - —Overpowering posterior muscles

Infection

- Syphillis
- Poliomyelitis

Idiopathic

- Must be considered

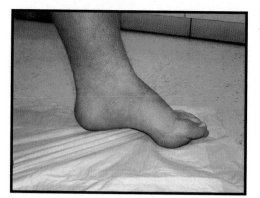

Figure 46-1. Clinical photo of cavus foot abnormality.

Differential Diagnosis

- Tarsal coalition
- Thorough evaluation for neuromuscular etiology (Box 46-1)

Making the Diagnosis

- Can be made clinically, but radiographs may be helpful to confirm the diagnosis.
- Cavovarus is defined by plantar flexion of the first ray (talo—first metatarsal angle greater than 15 degrees), seen on a *lateral, weight-bearing foot radiograph* (Figure 46-2).
- Because the cavus foot frequently results from a neuromuscular disease, thorough evaluation of motor strength, sensation, and reflexes is essential. *Family history and possibly a referral to a geneticist may be helpful* in the diagnostic workup because many neuromuscular diseases are hereditary.

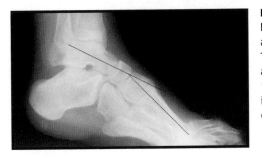

Figure 46-2. A line drawn through the long axis of the talus should be in line with a line drawn through the first metatarsal. This angle is called the talo first metatarsal angle or angle of Marie. Normal is 0 to 15 degrees of plantar flexion. Any sag in this angle (negative angle of Marie) is called pes planus.

Treatment

- The goals of treatment are to obtain a mobile, pain-free, stable, motor-balanced foot that fits in a shoe and allows weight-bearing function.
- For the minimally symptomatic patient, orthotics that pad the metatarsal heads and extra-depth shoes may be helpful.
- Ankle support splints may reduce the risk of ankle sprains in the child who wishes to remain active.
- Night splints can be helpful early in the pathogenesis of cavus to help prevent worsening contractures.
- An ankle-foot orthosis may be used for the foot drop because of ankle dorsiflexion weakness.
- Nonoperative measures are usually temporary, and surgical intervention often becomes necessary as nonoperative management becomes less effective.

Expected Outcomes/Prognosis

- Idiopathic: long-term prognosis is good for normal adult activities, even if surgical treatment is needed.
- Neurogenic: some etiologies may cause progressively worsening weakness, resulting in greater disability over time. Long-term results are much better for a cavus foot because of nonprogressive neuropathy.

When to Refer

- On presentation, refer to a pediatric orthopaedist to direct workup and treatment.

Relevant *International Classification of Diseases, Ninth Revision, Clinical Modification* Codes

- **736.73**   Pes cavus
- **736.75**   Pes cavovarus

CHAPTER 47

Calcaneal Valgus

Introduction/Etiology/Epidemiology

- The foot is positioned in extreme dorsiflexion with the dorsal surface touching the anterior shin.
- Commonly seen in the newborn nursery
- Intrauterine positioning generally causes this deformity.
- Mild calcaneal valgus is noted in up to 30% of newborns.
- Severe calcaneal valgus is seen in 1 per 1,000 newborns.

Signs and Symptoms

- Top of foot rests against the front of the shin (Figure 47-1).
- The ankle and hindfoot are flexible enough to easily correct the deformity.

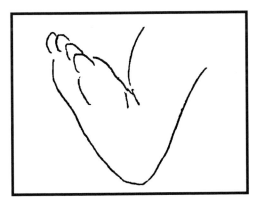

Figure 47-1. Calcaneal valgus.

Differential Diagnosis

- Lipomyelomeningocele or other neurologic cause
- If the hindfoot is rigid, consider the possibility of congenital vertical talus.

Making the Diagnosis

- Calcaneal valgus is a clinical diagnosis.
- Imaging is not necessary when the deformity is flexible.

- Evaluate motor function of the foot by gently stroking the top, bottom, medial, and lateral sides of the foot.
  — The foot should move actively in each direction.
  — If there is deficient activity of the plantar flexors, the workup should include evaluation of the spine for lipomyelomeningocele or other neurologic cause.

Treatment

- No treatment is necessary.
- Reassure families that the foot position improves spontaneously within a few days to a few weeks after birth.

Expected Outcomes/Prognosis

- Corrects spontaneously within a few weeks.
- By the time the child begins to walk the foot is generally normal or may have a mild, flexible flatfoot posture.
- Excellent long-term prognosis

When to Refer

- Referral to a pediatric orthopaedist or neurosurgeon is recommended if there is any question of neurologic cause or if the foot is not flexible.

Relevant *International Classification of Diseases, Ninth Revision, Clinical Modification* Code

- **754.62**   Calcaneal valgus

CHAPTER 48

Miscellaneous Conditions

Kohler Disease

INTRODUCTION/ETIOLOGY/EPIDEMIOLOGY

- Osteochondrosis of the tarsal navicular
- Most commonly presents from 4 to 9 years of age
- More common in males
- Multiple etiologic factors have been implicated, including macrotrauma or microtrauma and vascular insult, but most cases are considered idiopathic.
- Navicular begins to ossify at 3 to 4 years of age and irregularities in this process may be found in up to 20% to 30% of children.
- Some believe this may be a variation of normal development because many children with radiographic findings consistent with Kohler disease are asymptomatic.

SIGNS AND SYMPTOMS

- Insidious onset of medial midfoot pain, particularly after running or activity
- Tenderness over the navicular; there may also be swelling.
- Gait may be antalgic.

DIFFERENTIAL DIAGNOSIS

- Symptomatic accessory navicular bone (see Figure 41-2)
- Navicular stress fracture: tenderness of the navicular in adolescent athletes (particularly females) raises suspicion for navicular stress fracture.

MAKING THE DIAGNOSIS

- Diagnosis is based on physical examination and radiographs.
- Anteroposterior (AP), lateral, and oblique radiographs reveal sclerosis and collapse of the navicular (Figure 48-1).
- Because many asymptomatic children have radiographic irregularities of the navicular, diagnosis of Kohler disease depends on symptoms, not radiographic appearance alone.

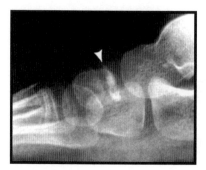

Figure 48-1. Kohler disease: Lateral radiograph of the foot showing a shattered, fragmented navicular (arrowhead). Reproduced with permission from Kasser JR (ed): *Orthopaedic Knowledge Update 5*. Rosemont, IL: American Academy of Orthopaedic Surgeons; 1996:503–514.

TREATMENT

- Goal is to achieve pain-free ambulation.
- Initial strategies include activity modification, changing shoe type, and custom-molded shoe orthoses with medial arch support.
- While symptoms may resolve sooner with casting for 6 to 8 weeks, casting does not seem to affect long-term outcome.
- Return to full activities and sports
  — Allowed as symptoms abate, usually within 8 to 10 weeks
  — Radiographic normalization may take several years and should not be used to determine return to activity.

EXPECTED OUTCOMES/PROGNOSIS

- Natural history is for complete resolution with time.
- Long-term outcome is universally favorable, regardless of treatment choice.
- There are usually no long-term sequelae.

WHEN TO REFER

- If activity modification does not relieve symptoms within 2 to 3 weeks, refer for shoe orthoses or to a pediatric orthopaedic specialist for possible casting.

RELEVANT *INTERNATIONAL CLASSIFICATION OF DISEASES, NINTH REVISION, CLINICAL MODIFICATION (ICD-9-CM)* CODE

- **732.5**   Kohler disease

Freiberg Infraction/Disease

INTRODUCTION/ETIOLOGY/EPIDEMIOLOGY

- Osteochondrosis of any of the lesser metatarsal heads
- Most commonly affects the second metatarsal.
- Presents between 11 and 17 years of age.
- Female-to-male ratio is up to 11:1.

- Multiple etiologic factors have been implicated, including repetitive microtrauma and vascular embarrassment.
- Feet with a second toe longer than the first (also known as a Morton toe) are at greater risk, probably because of increased mechanical stress across the longer toe.

SIGNS AND SYMPTOMS

- Insidious onset of forefoot pain and swelling that worsens with activity
- Tenderness over the involved metatarsophalangeal (MTP) joint
- Pain and limitation with passive MTP joint motion
- Gait may be antalgic.

DIFFERENTIAL DIAGNOSIS

- *Stress fractures* in the foot are most common in the second metatarsal and in feet with a long second ray but tend to produce pain and tenderness more proximally along the metatarsal, rather than directly over the MTP joint.
- *Morton neuroma* will be most tender in the intermetatarsal space, which may have a palpable nodule.
- *Metatarsalgia* is nonspecific pain of one or more metatarsals.

MAKING THE DIAGNOSIS

- Radiographs (AP, lateral, and oblique views) may reveal the deformity (Figure 48-2), although they are often normal during the first several weeks of symptoms.
- Bilateral AP views are helpful for comparison because findings may be subtle.
- Magnetic resonance imaging or bone scan may identify early subchondral changes.

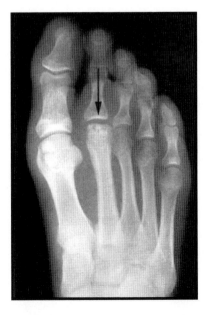

Figure 48-2. Radiograph showing Freiberg infraction. Note flattening and fragmentation at the head of the second metatarsal (arrow). Reproduced with permission from Griffin LY (ed): *Essentials of Musculoskeletal Care,* 3rd edition. Rosemont, IL: American Academy of Orthopaedic Surgeons; 2005.

TREATMENT

- Goal is pain-free ambulation.
- Activity modifications, followed by gradual increase in activity as symptoms allow
- Shoes with a wider toe box and rigid support under the forefoot, or shoe orthoses, such as a metatarsal bar or pad just proximal to the MTP joint, may help reduce pain with ambulation.
- Immobilization in a cast or boot, or a period of non-weight bearing, is sometimes required during the acute phase (6–12 weeks).
- Some experts consider surgical intervention after a 6-month trial of conservative treatment.

EXPECTED OUTCOMES/PROGNOSIS

- Long-term outcomes are variable and may include joint stiffness or persistent discomfort.
- Best results occur with early recognition and initiation of conservative or surgical treatments that may enhance remodeling of the MTP joint.
- Cases identified late may require resection rather than reconstruction of the joint, with outcomes that may be less favorable.

WHEN TO REFER

- If activity modification does not relieve symptoms within 2 to 3 weeks, refer for shoe orthoses or to a pediatric orthopaedic specialist for possible casting.
- Refer to a pediatric orthopaedic specialist for persistent symptoms after 6 months of nonoperative management.

PREVENTION

- Minimizing use of high heels and maintaining adequate calf muscle flexibility reduces mechanical stress across the forefoot and may help prevent symptoms in susceptible individuals.

RELEVANT *ICD-9-CM* CODE

- **732.5**　Freiberg infraction

Juvenile Bunions (Hallux Valgus)

INTRODUCTION/ETIOLOGY/EPIDEMIOLOGY

- Valgus deformity of the first MTP joint
- Tend to be bilateral and familial.
- Very common in pediatric and adult populations
- Juvenile bunions usually present in early to mid-adolescence and may be a different entity than those presenting in adults, with a more favorable natural history and less arthrosis.
- Female-to-male ratio is about 3:1.

- Commonly associated with flexible pes planus and generalized ligamentous laxity
- Activities that place increased stress across the MTP joint, such as dance and gymnastics, may contribute to bunion formation in susceptible individuals.

SIGNS AND SYMPTOMS

- Inspection in weight-bearing position reveals the characteristic medial prominence of the first MTP joint.
- There may be an overlying bursa with erythema or inflammation, but this is much less common in children than in adults.
- Metatarsal-phalangeal joint range of motion should be assessed but is usually preserved in adolescent bunions.

DIFFERENTIAL DIAGNOSIS

- Sesamoiditis or sesamoid stress fracture produces pain over plantar aspect of MTP joint.
- Turf toe (MTP joint sprain) is usually seen after a hyperextension or hyperflexion injury and is particularly painful with active or passive flexion or extension of the first MTP joint.

MAKING THE DIAGNOSIS

- Physical examination identifies valgus at first MTP joint.
- Imaging is generally not necessary in minor cases.
- If the deformity is severe or if there is concern about rapid progression, radiographs may be helpful (Figure 48-3).
  - — Weight-bearing AP radiographs are inspected for bony congruence of the MTP joint.
  - — Valgus angulation of the MTP joint and the intermetatarsal angle between the first and second metatarsal are measured.
  - — Angle measures serve as a marker for progression if serial radiographs are obtained.

TREATMENT

- Asymptomatic bunions do not require treatment.
- Patients with painful bunions should be advised to select shoes that do not compress the involved region and to avoid high heels.
- Medial arch supports (commonly sold over the counter as anti-pronation orthotics) may also help relieve MTP pressure in bunion patients with a flexible pes planus.
- For overlying hot spots, donut padding may help relieve any pressure over the region.
- Once appropriate shoes and protection are obtained, normal activities and athletic participation can often continue.
- Surgical correction may be considered for skeletally mature patients with significant symptoms despite compliance with this treatment.

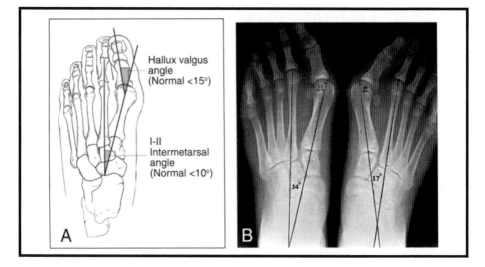

Figure 48-3. Hallux valgus severity is assessed by measuring the hallux valgus angle and the intermetarsal (IM) angle on a weight-bearing anteroposterior (AP) radiograph of the foot. A, Diagram showing the hallux valgus angle and the IM angle. B, AP radiograph of the feet of a patient with hallux valgus demonstrates valgus angulation of 14 degrees in the left foot and 17 degrees in the right foot. Part A is adapted with permission from Pedowitz W. Bunion deformity, in Pfeffer G, Frey C (eds): *Current Practice in Foot and Ankle Surgery.* New York, NY: McGraw Hill; 1993:219–242. Part B is reproduced with permission from Griffin LY (ed). *Essentials of Musculoskeletal Care* 3rd ed. Rosemont, IL: American Academy of Orthopaedic Surgeons; 2005.

EXPECTED OUTCOMES/PROGNOSIS

- Most respond to nonoperative treatment.
- Outcomes after surgery are highly variable. Athletes, and dancers in particular, may be unable to return to their previous level of performance after surgical intervention if MTP range of motion is compromised.

WHEN TO REFER

- Refer to a pediatric orthopaedic surgeon for significant pain despite compliance with conservative measures.

PREVENTION

- Symptoms can often be prevented by choosing footwear with toe boxes wide enough to accommodate the MTP joint without causing undue pressure over the region. However, this probably does not affect the development of the deformity itself.

RELEVANT *ICD-9-CM* CODE

- **735.0**   Hallux valgus

Congenital Toe Deformities

SIMPLE AND COMPLEX SYNDACTYLY OF THE TOES

Introduction/Etiology/Epidemiology

- Webbing or fusion between adjacent toes (see Figure 25-4)
- May be partial or complete.
- The second and third toes are most commonly involved.
- Found in up to 2 per 1,000 live births
- Frequently inherited as an autosomal-dominant trait with variable penetrance
- Usually an isolated finding, but may occur in conjunction with polydactyly (polysyndactyly) or with other genetic syndromes.

Signs and Symptoms

- Usually identified shortly after birth by its straightforward appearance

Making the Diagnosis

- Isolated syndactyly does not require imaging.
- Screen for stigmata of associated genetic syndromes, particularly if syndactyly involves the great toe.

Treatment

- Most do not require treatment.
- Surgical correction can be performed if angulation of the digits develops with growth, or for significant cosmetic concerns.

Expected Outcomes/Prognosis

- Usually remains asymptomatic without creating significant gait or footwear difficulties.

When to Refer

- Refer to a pediatric orthopaedic surgeon
  — If angulation of the digits develops with growth
  — For significant cosmetic concerns

Relevant ICD-9-CM Codes

- **755.10** Syndactyly of multiple and unspecified sites
- **755.13** Syndactyly of toes without fusion of bone
- **755.14** Syndactyly of toes with fusion of bone

TOE POLYDACTYLY

Introduction/Etiology/Epidemiology

- Extra digits on feet
- About one third of cases have a positive family history.
- In the United States polydactyly is more common in African Americans (11.1–13.5 per 1,000) than whites (0.4–2.3 per 1,000).
- Polydactyly of the toes is usually isolated but may be accompanied by polydactyly of the fingers or associated with one of several dozen genetic syndromes, most frequently trisomy 13, Meckel syndrome, and Down syndrome.
- Isolated polydactyly is often autosomal dominant.
- Syndromic polydactyly is usually autosomal recessive.
- Preaxial polydactyly (extra digit is medial to first ray) is most common type.
- Postaxial (extra digit lateral to fifth ray) is most easily treated (see Figure 25-4).
- Central polydactyly (extra digit medial or lateral to second, third, or fourth rays) is rare.

Signs and Symptoms

- Polydactyly is typically identified at birth or on prenatal ultrasound (see Figure 25-4).

Making the Diagnosis

- If identified on prenatal ultrasound, follow-up ultrasound is recommended between 17 and 34 weeks with biometric profile to determine if the polydactyly is isolated.
- Screen for commonly associated genetic syndromes (Box 48-1).
- Radiographs of the foot assist with treatment planning by identifying any bony articulations or presence of extra metatarsals.

Treatment

- Removal of extra digits is recommended due to frequent difficulties with footwear and ambulation, as well as psychosocial concerns.
- Surgery should be performed after the infant can tolerate anesthesia but before he or she is ambulatory, often between 9 and 12 months of age.
- If the extra digit is rudimentary and consists merely of soft tissue, it may be ligated in the nursery and allowed to auto-amputate.

When to Refer

- More fully formed digits and those with any corresponding metatarsal should be referred for surgical removal.

Expected Outcomes/Prognosis

- Postaxial polydactyly has best surgical results.
- Preaxial polydactyly and complex deformities are more likely to have poor surgical results.
- Central polydactyly frequently leads to permanent widening of the foot even after removal.

Box 48-1. Genetic Syndromes Associated With Polydactyly

Acrocallosal syndrome

Bardet-Biedl syndrome

Basal cell nevus syndrome

Biemond syndrome

Ectrodactyly-ectodermal dysplasias-cleft lip/palate syndrome

Ellis-van Creveld syndrome

McKusick-Kaufman syndrome

Meckel-Gruber syndrome

Mirror hand deformity (ulnar dimelia)

Mohr syndrome

Oral-facial-digital syndrome

Pallister-Hall syndrome

Rubinstein-Taybi syndrome

Short rib polydactyly

Vertebral (defects), (imperforate) anus, tracheoesophageal (fistula), radial, and renal (dysplasia) (VATER) association

Relevant ICD-9-CM Code

- **755.02**   Polydactyly of toes

CURLY TOES

Introduction/Etiology/Epidemiology

- Most common lesser toe deformity
- Result from congenital shortening of the flexor digitorum longus and brevis tendons.
- Typically results in rotated toes flexed at the proximal interphalangeal (PIP) joint with varus alignment.
- Fourth and fifth toes are most commonly involved.
- Often familial and bilaterally symmetric

Signs and Symptoms

- Physical examination reveals flexed and rotated digits.
- Passive dorsiflexion of the foot further shortens the flexor tendons and exaggerates the deformity.
- Passive plantarflexion allows the toes to straighten.

Making the Diagnosis

- If the examination is straightforward, imaging is not necessary.

Differential Diagnosis

• Hammer toes

Treatment

• Stretching of the toes, tape splinting, and spacers were previously recommended, but they probably do not significantly affect the natural history of the problem.
• Tenotomy may be considered for preschoolers with persistent significant deformities.
• Older children may require fusion of the PIP joint.

Expected Outcomes/Prognosis

• Most will resolve spontaneously.
• Persistence of the deformity may result in significant callus formation, which often requires flexor tendon release.

When to Refer

• Refer to a pediatric orthopaedic surgeon
— Preschoolers with persistence of significant deformities

Relevant ICD-9-CM Code

• **755.66**   Curly toes

HAMMER TOES

Introduction/Etiology/Epidemiology

• Congenital fixed flexion deformity of PIP joint
• May also be acquired by wearing shoes that are too short or narrow.
• Rotation is not present.
• The second toe is most commonly involved.

Signs and Symptoms

• Physical examination reveals flexed and rotated digits.
• A corn on the top of the toe and a callus on the sole of the foot may develop, which can make walking painful.
• Passive dorsiflexion of the foot further shortens the flexor tendons and exaggerates the deformity.
• Passive plantarflexion allows the toes to straighten.

Making the Diagnosis

• If the examination is straightforward, imaging is not necessary.

Differential Diagnosis

• Curly toes

Treatment

- Nonoperative treatment options include appropriately sized shoes with wide toe box, passive stretching, buddy taping, and corn pads.
- Surgery (interphalangeal joint fusion) may be necessary for adolescents with persistent pain or shoe-fitting problems.

Expected Outcomes/Prognosis

- Pain usually resolves with nonoperative treatment, although the deformity may persist.
- Surgery is rarely necessary.

When to Refer

- Refer adolescents with persistent pain or shoe-fitting problems to a pediatric orthopaedic surgeon.

Prevention

- Appropriately sized shoes
- Monitor children's shoe size frequently during periods of rapid growth.

Relevant ICD-9-CM Code

- **755.66**   Hammer toes

OVERLAPPING TOES

Introduction/Etiology/Epidemiology

- Common congential lesser toe deformity that is often bilateral and familial
- Contracture of the extensor digitorum longus results in an extended, adducted, and externally rotated toe, causing it to overlap the adjacent toe.

Signs and Symptoms

- Physical examination reveals the deformity.
- A dorsal callus is common in older patients.

Making the Diagnosis

- Diagnosis is made clinically; imaging is not necessary.

Treatment

- Initial management is expectant.
- For persistent pain or shoe-fitting problems, release of the tendon and accompanying contracture of the MTP joint may be performed.

Expected Outcomes/Prognosis

- Overlapping second, third, or fourth toes usually correct spontaneously.
- Overlapping fifth toe is more often permanent, and up to 50% will have callus formation and difficulty with shoe wear.

When to Refer

• Refer patients with persistent pain or shoe-fitting problems to a pediatric orthopaedic surgeon.

Relevant ICD-9-CM Code

• **755.66**   Overlapping toes

Bibliography

Berg EE. A reappraisal of metatarsus adductus and skewfoot. *J Bone Joint Surg Am.* 1986;68:1185–1196

Bertsch C, Unger H, Winkelmann W, Rosenbaum D. Evaluation of early walking patterns from plantar pressure distribution measurements. First year results of 42 children. *Gait Posture.* 2004;19:235–242

Betz RR, Kollmer CE, Clancy M, Steel HH. Relationship of congenital hip and foot deformities: a national Shriner's hospital survey. Paper presented at the annual meeting of the Pediatric Orthopaedic Society of North America; May 6–9, 1990; San Francisco, CA

Bleck EE. Metatarsus adductus: classification and relationship to outcomes of treatment. *J Pediatr Orthop.* 1983;3:2–9

Coleman SS. The cavus foot. In: Coleman SS. *Complex Foot Deformities in Children.* Philadelphia, PA: Lea & Febiger; 1983:147–165

Farsetti P, Weinstein SL, Ponseti IV. The long-term functional and radiographic outcomes of untreated and non-operatively treated metatarsus adductus. *J Bone Joint Surg Am.* 1994;76:257–265

Friedreich ataxia 1; FRDA. In: OMIM: Online Mendelian Inheritance in Man. Available at: http://www.ncbi.nlm.nih.gov/entrez/dispomim.cgi?id=229300. Accessed February 17, 2010

Geist ES. The accessory scaphoid bone. *J Bone Joint Surg Am.* 1925;7:570–574

Grogan DP, Gasser SI, Ogden JA. The painful accessory navicular: a clinical and histopathological study. *Foot Ankle.* 1989;10:164–169

Harris RI, Beath T. Etiology of peroneal spastic flat foot. *J Bone Joint Surg Am.* 1948;30B:624–634

Harris RI, Beath T. Hypermobile flat-foot with short tendon Achilles. *J Bone Joint Surg Am.* 1948;30A:116–140

Jacobs JE. Metatarsus varus and hip dysplasia. *Clin Orthop.* 1960;16:203–213

Kasser JR. The foot. In: Raymond T, Morrissy SLW, eds. *Lovell & Winter's Pediatric Orthopaedics.* 6th ed. Philadelphia, PA: Lippincott Williams & Wilkins; 2006:1257–1328

Kumar SJ, MacEwen GD. The incidence of hip dysplasia with metatarsus adductus. *Clin Orthop Relat Res.* 1982;164:234–235

Leonard MA. The inheritance of tarsal coalition and its relationship to spastic flat foot. *J Bone Joint Surg Br.* 1974;56B:520–526

Lysack JT, Fenton PV. Variations in calcaneonavicular morphology demonstrated with radiography. *Radiology.* 2004;230:493–497

Reimers J, Pedersen B, Brodersen A. Foot deformity and the length of the triceps surae in Danish children between 3 and 17 years old. *J Pediatr Orthop B.* 1995;4:71–73

Schwend RM, Drennan JC. Cavus foot deformity in children. *J Am Acad Orthop Surg.* 2003;11:201–211

Smith TWD, Kreibich DN. Freiberg's disease. In: Hetherington VJ, ed. *Hallux Valgus and Forefoot Surgery.* New York, NY: Churchill Livingstone; 1994:453–457

Staheli LT, Chew DE, Corbett M. The longitudinal arch. A survey of eight hundred and eighty-two feet in normal children and adults. *J Bone Joint Surg Am.* 1987;69:426–428

Sullivan JA. Ligament injuries of the foot/ankle in the pediatric athlete. In: DeLee JC, Drez D Jr, Miller MD, eds. *DeLee and Drez's Orthopaedic Sports Medicine: Principles and Practice.* 2nd ed. Philadelphia, PA: WB Saunders; 2003:2376–2391

Thompson GH, Simons GW. Congenital talipes equinovarus (clubfeet) and metatarsus adductus. In: Drennan JC, ed. *The Child's Foot and Ankle.* Philadelphia, PA: Lippincott Willians & Wilkins; 1992:123–127

Tsirikos AI, Riddle EC, Kruse R. Bilateral Köhler's disease in identical twins. *Clin Orthop Relat Res.* 2003;409:195–198

Volpon JB. Footprint analysis during the growth period. *J Pediatr Orthop.* 1994;14:83–85

Wenger DR. Metatarsus adductus and calcaneal valgus. In: Wenger DR, Rang M, eds. *The Art and Practice of Children's Orthopaedics.* Philadelphia, PA: Lippincott Williams & Wilkins; 1993:109–115

Wenger DR, Mauldin D, Speck G, Morgan D, Lieber RL. Corrective shoes and inserts as treatment for flexible flatfoot in infants and children. *J Bone Joint Surg Am.* 1989;71:800–810

Wheeless CR. Calcaneovalgus foot. *Wheeless' Textbook of Orthopaedics.* Available at: http://www.wheelessonline.com/ortho/calcaneovalgus_foot. Accessed February 17, 2010

Williams G, Cowell H. Köhler's disease of the tarsal navicular. *Clin Orthop Relat Res.* 1981;158:53–58

Part 14: Benign and Malignant Tumors

TOPICS COVERED

CHAPTER 49

Overview

Approach to the Evaluation of Benign and Malignant Musculoskeletal Tumors

HISTORY

- The most common presenting complaint is pain.
- Ask the patient to identify the site of pain precisely.
- Note the character of the pain (eg, achy, dull, intermittent, constant, radicular) and if the pain is worse at night or awakens the child from sleep.
- Note how long has the pain been present, and whether the pain is getting better, getting worse, or staying the same.
- Ask about interventions to relieve pain (eg, rest, nonsteroidal anti-inflammatory drugs, ice) and if the measures were helpful.
- Review of systems—history of fevers, malaise or night sweats, weight loss, poor appetite, abdominal pain, vomiting or diarrhea, and other joint pain or swelling.

PHYSICAL EXAMINATION

- Perform a general physical examination and detailed musculoskeletal examination of the affected region.
- Evaluate for muscle atrophy, which suggests the pain has been present for an extended period.
- If a mass is found, note the size, shape, location, consistency, mobility, tenderness, temperature, and character of the overlying skin. Transilluminate if possible—cysts transmit light better than the surrounding tissue.
- Perform neurologic, skin, abdominal, and lymph system examinations.
- Box 49-1 lists characteristics of malignant tumors.

RADIOGRAPHS

- Radiographs are the initial diagnostic test for patients with suspected musculoskeletal injury or neoplasm.
  - Obtain anteroposterior and lateral views of the affected extremity or joint.

Box 49-1. Characteristics of Malignant Tumors

While it is not always possible to determine whether a lesion is benign or malignant based solely on history and physical examination, malignancy is more likely when the following characteristics are present:

- Systemic symptoms (fever and malaise)
- Pain that is unrelated to physical activity
- Pain that is constant or progressive
- Deep, firm, non-movable, tender mass
- Adjacent lymphadenopathy

- When interpreting the radiographs, note the location, size, and character of the lesion and the response of the adjacent bone (figures 49-1 and 49-2).
  — Determine whether the lesion is in the spine, a long bone, or a flat bone.
  — Note whether it is in the metaphysis, diaphysis, or epiphysis.
  — Establish whether it is in the medullary canal, in the cortex, or on the surface of the bone.
  — Note whether it is centrally or eccentrically located.
  — Note whether it appears radiolucent or radiodense.
    ▪ If the lesion is radiolucent, note areas of increased density and calcifications within the lesion, or if it is completely radiolucent.
  — Note if the lesion has well-circumscribed, sclerotic borders, or if the borders are indistinct from the surrounding bone.
  — Note if the lesion is causing cortical destruction or erosions in the bone.
  — Note the bone response to the lesion (eg, periosteal reaction).
- *Benign lesions* are well defined with sclerotic margins.
- *Malignant lesions* have less distinct borders and cause cortical destruction, erosions, and periosteal reaction.

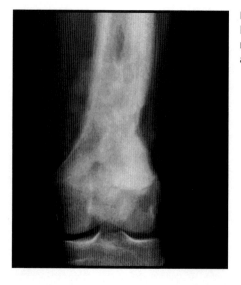

Figure 49-1. Central radiodense lesion with lucent areas, indistinct borders, periosteal reaction, and bone destruction in diaphysis and metaphysis of distal femur.

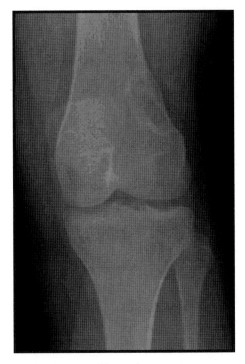

Figure 49-2. Well-circumscribed, cortical, eccentric, radiolucent lesion with sclerotic borders in lateral distal femur mataphysis.

- Patient age and lesion location can suggest a preliminary differential diagnosis.
  — *Benign spine tumors* in children are usually noted in the posterior elements and include aneurysmal bone cyst, osteoid osteoma, and osteoblastoma.
  — *Malignant spine tumors* are usually noted in the vertebral bodies, including Ewing sarcoma and osteosarcoma (rare), both of which can cause vertebra plana (flattening of the vertebral body). An exception is Langerhans cell histiocytosis, a benign tumor that can occur in the vertebral body, also causing vertebra plana.
  — *Long bone lesions*
    - *Diaphyseal:* Ewing sarcoma, fibrous dysplasia, aneurysmal bone cyst, enchondroma, Langerhans histiocytosis, and chondromyxoid fibroma
    - *Metaphyseal:* Nonossifying fibroma and osteosarcoma
    - *Epiphyseal:* Chondroblastoma and simple bone cyst
    - Note: Enchondromas are found in short tubular bones.

ADVANCED IMAGING

- *Bone scans* are useful for screening the entire skeleton for metastatic lesions.
- *Computed tomography scan* is used to define morphology of bone tumors and to guide needle biopsy.
- *Magnetic resonance imaging* determines size and extent of soft tissue and bone lesions.

CHAPTER 50

Common Benign Tumors

Osteoid Osteoma

INTRODUCTION/ETIOLOGY/EPIDEMIOLOGY

- Osteoid osteoma is a common benign bone tumor (Figure 50-1).
- It comprises about 11% of all benign bone tumors in children.
- Male-to-female predominance of about 3:1
- Most commonly found in the femur and tibia, but also found elsewhere in the skeleton, including the posterior elements of the spine

SIGNS AND SYMPTOMS

- Constant pain that may be worse at night
  — Usually, nonsteroidal anti-inflammatory drugs (NSAIDs) or aspirin provide complete or nearly complete pain relief.
  — Physical activity does not affect pain.
- Physical examination may reveal a limp and disuse atrophy of the affected extremity.
- Joint examination, including range of motion, will be normal.
- Palpation may reveal the site of the lesion if it is located in an area without significant overlying soft tissue, such as the proximal tibia.
- Scoliosis may be observed with spinous process lesions.

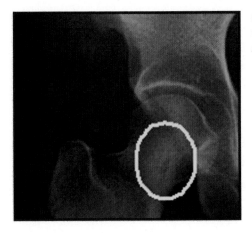

Figure 50-1. Osteoid osteoma of the femoral neck in an 18-year-old college runner presenting with right groin pain.

MAKING THE DIAGNOSIS

- Radiographs may be diagnostic, revealing an area of dense reactive bone surrounding a radiolucent nidus (Figure 50-1).
- Computed tomography (CT), magnetic resonance imaging (MRI), or bone scan
  — May be necessary to identify lesions in the proximal femur or posterior spine.
  — Useful for identifying early lesions because onset of pain may precede findings on plain radiographs
- Biopsy may performed to confirm the diagnosis.

DIFFERENTIAL DIAGNOSIS

- Biopsy will differentiate osteoid osteoma from *infection* and *malignant bone tumor*. Also, patients with osteoid osteoma are unlikely to have fever, which is common in Brodie abscess and osteomyelitis.
- Histologically, *osteoblastoma* appears the same as osteoid osteoma; differentiation is based on the size of the lesion, with osteoid osteoma being smaller than 2 cm.

TREATMENT

- The preferred therapy is percutaneous radiofrequency ablation (RFA). This eliminates months of pain and chronic NSAID therapy for patients.
- Biopsy is performed to confirm the diagnosis prior to RFA.

EXPECTED OUTCOMES/PROGNOSIS

- Spontaneous resolution of osteoid osteoma lesions may occur over 30 to 40 months.
- After RFA, children can resume activity as tolerated, without restriction.
- Treatment of spine lesions that cause scoliosis leads to resolution of scoliosis if treated before symptoms have been present for 15 months.

WHEN TO REFER

- Refer to a pediatric orthopaedic surgeon for treatment when the lesion is identified.

RELEVANT *INTERNATIONAL CLASSIFICATION OF DISEASES, NINTH REVISION, CLINICAL MODIFICATION (ICD-9-CM)* CODE

- **213.9**   Osteoid osteoma

Osteoblastoma

INTRODUCTION/ETIOLOGY/EPIDEMIOLOGY

- Osteoblastoma is a rare benign bone tumor histologically identical to osteoid osteoma.
- Comprises 1% of primary bone tumors and 3.5% of benign bone tumors.
- Male-to-female predominance of 2–3:1
- Most patients present between 10 and 20 years of age.

SIGNS AND SYMPTOMS

- Pain is the primary symptom.
  - — Nonsteroidal anti-inflammatory drugs and aspirin therapy may provide pain relief, but it may not be as dramatic as in osteoid osteoma.
- Soft tissue swelling may be present.
- Occasionally, patients may notice a mass.
- Lesions in extremities may cause limp and disuse atrophy.
- About 50% of osteoblastoma lesions are located in the spine and may cause a decreased range of motion, painful scoliosis, or neurologic signs and symptoms (Figure 50-2).

DIFFERENTIAL DIAGNOSIS

- Osteoblastoma is histologically identical to *osteoid osteoma*, but osteoblastoma is larger, and pain from osteoblastoma is not as readily relieved with NSAIDs.
- *Aneurysmal bone cyst* is clinically and radiographically similar to osteoblastoma; biopsy will differentiate the two.
- On radiographs, *osteosarcoma* is more invasive than osteoblastoma, causing cortical destruction and significant periosteal reaction; biopsy rules out malignancy.

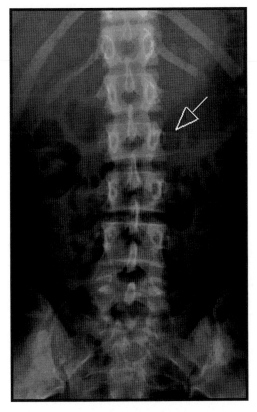

Figure 50-2. Osteoblastoma of the spine may cause mild scoliosis.

MAKING THE DIAGNOSIS

- Laboratory studies are usually normal.
- Plain radiographs are often nonspecific.
  — The lesion is usually diaphyseal or metaphyseal and may be cortical or intramedullary.
  — Cortical lesions expand the cortex and have a thin rim of reactive bone.
  — The lesion has mixed qualities with radiodense and radiolucent areas.
  — Typical findings in the spine include enlargement of the spinous process, decreased pedicle definition, and irregular cortex.
- *Bone scan* or *CT scan* may be necessary to locate and further evaluate spinous process lesions, which may be difficult to identify on radiographs.
- *Computed tomography scan* may also help to differentiate from malignant lesions, which is sometimes difficult on radiographs.

TREATMENT

- Some smaller lesions may be followed with serial radiographs.
- Lesions are often locally aggressive and require wide surgical resection to prevent damage to surrounding structures.

EXPECTED OUTCOMES/PROGNOSIS

- As with osteoid osteoma, if spine lesions are identified and treated within 15 months after the onset of symptoms, associated scoliosis will resolve or decrease significantly.
- Rarely, sarcomatous degeneration of osteoblastoma lesions has been reported.

WHEN TO REFER

- Refer to a pediatric orthopaedic oncologist once the lesion is identified.

RELEVANT *ICD-9-CM* CODE

- **213.9**   Osteoblastoma

Exostosis

INTRODUCTION/ETIOLOGY/EPIDEMIOLOGY

- Exostosis, or *osteochondroma*, is a common benign lesion, accounting for 10% of all tumors and 30% of all benign bone tumors (Figure 50-3).

SIGNS AND SYMPTOMS

- Most patients present with a painless mass.
- Some patients may complain of pain because of repeated trauma of the exostosis or present with a pathologic fracture.
- In asymptomatic patients, lesions are identified on radiographs obtained for other reasons.

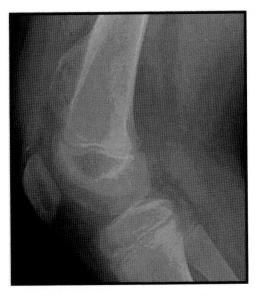

Figure 50-3. Sessile exostosis of the distal femur, presenting as a painless mass in a 10-year-old boy.

- Large lesions may limit joint range of motion, cause neural or vascular compression, or irritate overlying muscle.
- Physical examination reveals a non-tender, fixed mass.
- Range of motion of the adjacent joint may be limited.
- If nerve compression is present, isolated peripheral neurologic signs will be noted.

DIFFERENTIAL DIAGNOSIS

- Multiple hereditary exostoses (MHE) is an autosomal-dominant syndrome in which patients have *multiple exostoses.*
  — Lesions may cause growth disturbance, loss of joint motion, and joint deformity.
  — Deformity of the radius and ulna and short stature are common.

MAKING THE DIAGNOSIS

- The diagnosis can usually be made with plain radiographs.
  — The exostosis may be pedunculated or sessile and is in continuity with the medullary canal of the bone (Figure 50-3).
- Advanced imaging is not usually needed, but if the diagnosis is not clear on plain radiograph, MRI or CT can establish the diagnosis.

TREATMENT

- Surgical intervention in the pediatric age group is indicated if the lesion restricts joint mobility, irritates the overlying muscle, or causes pain due to nerve compression, fracture, or repeated trauma.
- Yearly radiographic evaluation of lesions is recommended.

EXPECTED OUTCOMES/PROGNOSIS

- Exostoses grow until skeletal maturity.
- Malignant degeneration is rare.
- Pathologic fractures may occur during physical activity.
- Patients with MHE have increased risk for secondary chondrosarcoma as adults (rare).

WHEN TO REFER

- Refer to a pediatric orthopaedic surgeon once the lesion is identified.

RELEVANT *ICD-9-CM* CODE

- **213.9**   Exostosis

Enchondroma

INTRODUCTION/ETIOLOGY/EPIDEMIOLOGY

- Common benign tumor, comprising 11% of benign bone tumors (Figure 50-4)
- Most commonly found in the phalanges of the hands and feet; other common locations include the proximal humerus and distal femur.

SIGNS AND SYMPTOMS

- May be asymptomatic or may present with pain or pathologic fracture.
- Physical examination may reveal tenderness at the site of the lesion and the affected digit, or extremity may appear swollen.

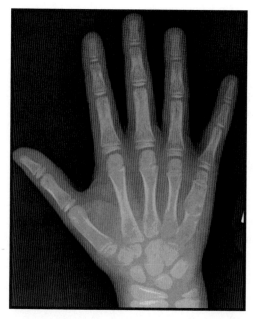

Figure 50-4. Enchondroma of the fifth metacarpal. It is a centrally located, metaphyseal, lucent expansile lesion causing thinning of the cortex. It presented as a painless finger mass in an 8-year-old boy.

DIFFERENTIAL DIAGNOSIS

- *Chondrosarcoma* appears more aggressive on radiograph with cortical destruction—biopsy may be needed to definitively distinguish the two.
- *Fibrous dysplasia* is diaphyseal rather than metaphyseal and in long bones has a more ground-glass appearance, while enchondroma has a more lytic appearance.
- *Multiple enchondroma,* also called *Ollier disease,* are less common than solitary enchondroma and are usually diagnosed at a younger age, typically younger than 10 years.
  — Lesions may be bilateral but are usually worse on one side.
  — Angular and shortening deformities of the extremities are common and may require surgical intervention.

MAKING THE DIAGNOSIS

- Plain radiographs
  — Enchondromas are usually found in the metaphysis within the medullary canal, but epiphyseal lesions have been reported.
  — Lesions are lucent, expansile, and may cause thinning of the cortex.
  — Periosteal reaction is not usually present.
- Magnetic resonance imaging may be used to confirm the diagnosis.
  — Lesions are well-circumscribed and have a high intensity signal on T2-weighted images and intermediate signal on T1.

TREATMENT

- Asymptomatic enchondromas do not require treatment.
- Symptomatic enchondromas and those associated with fracture should be excised.

EXPECTED OUTCOMES/PROGNOSIS

- Unlike with solitary enchondroma, patients with multiple enchondroma are at risk for secondary chondrosarcoma over time, particularly in the shoulder and pelvis.

WHEN TO REFER

- Refer symptomatic enchondromas and those associated with fractures to a pediatric orthopaedic surgeon for excision.

RELEVANT *ICD-9-CM* CODES

- **213.9**   Enchondroma
- **756.4**   Ollier disease

Chondroblastoma

INTRODUCTION/ETIOLOGY/EPIDEMIOLOGY

* Uncommon, benign bone tumor; comprises 1% of bone tumors (Figure 50-5 a, b).
* Commonly affects children with open physes between 10 and 19 years of age.
* The humerus, tibia, and femur are common sites of involvement.

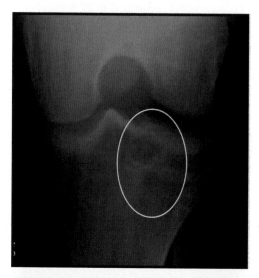

Figure 50-5a. Chondroblastoma of the proximal tibia. An epiphyseal lesion that is lucent, well-circumscribed, and centrally located. This lesion presented in a 16-year-old boy as knee pain.

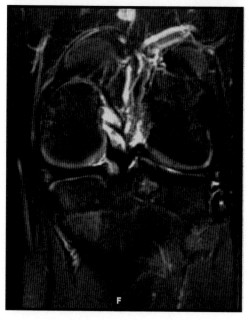

Figure 50-5b. Magnetic resonance imaging of the same well-circumscribed lesion showing enhancement on T2-weighted images.

SIGNS AND SYMPTOMS

- Presents with pain, tenderness, and limited range of motion of an adjacent joint.
- Joint effusion may be present, particularly with lesions in distal femur or proximal tibia.

DIFFERENTIAL DIAGNOSIS

- Chronic synovitis
- Osteochondritis dissecans
- Osteomyelitis

MAKING THE DIAGNOSIS

- Plain radiographs reveal a radiolucent lesion with central calcifications.
  - — Reactive bone surrounds the lesion and periosteal reaction may be present.
  - — Lesions are usually epiphyseal but may cross the physis into metaphysis.
- Chest CT should be obtained because chondroblastoma may cause lung implants even though it is thought to be a benign lesion.

TREATMENT

- Curettage with or without bone grafting

EXPECTED OUTCOMES/PROGNOSIS

- Chondroblastomas tend to enlarge.
- Growth disturbance is rare, even when the tumor crosses the physis.

WHEN TO REFER

- Refer to a pediatric orthopaedic surgeon when the lesion is identified.

RELEVANT *ICD-9-CM* CODE

- **213.9**   Chondroblastoma

Nonossifying Fibroma

INTRODUCTION/ETIOLOGY/EPIDEMIOLOGY

- Nonossifying fibroma (fibrous cortical defect) is the most common bone lesion in children, occurring in *up to 35% to 40%* of all children (Figure 50-6).
- Most lesions are found in the distal femur.

SIGNS AND SYMPTOMS

- Nonossifying fibromas are asymptomatic; they are diagnosed when found incidentally on radiographs obtained for other reasons.
- Rarely, children present with symptoms caused by pathologic fracture.

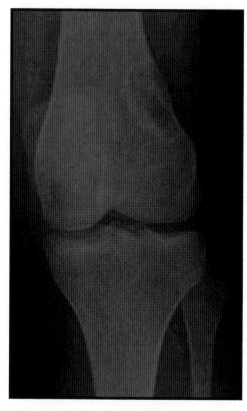

Figure 50-6. Nonossifying fibroma of the distal femur. A well-circumscribed, metaphyseal lesion with sclerotic borders. This lesion was found incidentally in a 15-year-old boy who had these films taken after a knee injury during a football game.

DIFFERENTIAL DIAGNOSIS

- Distinguish from *fibrous dysplasia* by size and location. Fibrous dysplasia lesions are larger and intramedullary compared with nonossifying fibromas, which are smaller and cortical.

MAKING THE DIAGNOSIS

- Radiographs are usually diagnostic, revealing a well-circumscribed, eccentrically located lesion originating from the medullary canal (Figure 50-6).
- No further imaging or evaluation is needed.

TREATMENT

- Lesions less than 50% of the diameter of the bone can be followed by the primary care provider with serial radiographs every 3 to 6 months.
- Lesions exceeding 50% of the diameter of the bone are at increased risk for pathologic fracture and may require curettage and bone graft.
- Pathologic fracture is treated like other fractures; healing within a normal length of time can be expected.

EXPECTED OUTCOMES/PROGNOSIS

- Lesions resolve spontaneously over time.
- Large lesions (greater than 50% of the diameter of the bone) are at increased risk for pathologic fracture.

WHEN TO REFER

- Refer lesions exceeding 50% of the diameter of the bone to a pediatric orthopaedic surgeon.

RELEVANT *ICD-9-CM* CODE

- **733.99**   Nonossifying fibroma

Fibrous Dysplasia

INTRODUCTION/ETIOLOGY/EPIDEMIOLOGY

- Fibrous dysplasia is common, representing 5% to 7% of benign tumors (Figure 50-7).
- Fibrotic lesions replace and weaken the bone.
- There are 2 types of fibrous dysplasia.
  — Monostotic (single lesion) is more common.
  — Polyostotic (multiple lesions) is more severe.

SIGNS AND SYMPTOMS

- Monostotic
  — Majority are asymptomatic, presenting as an incidental finding on radiographs obtained for other reasons.
  — Large lesions may present with pain and swelling or pathologic fracture, which is the presenting feature in about 30% to 50% of cases.
  — Angular deformity and leg-length discrepancy are less common presenting complaints.
- Polyostotic
  — Much more likely to present with limb-length discrepancy or angular deformity
    ▪ Shepherd crook deformity (varus deformity of the femoral neck) is the most common.
  — Scoliosis is occasionally found.
  — Rarely, polyostotic fibrous dysplasia is associated with McCune-Albright syndrome, a genetic disease characterized by the triad of polyostotic fibrous dysplasia, café au lait spots, and precocious puberty.

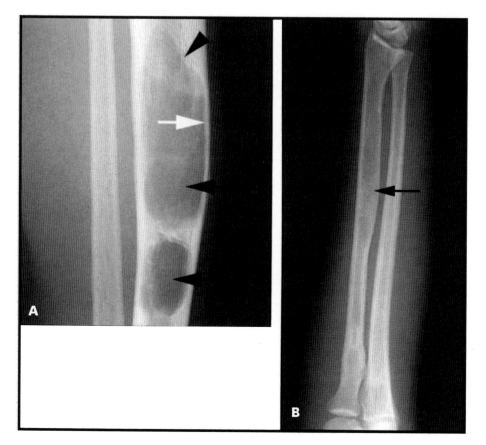

Figure 50-7. Fibrous dysplasia. A, Lateral view of the lower leg of a young woman, taken after an injury. The patient reported no preinjury pain. Note the large, multiloculated geographic lytic lesion located centrally in the middiaphysis of the tibia (black arrows). The surrounding cortex is chronically thinned and slightly dilated, with a sharply defined sclerotic narrow zone of transition (white arrow) typical of a benign tumor. The "smoky" appearance of the upper portion of the lesion (arrowhead) is caused by fibro-osseous tissue typically found in the lytic core of fibrous dysplastic lesions. This feature is not seen in solitary bone cysts, which appear darker because of the lack of such tissue. B, Anteroposterior view showing fibrous dysplasia involving the entire radius of a young woman who reported no pain. Note the "smoky" area of fibro-osseous matrix calcification surrounded by a thinly dilated cortex (arrow). Reproduced with permission from Johnson TR, Steinbach LS (eds): *Essentials of Musculoskeletal Imaging.* Rosemont, IL: American Academy of Orthopaedic Surgeons; 2004.

DIFFERENTIAL DIAGNOSIS

- *Nonossifying fibroma*: smaller and cortical (rather than intramedullary), distinguishing it from fibrous dysplasia
- *Low-grade osteosarcoma*: comparatively, fibrous dysplasia lesions appear less aggressive with no reactive shell or permeative borders.

MAKING THE DIAGNOSIS

- Plain radiographs (Figure 50-7)
  - — The lesions are diaphyseal and intramedullary with a *ground-glass appearance.*
  - — The diaphysis appears enlarged and the cortex is thinned.
  - — The border between the medullary canal and cortex may be less distinct.
  - — Over time, the lesion may take on a cystic or radiodense appearance.
  - — In polyostotic type, the lesions are usually unilateral but may be bilateral.
- Bone scan should be performed to evaluate for polyostotic dysplasia.
- Computed tomography and MRI can be used to further evaluate lesions for diagnosis and surgical planning. On MRI, the lesions are hypodense on T1- and T2-weighted images.

TREATMENT

- Asymptomatic lesions should be evaluated with radiographs to monitor growth every 3 to 6 months until skeletal maturity is achieved.
- If the lesion is large, painful, or located in the femoral neck, curettage and bone grafting may be necessary.

EXPECTED OUTCOMES/PROGNOSIS

- Monostotic lesions enlarge during periods of skeletal growth and stabilize with skeletal maturity.
- Patients with polyostotic fibrous dysplasia are more likely to experience progressive deformity; lesions may continue to grow even after skeletal maturity.
- Malignant transformation of fibrous dysplasia lesions is rare.

WHEN TO REFER

- Patients with polyostotic fibrous dysplasia should be referred to a pediatric orthopaedic surgeon and an endocrine specialist at the time of diagnosis.

RELEVANT *ICD-9-CM* CODES

- **733.29** Monostotic fibrous dysplasia
- **756.54** Polyostotic fibrous dysplasia
- **756.59** McCune-Albright syndrome

Aggressive Fibromatosis

INTRODUCTION/ETIOLOGY/EPIDEMIOLOGY

• Aggressive fibromatosis, or extra-abdominal desmoid, is a benign fibrous lesion.
• Uncommon, comprising 3% of all soft tissue tumors with an incidence of 2 to 4 per million
• Extremity lesions are common in children.
• Lesions are also found in the abdominal wall, trunk, head, neck, and breast.
• More common in females
• Frequently found in patients with familial adenomatous polyposis (FAP) or Gardner syndrome, which is characterized by colorectal polyposis, epidermal cysts, and osteomata.

SIGNS AND SYMPTOMS

• Painless swelling in an extremity
• Large lesions may present with loss of joint range of motion or neurologic symptoms such as numbness, paresthesias, or radiating pain caused by nerve impingement.
• Physical examination may reveal a mildly tender, growing mass that is firm and tends to be deep to the surface.

MAKING THE DIAGNOSIS

• Plain radiographs may help with diagnosis.
— Soft tissue mass may be noted and rarely may cause bony erosions.
• Magnetic resonance imaging is useful for defining the extent of the lesion and following progression.
— The lesion may be hypo-intense or hyperintense compared with adjacent muscle.
— It tends to have low signal on T1 and T2.

DIFFERENTIAL DIAGNOSIS

• Aggressive fibromatosis can be distinguished from other soft tissue sarcomas on MRI by its lower signal intensity on T2-weighted images.

TREATMENT

• Surgical excision is recommended because, while benign, these lesions may be locally invasive and destructive.
• Complete excision is difficult because the lesion tends to be infiltrative.
• Wide resection is usually not indicated if it will lead to dysfunction.
• If pathology reveals positive margins, patients are followed for local recurrence.
— Irradiation has been used when margins are positive or for recurrent disease.
— Adjuvant chemotherapy may also be employed.

EXPECTED OUTCOMES/PROGNOSIS

• Lesions may spontaneously regress or stop growing over time.

WHEN TO REFER

• At the time of diagnosis, refer to a pediatric orthopaedic surgeon for treatment and to a gastroenterologist to evaluate for FAP and Gardner syndrome.

RELEVANT *ICD-9-CM* CODE

• **238.1**   Aggressive fibromatosis

Osteofibrous Dysplasia

INTRODUCTION/ETIOLOGY/EPIDEMIOLOGY

• Benign lesion found in the anterior tibia (may also occur in mandible)
• Rare

SIGNS AND SYMPTOMS

• Typically presents as a painless deformity, usually with anterior bowing of tibia.
• Some may present with pathologic fracture.

DIFFERENTIAL DIAGNOSIS

• *Adamantinoma:* patients are significantly older, presenting in their 20s, and the lesions tend to be more progressive and appear more aggressive on radiographs.

MAKING THE DIAGNOSIS

• Radiographs are usually diagnostic (Figure 50-8).
— The lesion is found in the anterior cortex of the diaphysis of the tibia.
— There is bowing of the bone and intracortical osteolysis with an adjacent sclerotic band.

TREATMENT

• Surgical intervention is not always needed.
• The patient will be followed with radiographs every 6 months.
• Biopsy and resection are performed for progressive lesions.

EXPECTED OUTCOMES/PROGNOSIS

• Lesions may progress until puberty or spontaneously regress.

WHEN TO REFER

• Refer to a pediatric orthopaedic surgeon or orthopaedic oncologist.

RELEVANT *ICD-9-CM* CODE

• **756.59**   Osteofibrous dysplasia

Unicameral Bone Cyst (Simple Bone Cyst)

INTRODUCTION/ETIOLOGY/EPIDEMIOLOGY

• Unicameral bone cysts (UBCs) are common, benign, fluid-filled bone lesions frequently found in children and adolescents (Figure 50-8).
• The proximal humerus and femur are the most common sites.
• Male-to-female predominance is 2:1.

SIGNS AND SYMPTOMS

• Usually asymptomatic unless pathologic fracture occurs.
• Often identified as an incidental finding on a radiograph obtained for unrelated reasons

MAKING THE DIAGNOSIS

• Radiographs are diagnostic.
  — Unicameral bone cysts originate from the epiphysis and extend into the metaphysis.
  — Unicameral bone cyst borders are well circumscribed with a thin rim of bone.
  — Some UBCs have fallen leaf sign—fragment of bone at the bottom of the cyst cavity.
• Magnetic resonance imaging may be obtained to establish the diagnosis, if needed.

TREATMENT

• For large lesions or those in high-stress anatomic sites, which are at increased risk for pathologic fracture, surgical intervention is appropriate.
  — Treatment with intralesional injection of corticosteroids may be sufficient, but serial injections may be required.
  — For lesions that do not respond to injection, curettage and bone graft or intramedullary nailing can be performed.
• While lesions often heal after pathologic fracture, surgical intervention may be necessary for lesions associated with multiple pathologic fractures.

EXPECTED OUTCOMES/PROGNOSIS

• Unicameral bone cysts usually move away from the epiphysis with growth and resolve spontaneously.
• Possible complications include recurrence and growth arrest.

WHEN TO REFER

• Refer UBCs to a pediatric orthopaedic surgeon for management.

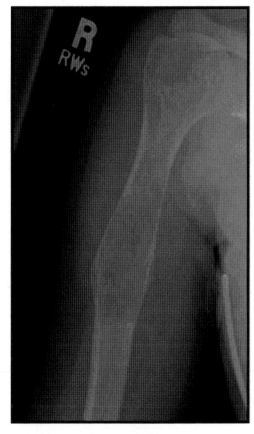

Figure 50-8. Unicameral bone cyst (simple bone cyst) found in a 17-year-old swimmer when she presented with pathologic fracture.

RELEVANT *ICD-9-CM* CODE

● **733.21**   Unicameral bone cyst

Aneurysmal Bone Cyst

INTRODUCTION/ETIOLOGY/EPIDEMIOLOGY

● Aneurysmal bone cyst (ABC) is a relatively rare, blood-filled bone cyst in children.
● Comprises 1% of all bone tumors; 1 per 1.4 per million.
● Slightly more common in females than males

SIGNS AND SYMPTOMS

● Often asymptomatic; identified on radiographs obtained for other reasons
● Some patients may present with chronic, dull, achy pain and swelling.
● Rarely, patients present with pathologic fracture.
● Physical examination is usually normal, unless pathologic fracture has occurred.
● In spinal lesions, patients may present with scoliosis or neurologic symptoms secondary to cord or nerve root compression.

MAKING THE DIAGNOSIS

- *Radiographic findings* depend on the anatomic site of the lesion.
  - — In long bones, ABC is metaphyseal or diaphyseal, eccentrically located, and arising from the medullary canal. It expands the bone and thins the cortex.
  - — In the spine, ABC arises in the posterior elements and may extend into the body of the vertebra or adjacent rib.
- *Computed tomography* and *MRI* can identify fluid levels and are often necessary to establish the diagnosis, especially for spinal lesions.

DIFFERENTIAL DIAGNOSIS

- The metaphyseal/diaphyseal location of ABC distinguishes it from UBC, which is an epiphyseal lesion extending into the metaphysis.
- Aneurysmal bone cyst is usually less aggressive than osteosarcoma and Ewing sarcoma.

TREATMENT

- Curettage and packing with bone graft or polymethylmethacrylate
- For lesions not accessible to curettage, packing with demineralized bone and autogenous bone marrow may be used to induce healing of the lesion.

EXPECTED OUTCOMES/PROGNOSIS

- Recurrence is common in younger patients.
- Proximal femoral lesions are at high risk for pathologic fracture.

WHEN TO REFER

- Refer immediately to a pediatric orthopaedic surgeon for definitive evaluation and management.

RELEVANT *ICD-9-CM* CODE

- **733.22**   Aneurysmal bone cyst

Langerhans Cell Histiocytosis

INTRODUCTION/ETIOLOGY/EPIDEMIOLOGY

- Also called histiocytosis X or eosinophilic granuloma (Figure 50-9 a,b)
- Develops in patients between 5 and 15 years of age.
- Commonly presents as a painless mass in the skull, but may also manifest in the long bones, spine, and pelvis.

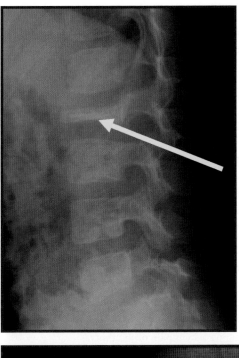

Figure 50-9a. Langerhans histiocytosis of the vertebral body causing vertebra plana.

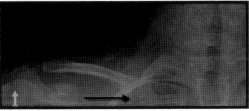

Figure 50-9b. Langerhans histiocytosis of the proximal clavicle presenting as shoulder pain in a 12-year-old female swimmer.

- Severe forms of Langerhans histiocytosis have been identified.
  - *Letterer-Siwe disease* refers to disseminated Langerhans and is associated with multiple lesions, wasting, and hepatosplenomegaly.
  - Langerhans with skull lesions, diabetes insipidus, and exophthalmos is called *Hand-Schüller-Christian disease.*

SIGNS AND SYMPTOMS

- Presenting symptoms include pain at the site of the lesion and fever.
- Patients with long bone lesions may present with pathologic fracture.
- Patients with spine lesions may have neurologic symptoms such as radicular pain or gait abnormalities.
- Physical examination reveals tenderness to palpation at the site of the lesion.
- Neurologic deficits such as altered gait may be observed with spine lesions.

DIFFERENTIAL DIAGNOSIS

- For long bone lesions, osteomyelitis, Ewing sarcoma, and lymphoma
- For spine lesions, Ewing sarcoma, lymphoma, leukemia, aneurysmal bone cyst, and infection

MAKING THE DIAGNOSIS

- Laboratory studies may show elevated erythrocyte sedimentation rate and C-reactive protein.
- Radiographic findings depend on the location of the lesion.
  - In the spine, vertebra plana—flattening of the vertebral body (Figure 50-9a)
  - In flat bones, punched out, lytic lesions will be seen (Figure 50-9b).
  - Magnetic resonance imaging may be necessary to further evaluate extent of the lesion.
- Biopsy may be necessary for definitive diagnosis.
- A bone scan should be performed to evaluate for multiple skeletal lesions.

TREATMENT

- Because lesions will usually resolve spontaneously, observation and splinting for comfort is often sufficient.
- Surgery may be required for lesions causing persistent pain or disability.
- Intralesional steroid injection may be used for painful lesions not easily accessible surgically.
- Pathologic fractures are treated with appropriate immobilization and may require bone graft.
- Some children may be treated with radiation or chemotherapy, especially those with spine lesions or multiple lesions.
- Some children with spine lesions may require surgery for deformity.

EXPECTED OUTCOMES/PROGNOSIS

- Children with isolated skeletal lesions have a good prognosis because the lesions will usually resolve spontaneously over several months.

WHEN TO REFER

- Lesions in the spine causing neurologic signs should be referred to a neurosurgeon or an orthopaedic spine surgeon.
- Lesions in the long bones or pelvis should be referred to an orthopaedic surgeon.

RELEVANT *ICD-9-CM* CODES

- **277.89**   Langerhans cell histiocytosis, chronic
- **202.5**   Langerhans cell histiocytosis, acute

Popliteal (Baker) Cyst

INTRODUCTION/ETIOLOGY/EPIDEMIOLOGY

- Benign swelling of the bursa between the gastrocnemius and semi-membranous tendons (medial aspect of popliteal fossa)
- Common in children between 4 and 12 years of age
- More frequent in boys
- Unlike in adults, popliteal cysts in children rarely communicate with the joint and are rarely associated with intra-articular pathology.

SIGNS AND SYMPTOMS

- Painless swelling in the back of the knee
- Cyst is non-tender, smooth, and distensible.
- Remainder of knee examination is normal.

DIFFERENTIAL DIAGNOSIS

- Solid tumors: lipomas, xanthomas, vascular tumors, fibrosarcomas

MAKING THE DIAGNOSIS

- The diagnosis can be made by history and physical examination.
  — Unlike a solid tumor, the popliteal cyst will transilluminate.
- If there is any uncertainty, ultrasound can distinguish a fluid-filled popliteal cyst from a solid tumor.

TREATMENT

- Reassurance that the cyst will resolve spontaneously with time
- Aspiration is not recommended because of the high rate of recurrence.
- In children, surgical excision of popliteal cysts is rarely indicated.
  — Excision may be considered for very large or painful cysts.
  — Recurrence after excision is common.

EXPECTED OUTCOMES/PROGNOSIS

- The natural history is for spontaneous resolution, but this may take several months to several years.

WHEN TO REFER

- Children with painful cysts or large cysts that limit joint motion should be referred to a pediatric orthopaedic surgeon.

RELEVANT *ICD-9-CM* CODE

- **727.51** Popliteal cyst

CHAPTER 51

Malignant Tumors

Leukemia

INTRODUCTION/ETIOLOGY/EPIDEMIOLOGY

- Comprises 25% to 30% of cancer in the pediatric age group
- More common in white children than in black children

SIGNS AND SYMPTOMS

- Twenty-five percent of children with leukemia will present with bone pain, usually in the extremities; a few may also complain of joint pain, swelling, or limp.
- Musculoskeletal symptoms are less common than systemic symptoms, which include fatigue, easy bruising or bleeding, infection, or fever.
- Physical examination may reveal diffuse lymphadenopathy, hepatosplenomegaly, and tenderness to palpation of affected long bones of the extremities.
- Bruises in multiple stages of healing may also be found.

DIFFERENTIAL DIAGNOSIS

- Laboratory studies and radiographs will differentiate bone pain caused by leukemia from *osteomyelitis* or *primary bone tumor*.

MAKING THE DIAGNOSIS

- In those with musculoskeletal symptoms, *radiographic findings* may include
  — Osteopenia
  — Periosteal reaction
  — Metaphyseal bands
  — Sclerosis with or without lytic areas
- Complete blood count will show bone marrow failure, usually with anemia and thrombocytopenia.
- Leukemic cells may or may not be seen on peripheral blood smear.
- *Bone marrow biopsy* provides definitive diagnosis.

TREATMENT

- Treatment involves chemotherapy.

EXPECTED OUTCOMES/PROGNOSIS

- Prognosis is better for children with the following factors:
  — Age at presentation between 1 and 9 years of age (B-cell acute lymphoblastic leukemia [ALL] only)
  — White blood cell count at presentation less than 100,000
  — White race
  — Female gender
  — Pre-B or early pre–B-cell ALL (vs T-cell and mature B-cell ALL)
  — Only one chemotherapy cycle needed to achieve remission
  — No spread to liver, spleen, spinal fluid, or testicles

WHEN TO REFER

- Refer immediately to a pediatric oncologist for definitive diagnosis and treatment.

RELEVANT *INTERNATIONAL CLASSIFICATION OF DISEASES, NINTH REVISION, CLINICAL MODIFICATION (ICD-9-CM)* CODE

- **208.9** ·Leukemia

Neuroblastoma

INTRODUCTION/ETIOLOGY/EPIDEMIOLOGY

- Neuroblastoma is a cancer of the peripheral sympathetic nervous system, accounting for 8% of cancers in children.

SIGNS AND SYMPTOMS

- Symptoms include abdominal pain and swelling.
- If metastatic disease is present, children may complain of bone pain, fever, weight loss, subcutaneous nodules, orbital proptosis, and periorbital ecchymoses.
- Paraspinal lesions may cause back pain with radicular symptoms.

DIFFERENTIAL DIAGNOSIS

- Abdominal rhabdomyosarcoma
- Wilms tumor

MAKING THE DIAGNOSIS

- Radiographs of the extremities (obtained for bone pain) are expected to be normal; however, an intra-abdominal mass may be seen on radiographs or computed tomography (CT).
- *Bone scan* will identify metastatic bone lesions.
- *Biopsy* is usually required for definitive diagnosis.

TREATMENT

- Surgical excision, chemotherapy, and possibly radiation therapy may be indicated.

EXPECTED OUTCOMES/PROGNOSIS

- Depends on age, stage, and certain biologic characteristics of the tumor.

WHEN TO REFER

- Refer immediately to a pediatric oncologist for definitive diagnosis and treatment.

RELEVANT *ICD-9-CM* CODE

- **171.9**   Neuroblastoma

Osteosarcoma

INTRODUCTION/ETIOLOGY/EPIDEMIOLOGY

- Common primary malignancy of bone in patients younger than 30 years
- Comprises 56% of all malignant bone tumors.
- Annual incidence is 4.8 per million.
- Incidence is slightly higher in boys versus girls and black versus white children.
- Children with a history of hereditary retinoblastoma, Li-Fraumeni syndrome, and Rothmund-Thomson syndrome are at increased risk for osteosarcoma.
- Osteosarcoma is found in the long bones of the upper and lower extremities, and the central axis (ie, flat bones of the shoulder, chest, and pelvis, and soft tissues).
- The distal femur is the most common site, followed by the proximal tibia and proximal humerus.

SIGNS AND SYMPTOMS

- *Pain* and mass are the most common presenting symptoms.
  - — Onset of pain is insidious but progressive.
  - — Patients wait an average of 6 weeks before presenting for evaluation.
  - — Twenty percent report nighttime pain.
  - — Fifty-five percent report intermittent pain at rest.
- At the first visit, 40% have a *palpable mass* that is typically tender and firm.
- There may be *limited range of motion* of the adjacent joint.
- *Swelling* of the affected limb may be noted when a distinct mass is not palpable.
- *Paresthesia* related to peripheral nerve compression by tumor is rare.
- If *pathologic fracture* has occurred, the child may complain of sudden onset of pain and swelling.

DIFFERENTIAL DIAGNOSIS

• Osteomyelitis
• Symptoms may resemble *musculoskeletal injury* early in the course of disease; maintain a high index of suspicion for osteosarcoma in patients whose symptoms persist or worsen despite conservative therapy.

MAKING THE DIAGNOSIS

• *Radiographs* usually establish the diagnosis but do not always demonstrate the full involvement of the primary tumor.
  — Typically manifests as a metaphyseal lesion with poorly defined borders that has lytic and blastic components (Figure 51-1).
  — Periosteal reaction may have a sunburst appearance or Codman triangle.
• *Chest radiographs* are performed to rule out skeletal and pulmonary metastases.
• *Laboratory studies* may demonstrate elevated alkaline phosphatase or lactate dehydrogenase (LDH) levels, but are often normal.

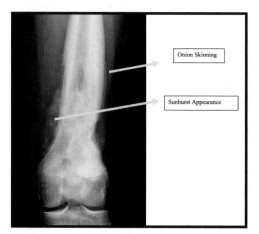

Figure 51-1. Osteosarcoma—anteroposterior (AP) view of proximal humerus. AP view of the proximal humerus of a teenaged boy showing a large, aggressive-appearing, osteoblastic, centrally located, metaphyseal lesion that has broken out circumferentially for a great distance under the periosteum.

TREATMENT

• Treatment includes adjuvant and neoadjuvant chemotherapy and surgical resection of the primary tumor.
  — Neoadjuvant chemotherapy reduces tumor size, allowing for easier excision and assessment of tumor response to chemotherapy.
  — Limb sparing procedures are possible in up to 80% of children.

EXPECTED OUTCOMES/PROGNOSIS

• Patients with localized osteosarcoma have 3- to 5-year event-free survival of 60% to 70%.
• Patients who have pulmonary metastases at the time of diagnosis do not fare as well and have a 20% to 30% survival rate.

- Patients with skip metastases in the bone, synchronous regional bone metastases, have a worse prognosis.
- Functional outcome depends on tumor location, size, and soft tissue involvement.
  — For the proximal humerus, patients report 70% to 90% of normal function on the Musculoskeletal Tumor Society functional assessment tool.
  — For the distal femur, functional scores of 77% of normal are reported.

WHEN TO REFER

- Refer immediately to an orthopaedic surgeon for biopsy and definitive surgery.

RELEVANT *ICD-9-CM* CODE

- **170.9**   Osteosarcoma

Ewing Sarcoma

INTRODUCTION/ETIOLOGY/EPIDEMIOLOGY

- Most common bone tumor in patients younger than 10 years
- Second most common bone tumor in adolescents
- Accounts for 34% of bone tumors in children.
- Annual incidence is 2.9 per million.
- Boys are more commonly affected than girls.
- Rare in black population; white children are 6 times more likely to have Ewing sarcoma.
- Central axis is the most common site of involvement (ie, the flat bones of the shoulder, chest, and pelvis, and soft tissues).
- The femur is the most common site for extremity involvement.

SIGNS AND SYMPTOMS

- Pain is the most common presenting symptom.
  — Because the onset of pain is insidious, patients typically delay seeking medical care for an average of 15 weeks, with a total delay from time of symptom onset to diagnosis as long as 6 months.
- Soft tissue swelling or erythema may be reported.
- A palpable mass may be noted in 34% of patients.
- Range of motion of adjacent joints may be limited.
- Twenty percent of parents will report that the child has been limping.
- Thirty percent of patients have unexplained fevers.
- Spine and pelvic lesions, which are more common in Ewing sarcoma than in osteosarcoma, are more difficult to palpate and view on radiographs.

DIFFERENTIAL DIAGNOSIS

- Osteomyelitis and cellulitis
  — Because of the erythema and history of fever, patients may be initially misdiagnosed with bone or soft tissue infection.
- Musculoskeletal injury
  — As with osteosarcoma, symptoms may resemble musculoskeletal injury early in the course of disease; maintain a high index of suspicion in patients whose symptoms persist or worsen despite conservative therapy.

MAKING THE DIAGNOSIS

- Diagnosis can usually be made with *plain radiographs.*
  — Destructive metaphyseal or diaphyseal lesion with periosteal reaction and a soft tissue mass
  — The periosteal reaction may have the typical onion skin appearance or form a Codman triangle.
- *Magnetic resonance imaging* may be used to determine the full extent of the primary lesion and associated soft tissue mass.
- *Chest radiograph* and *CT* are obtained to look for pulmonary metastases—the most common site for metastases.
- A *bone scan* is performed to identify skeletal metastases.
- *Laboratory findings* include an increased white blood cell count, sedimentation rate or LDH, and anemia.
  — Increased LDH and anemia are associated with an unfavorable prognosis.

TREATMENT

- Neoadjuvant and adjuvant chemotherapy followed by resection of the primary tumor as indicated
  — Neoadjuvant chemotherapy may shrink the tumor, allowing for safer excision and an assessment of tumor response to chemotherapy.
- If the primary tumor site is not accessible to resection, as in spine or pelvis lesions, radiation therapy may be performed instead of surgical resection.

EXPECTED OUTCOMES/PROGNOSIS

- Long-term survival rates range from 50% to 70%.
- Those with extremity lesions have improved survival rates compared with those with pelvic-sacral lesions.
- Those with metastatic disease at the time of diagnosis have poor outcomes.

WHEN TO REFER

- Refer immediately to an orthopaedic oncologist.

RELEVANT *ICD-9-CM* CODE

* **170.9**   Ewing sarcoma

Rhabdomyosarcoma

INTRODUCTION/ETIOLOGY/EPIDEMIOLOGY

* Soft tissue sarcoma of childhood that accounts for 3.5% of all childhood malignancies
* Represents 50% to 60% of all soft tissue sarcomas in children younger than 5 years and 23% to 25% in 15- to 19-year-olds.
* Annual incidence is 4.6 per million children.
* Slightly more common in males than females with a ratio of 1.6:1
* Children with a history of retinoblastoma, neurofibromatosis-1, and Li-Fraumeni syndrome are at increased risk.
* Can occur in any part of the body. Extremity lesions, which may present as an orthopaedic problem, make up about 20% of all rhabdomyosarcomas.

SIGNS AND SYMPTOMS

* Rhabdomyosarcoma in the extremity manifests as a *painless* mass.
* There may be palpable lymphadenopathy in the affected limb because lymph node metastasis is common.

MAKING THE DIAGNOSIS

* *Radiographs* demonstrate a soft tissue mass.
* *Magnetic resonance imaging* or *CT* are performed to establish the extent of the primary lesion and should include the regional lymph nodes to look for metastases.
* *Biopsy* confirms the diagnosis.
* *Bone marrow biopsy* may be performed for staging.
* *Bone scan* and *chest CT* will help in searching for distant metastases.

DIFFERENTIAL DIAGNOSIS

* Biopsy will differentiate rhabdomyosarcoma from *other soft tissue sarcomas.*
* Rhabdomyosarcoma is histologically similar to *other round blue cell tumors* (eg, Ewing sarcoma, neuroblastoma, lymphoma); molecular testing can differentiate these.

TREATMENT

* Surgical resection with wide margins, neoadjuvant and adjuvant chemotherapy
* Radiation may be used before resection in cases where amputation might otherwise be needed to obtain a wide margin on resection. Radiation may also be used after resection if the margins are not clear.

EXPECTED OUTCOMES/PROGNOSIS

- Children who present with rhabdomyosarcoma of the extremities have a poor prognosis compared with those who present with genitourinary or head and neck tumors.
- *Early diagnosis and immediate referral* are imperative.
  - Tumors that are more than 5 cm in diameter at the time of diagnosis have a poor prognosis compared with smaller tumors.
  - Young children have a higher 5-year survival rate (75%–81%) compared with adolescents and young adults (20%–40%).

WHEN TO REFER

- Refer immediately to an orthopaedic oncologist for biopsy.

RELEVANT *ICD-9-CM* CODE

- **171.9**   Rhabdomyosarcoma

Synovial Cell Sarcoma

INTRODUCTION/ETIOLOGY/EPIDEMIOLOGY

- Usually found in the extremities
- Account for about 10% of all soft tissue sarcomas in children.
- Annual incidence is 0.4 per million children.
- Occur more often in adolescents

SIGNS AND SYMPTOMS

- Presents as a *painful* mass that is usually tender and firm.
- Onset of pain may precede development of a palpable mass.
- If metastasis has occurred, regional lymphadenopathy may be palpable.

DIFFERENTIAL DIAGNOSIS

- Biopsy and molecular testing will differentiate synovial cell sarcoma from *other soft tissue sarcomas* and *round blue cell tumors* (eg, Ewing sarcoma, neuroblastoma, lymphoma).

MAKING THE DIAGNOSIS

- *Radiographs* demonstrate a soft tissue mass and calcifications or ossification within the tumor.
- *Magnetic resonance imaging, including regional lymph nodes,* demonstrates the full extent of the lesions and identifies regional lymph node metastasis.
- *Biopsy* confirms the diagnosis.
- *Computed tomography scan of the chest* is performed to evaluate for pulmonary metastasis.

TREATMENT

- Surgical resection
- Chemotherapy and radiation may also be used as part of the treatment.

EXPECTED OUTCOMES/PROGNOSIS

- Prognosis depends on the size of tumor at diagnosis.
  — Eighty-five percent of patients with tumors that are less than 5 cm in diameter and completely resectable are expected to survive long term.
  — Fifty percent of patients with tumors that are larger than 5 cm in diameter or are not resectable survive long term.
- If metastatic disease is present at time of diagnosis, fewer than 10% survive 5 years.

WHEN TO REFER

- Refer immediately to an orthopaedic oncologist.

RELEVANT *ICD-9-CM* CODE

- **171.9**   Synovial cell sarcoma

Bibliography

Arata MA, Peterson HA, Dahlin DC. Pathologic fractures through non-ossifying fibromas. Review of the Mayo Clinic experience. *J Bone Joint Surg Am.* 1981;63:980–988

Capanna R, Campanacci DA, Manfrini M. Unicameral and aneurysmal bone cysts. *Orthop Clin North Am.* 1996;27:605–614

Capanna R, Springfield DS, Ruggieri P, et al. Direct cortisone injection in eosinophilic granuloma of bone: a preliminary report on 11 patients. *J Pediatr Orthop.* 1985;5:339–342

Carnesale PG. Benign bone tumors. In: Canale ST, ed. *Canale: Campbell's Operative Orthopedics.* 10th ed. St Louis, MO: Mosby; 2003:793–811

Carpintero P, Leon F, Zafra M, Montero M, Berral FJ. Fractures of osteochondroma during physical exercise. *Am J Sports Med.* 2003;31:1003–1006

Crandall BF, Field LL, Sparkes RS, Spence MA. Hereditary multiple exostoses. Report of a family. *Clin Othop Relat Res.* 1984;190:217–219

de Sanctis N, Andreacchio A. Elastic stable intramedullary nailing is the best treatment of unicameral bone cyst of the long bones in children? Prospective long-term follow-up study. *J Pediatr Orthop.* 2006;26:520–525

DiCaprio MR, Enneking WF. Fibrous dysplasia. Pathophysiology, evaluation, and treatment. *J Bone Joint Surg Am.* 2005;87:1848–1864

Docquier PL, Delloye C. Treatment of aneurysmal bone cysts by introduction of demineralized bone and autogenous bone marrow. *J Bone Joint Surg Am.* 2005;87:2253–2258

Easley ME, Kneisl JS. Pathologic fractures through nonossifying firbromas: is prophylactic treatment warranted? *J Pediatr Orthop.* 1997;17:808–813

Eich GF, Hoeffel JC, Tschappeler H, Gassner I, Willi UV. Fibrous tumours in children: imaging features of a heterogeneous group of disorders. *Pediatr Radiol.* 1998;28:500–509

Faulkner LB, Hajdu SI, Kher U, et al. Pediatric desmoid tumor: retrospective analysis of 63 cases. *J Clin Oncol.* 1995;13:2813–2818

Garg S, Mehta S, Dormans JP. Langerhans cell histiocytosis of the spine in children. Long-term follow-up. *J Bone Joint Surg Am.* 2004;86:1740–1750

Golant A, Dormans JP. Osteoblastoma: a spectrum of presentation and treatment in pediatric population. *Univ Penn Orthop J.* 2003;16:9–17

Golding JS. The natural history of osteoid osteoma; with a report of twenty cases. *J Bone Joint Surg Br.* 1954;36-B:218–229

Green P, Whittaker RP. Benign chondroblastoma. Case report with pulmonary metastasis. *J Bone Joint Surg Am.* 1975;57:418–420

Harris WH, Dudley HR Jr, Barry RJ. The natural history of fibrous dysplasia. An orthopaedic, pathological, and roentgenographic study. *J Bone Joint Surg Am.* 1962;44:207–233

Hecht AC, Gebhardt MC. Diagnosis and treatment of unicameral and aneurysmal bone cysts in children. *Curr Opin Pediatr.* 1998;10:87–94

Hosalkar HS, Fox EJ, Delaney T, Torbert JT, Ogilvie CM, Lackman RD. Desmoid tumors and current status of management. *Othop Clin North Am.* 2006;37:53–63

Ippolito E, Bray EW, Corsi A, et al. Natural history and treatment of fibrous dysplasia of bone: a multi-center clinicopathologic study promoted by the European Pediatric Orthopaedic Society. *J Pediatr Orthop B.* 2003;12:155–177

Kilpatrick SE, Wenger DE, Gilchrist GS, Shives TC, Wollan PC, Unni KK. Langerhans' cell histiocytosis (histiocytosis X) of bone. A clinicopathologic analysis of 263 pediatric and adult cases. *Cancer.* 1995;76:2471–2484

Kneisl JS, Simon MA. Medical management compared with operative treatment for osteoid-osteoma. *J Bone Joint Surg Am.* 1992;74:179–185

Kransdorf MJ, Sweet DE. Aneurysmal bone cyst: concept, controversy, clinical presentation, and imaging. *AJR Am J Roentgenol.* 1995;164:573–580

Leithner A, Windhager R, Lang S, Haas OA, Kainberger F, Kotz R. Aneurysmal bone cyst. A population based epidemiologic study and literature review. *Clin Orthop Relat Res.* 1999;363:176–179

Lichtenstein L. Benign osteoblastoma; a category of osteoid- and bone-forming tumors other than classical osteoid osteoma, which may be mistaken for giant-cell tumor or osteogenic sarcoma. *Cancer.* 1956;9:1044–1052

Mankin HJ, Hornicek FJ, Ortiz-Cruz E, Villafuerte J, Gebhardt MC. Aneurysmal bone cyst: a review of 150 patients. *J Clin Oncol.* 2005;23:6756–6762

Marsh BW, Bonfiglio M, Brady LP, Enneking WF. Benign osteoblastoma: range of manifestations. *J Bone Joint Surg Am.* 1975;57:1–9

Mendenhall WM, Zlotecki RA, Morris CG, Hochwald SN, Scarborough MT. Aggressive fibromatosis. *Am J Clin Oncol.* 2005;28:211–215

Pettine KA, Klassen RA. Osteoid-osteoma and osteoblastoma of the spine. *J Bone Joint Surg Am.* 1986;68:354–361

Ponseti IV, Friedman B. Evolution of metaphyseal fibrous defects. *J Bone Joint Surg Am.* 1949;31A:582–585

Potter BK, Freedman BA, Lehman RA, Shawen SB, Kuklo TR, Murphey MD. Solitary epiphyseal enchondromas. *J Bone Joint Surg Am.* 2005;87:1551–1560

Ramappa A, Lee FY, Tang P, Carlson JR, Gebhardt MC, Mankin HJ. Chondroblastoma of bone. *J Bone Joint Surg Am.* 2000;82-A:1140–1145

Raney RB Jr. Chemotherapy for children with aggressive fibromatosis and Langerhans' cell histiocytosis. *Clin Orthop Relat Res.* 1991;262:58–63

Schmale GA, Conrad EU, Rasking WH. The natural history of hereditary multiple exostoses. *J Bone Joint Surg Am.* 1994;74:986–992

Schwartz HS, Zimmerman NB, Simon MA, Wroble RR, Millar EA, Bonfiglio M. The malignant potential of enchondromatosis. *J Bone Joint Surg Am.* 1987;69:269–274

Seki T, Fukuda H, Ishii Y, Hanoaka H, Yatabe S. Malignant transformation of benign osteoblastoma. A case report. *J Bone Joint Surg Am.* 1975;57:424–426

Sessa S, Sommelet D, Lascombes P, Prevot J. Treatment of Langerhans-cell histiocytosis in children. Experience at the Children's Hospital of Nancy. *J Bone Joint Surg Am.* 1994;76:1513–1525

Springfield DS, Capanna R, Gherlinzoni F, Picci P, Campanacci M. Chondroblastoma. A review of seventy cases. *J Bone Joint Surg Am.* 1985;67:748–755

Springfield DS, Gebhardt MC. Bone and soft tissue tumors. In: Morrissey RT, Weinstein SL, eds. *Lovell and Winters Pediatric Orthopedics.* 6th ed. Philadelphia, PA: Lippincott Williams and Wilkins; 2006:493–549

van der Woude HJ, Bloem JL, Pope TL Jr. Magnetic resonance imaging of the musculoskeletal system. Part 9. Primary tumors. *Clin Orthop Relat Res.* 1998;347:272–286

Part 15: Limb-Length Discrepancy/Congenital Lower Extremity

TOPICS COVERED

CHAPTER 52

Leg-Length Discrepancy

Introduction/Etiology/Epidemiology

- Incidence of limb-length inequality, or anisomelia, is unknown. Studies estimate up to 35% of adults have discrepancies between 0.5 and 1.5 cm^2.
- Underdiagnosis of small discrepancies is common.
- Misdiagnosis of discrepancies is also common.
- Discrepancies may be acquired, congenital, or idiopathic (common) (Box 52-1).
- Clinically significant leg-length discrepancies usually have an identifiable cause.
- The behavior of a limb-length discrepancy depends on its etiology.
- *Acquired leg-length discrepancy* is most commonly caused by trauma or infection.
  — *Trauma to the growth plates:* the potential resultant discrepancy depends on the affected bone, the amount of growth remaining, and the extent of injury to the growth plate.
    - A Salter-Harris type II injury of the distal femoral physis has a reported rate of growth arrest as high as 37%.
    - A Salter-Harris type II injury of the distal radius may lead to growth arrest only 4% of the time.
    - A distal femoral physeal fracture in a boy with a skeletal age of 10 years with 6½ years of growth remaining could result in a 6-cm (0.9 cm/year × 6.5 years = 5.85 cm) discrepancy. The same fracture in the distal tibial physis would only result in a 2-cm (0.3 cm/year × 6.5 years = 1.95 cm) discrepancy that may not require any intervention.
    - The diaphysis may be shortened by trauma or stimulated to overgrow after a fracture.
    - The fractured femoral diaphysis in a child aged 2 to 10 years may overgrow the opposite side by up to 2 cm. Average overgrowth is 78% and occurs in the first 15 months after fracture.
  — *Osteomyelitis:* bacterial enzymes and inflammation can injure the growth plate.
- *Congenital leg-length discrepancies* tend to worsen with time.

Signs and Symptoms

- The most common presenting complaints are abnormal gait, toe walking, scoliosis, hip pain, or back pain.

Box 52-1. Etiology of Leg-Length Discrepancy

Acquired

Trauma
Acute bone loss
Physeal fracture
Posttraumatic overgrowth
Burns
Irradiation
Iatrogenic (surgical)
Infection
Osteomyelitis
Septic arthritis
Bacteremic
Inflammation
Juvenile rheumatoid arthritis
Hemophilia
Pigmented villonodular synovitis
Neurologic
Closed head injury
Poliomyelitis
Cerebral palsy
Myelomeningocele
Vascular
Congenital heart disease
Thromboembolic

Congenital

Developmental dysplasia of the hip
Limb hypoplasia
Proximal focal femoral deficiency
Congenital short femur/tibia
Hypoplastic femur
Fibular hemimelia
Tibial hemimelia
Congenital pseudarthrosis of tibia
Amniotic band syndrome
Hemihypertrophy/atrophy
Idiopathic
Klippel-Trenauney syndrome
Beckwith-Wiedemann syndrome
Proteus syndrome
Russell-Silver syndrome
Neurofibromatosis-1
Skeletal dysplasia
Ollier disease
Fibrous dysplasia
Multiple hereditary exostoses

Differential Diagnosis

- Leg-length discrepancies may be real or apparent (Figure 52-1). Muscle contractures or bony deformities around the hip may produce a pelvic tilt that causes an *apparent leg-length discrepancy.*

Making the Diagnosis

- *History* may reveal one or more of the following causes or risk factors:
  — History of trauma, infection, burn, or other injury to the limbs
  — History of clubfeet, bowing of the tibia, café au lait spots (eg, neurofibromatosis), and overgrowth or "swelling" of the leg (Figure 52-2)
  — Personal or family history of skeletal dysplasias
- *Physical examination*
  — Leg-length assessment can be simply and rapidly performed.
  — Leg lengths should be assessed at the annual well-child care visit and whenever a gait abnormality, hip pain, or spinal asymmetry is identified.

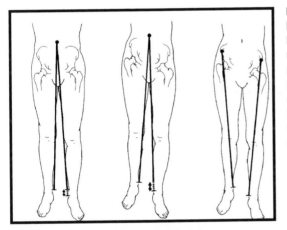

Figure 52-1. Real versus apparent leg-length discrepancy. The apparent leg length is measured from the umbilicus to the tip of the medial malleolus. This will take into account pelvic obliquity due to muscle contracture around the pelvis. Real leg length may be measured form the anterior superior iliac spine to the tip of the medial malleolus.

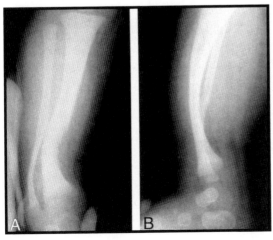

Figure 52-2. Anteroposterior (A) and lateral (B) radiographs showing anterolateral bowing of the tibia. Reproduced with permission from Griffin LY (ed): *Essentials of Musculoskeletal Care,* 3rd edition. Rosemont, IL: American Academy of Orthopaedic Surgeons; 2005.

— Observe posture and gait from behind, focusing on the pelvis.

  ▪ Limp resulting from limb-length discrepancy is associated with a decreased stance time on the shorter side, decreased walking velocity, increased cadence, and decreased step length on the shorter side.

— Leg lengths may be measured directly with a tape measure (Figure 52-3).

— Blocks of varying heights to level the pelvis may be used to measure leg length.

— Some patients develop a *lumbar curvature* because of the pelvic tilt that results from leg-length discrepancy.

  ▪ Cobb angle of the curvature will be proportional to the amount of limb-length discrepancy.

  ▪ Lumbar curves improve or normalize when the leg-length discrepancy is corrected with blocks or a shoe lift.

• *Radiographic assessment*

— *A weight-bearing anteroposterior (AP) radiograph of both lower extremities* can show relative lengths and alignment of the femora and tibiae.

  ▪ When a ruler is added to assess leg length, this technique is called *teleoroentgenography*.

  ▪ The shortcoming of this technique is magnification at the upper and lower ends of the studied area because of an angled x-ray beam.

— *Orthoroentgenography* involves imaging the entire limb with 3 exposures onto the same long-film cassette (Figure 52-4a). The smaller aperture of the x-ray beam source limits the angular magnification for each segment of the limb.

— A *scanogram* (Figure 52-4b) is the most popular technique used by orthopaedists, but it does not image the entire limb and often omits the portion of the bone that may create the deformity. It is similar to an orthoroentgenogram, except it is taken on a standard 14″ x 17″ cassette focusing on just the hip, knee, and ankle joints.

— *Computed tomography scanography* has comparable accuracy to standard scanogram and can eliminate the error produced in standard radiographs when there are knee or hip flexion contractures.

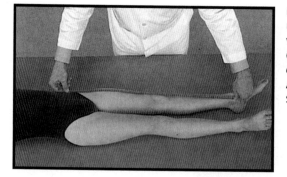

Figure 52-3. Measuring leg length using a tape measure. Reproduced with permission from Griffin LY (ed): *Essentials of Musculoskeletal Care,* 3rd edition. Rosemont, IL: American Academy of Orthopaedic Surgeons; 2005.

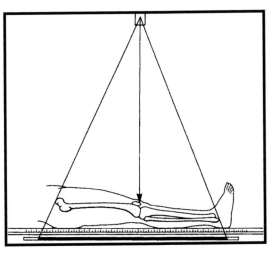

Figure 52-4a. Orthoroentgenogram. A single image of both legs is created on a 3-foot cassette. A ruler is placed adjacent to both legs for measurement. A standing version of this technique demonstrates the alignment of the legs.

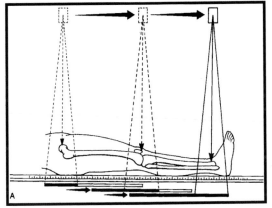

Figure 52-4b. A scanogram is performed on a standard 14" X 17" cassette. Three narrow aperture images are created with the source centered over the hip, knee, and ankle to minimize magnification. A radiographic ruler is placed next to each leg to permit measurement.

- *Assessment of skeletal maturity*
  - In the serial analysis of limb-length discrepancy and in planning for correction, accurate assessment of skeletal maturity is required.
  - Greulich and Pyle atlas is frequently used to determine skeletal age.
    - The atlas includes radiographs of the hand and wrist of children from birth to 15 years of age for girls and 17 years of age for boys.
    - The patient's left hand and wrist AP image is compared to the standard images to determine the closest match.
    - The calculated standard deviation of skeletal age between standards may vary up to 11 months.
- *Abdominal ultrasound* is recommended for patients with *hemihypertrophy* and *hemiatrophy* to allow early detection and treatment of tumors.
  - Patients with hemihypertrophy and Beckwith-Wiedemann syndrome have an aggregate 5.9% risk of developing visceral malignancy, specifically Wilms tumor and hepatoblastoma.

— Associated adrenal cell carcinoma and leiomyosarcoma may occur in up to 4% of patients with idiopathic hemihypertrophy and in 20% of patients with Beckwith-Wiedemann syndrome.
— There is debate about the ideal interval and duration of screening. The First International Conference on Molecular and Clinical Genetics of Childhood Renal Tumors suggests ultrasound be performed every 3 months until 7 years of age, followed by physical examinations of the abdomen every 6 months until the completion of growth.

Treatment

- Treatment of limb-length discrepancy depends on the discrepancy and ranges from observation to amputation and prosthetic fitting (Table 52-1).
- *Rule of thumb:* a patient with a projected leg-length discrepancy of 2 cm or more will probably benefit from intervention.
- A new complaint of gait alteration, back pain, knee pain, hip pain, or increasing fatigue with activity should trigger a reassessment for a change in the discrepancy or a new functional effect of a small discrepancy.
- *Shoe lifts*
  — In-shoe orthotics are limited to ⅜" (approximately 1 cm) or less.
  — Shoe lifts larger than ⅜" must be incorporated into the shoe.
  — Lifts bigger than 8 cm are associated with ankle sprains.
  — A shoe lift may be used on a trial basis. If symptoms improve, the lift can become the permanent form of treatment, or a surgical means of correction can be sought.
- *Limb shortening*
  — For discrepancies ranging from 2 to 5 cm, shortening of the longer limb may be performed to achieve equalization of the limb lengths.
  — Three options for shortening include *epiphysiodesis*, surgical closure of an open growth plate, and acute surgical shortening.
- *Limb lengthening*
  — Surgical lengthening of the long bones is a difficult undertaking, although many advances have been made in the biology and technology of limb lengthening.
  — Lengthening is recommended for projected discrepancies greater than 5 cm and less than 15 to 20 cm.

Table 52-1. Recommended Treatment for Limb-Length Discrepancy

Discrepancy	Treatment
<2 cm	Observation. Shoe lift if patient develops limp or back pain. Refer to orthopaedist if symptoms develop.
2–6 cm	Epiphysiodesis to shorten limb. Shoe lift may temporize until timing of epiphysiodesis appropriate. Surgical lengthening or shortening an option.
5–20 cm	Lengthening of shortened limb alone or with epiphysiodesis of longer limb
>20 cm	Amputation or early prosthetic fitting

Expected Outcomes/Prognosis

- Leg-length discrepancies affect people differently. There is evidence for and against leg-length discrepancy as a cause of back pain, knee pain, and hip pain.
- There is no proven direct correlation between small leg-length discrepancies (less than 2 cm) and low back pain.
- In persons who walk on their toes to compensate for a leg-length discrepancy, an Achilles tendon contracture may develop.

Prevention

- Early recognition and treatment of infections may prevent a growth arrest.
- Early recognition of posttraumatic growth arrest will lead to optimal results.

When to Refer

- Leg-length discrepancies that are nonprogressive can be observed. These include idiopathic leg-length discrepancies and those associated with temporary growth arrests after trauma.
- Progressively worsening leg-length discrepancies that occur following trauma or infection or from an undetermined source should be referred to an orthopaedist as soon as they are recognized.

Relevant *International Classification of Diseases, Ninth Revision, Clinical Modification* Codes

- **736.81**   Leg-length discrepancy, acquired
- **755.30**   Leg-length discrepancy, congenital
- **755.33**   Leg-length discrepancy, congenital, combined femur, tibia, and fibula
- **755.34**   Leg-length discrepancy, congenital, femur
- **755.35**   Leg-length discrepancy, congenital, combined tibia and fibula
- **755.36**   Leg-length discrepancy, congenital, tibia
- **755.37**   Leg-length discrepancy, congenital, fibula
- **759.89**   Beckwith-Wiedemann syndrome
- **759.89**   Hemihypertrophy

Bibliography

Abraham P. What is the risk of cancer in a child with hemihypertrophy? *Arch Dis Child.* 2005;90:1312–1313

Antoci V, Ono CM, Antoci V Jr, Raney EM. Bone lengthening in children: how to predict the complications rate and complexity? *J Pediatr Orthop.* 2006;26:634–640

Ballock RT, Wiesner GL, Myers MT, Thompson GH. Hemihypertrophy. Concepts and controversies. *J Bone Joint Surg Am.* 1997;79:1731–1738

Bhave A, Paley D, Herzenberg JE. Improvement in gait parameters after lengthening for the treatment of limb-length discrepancy. *J Bone Joint Surg Am.* 1999;81:529–534

Bowen JR, Kumar SJ, Orellana CA, Andreacchio A, Cardona JI. Factors leading to hip subluxation and dislocation in femoral lengthening of unilateral congenital short femur. *J Pediatr Orthop*. 2001;21:354–359

Epps CH Jr. Proximal femoral focal deficiency. *J Bone Joint Surg Am*. 1983;65:867–870

Friberg O. Clinical symptoms and biomechanics of lumbar spine and hip joint in leg length inequality. *Spine (Phila Pa 1976)*. 1983;8:643–651

Gillespie R, Torode IP. Classification and management of congenital abnormalities of the femur. *J Bone Joint Surg Br*. 1983;65:557–568

Greulich M. *Beiträge zur Geschichte des Streichinstrumentenspiels im 16. Jahrhundert*. Saalfeld,: Ostpr.; 1933.

Griffith SI, McCarthy JJ, Davidson RS. Comparison of the complication rates between first and second (repeated) lengthening in the same limb segment. *J Pediatr Orthop*. 2006;26:534–536

Gross RH. Leg length discrepancy: how much is too much? *Orthopedics*. 1978;1:307–310

Hellsing AL. Leg length inequality. A prospective study of young men during their military service. *Ups J Med Sci*. 1988;93:245–253

Herring JA. *Tachdjian's Pediatric Orthopaedics*. 3rd ed. Philadelphia, PA: WB Saunders; 2002

Hult L. The Munkfors investigation; a study of the frequency and causes of the stiff neck-brachialgia and lumbago-sciatica syndromes, as well as observations on certain signs and symptoms from the dorsal spine and the joints of the extremities in industrial and forest workers. *Acta Orthop Scand Suppl*. 1954;16:1–76

Ilizarov GA. The tension-stress effect on the genesis and growth of tissues: Part II. The influence of the rate and frequency of distraction. *Clin Orthop Relat Res*. 1989;239:263–285

Lovell WW, Winter RB, Morrissy RT, Weinstein SLV. *Lovell and Winter's Pediatric Orthopaedics*. 4th ed. Philadelphia, PA: Lippincott Williams & Wilkins; 1996

Menelaus MB. Correction of leg length discrepancy by epiphysial arrest. *J Bone Joint Surg Br*. May 1966;48: 336–339

Papaioannou T, Stokes I, Kenwright J. Scoliosis associated with limb-length inequality. *J Bone Joint Surg Am*. 1982;64:59–62

Patel M, Paley D, Herzenberg JE. Limb-lengthening versus amputation for fibular hemimelia. *J Bone Joint Surg Am*. 2002;84-A:317–319

Sanders JO, Browne RH, McConnell SJ, Margraf SA, Cooney TE, Finegold DN. Maturity assessment and curve progression in girls with idiopathic scoliosis. *J Bone Joint Surg Am*. 2007;89:64–73

Shapiro F. Developmental patterns in lower-extremity length discrepancies. *J Bone Joint Surg Am*. 1982;64:639–651

Song KM, Halliday SE, Little DG. The effect of limb-length discrepancy on gait. *J Bone Joint Surg Am*. 1997; 79:1690–1698

Soukka A, Alaranta H, Tallroth K, Heliovaara M. Leg-length inequality in people of working age. The association between mild inequality and low-back pain is questionable. *Spine (Phila Pa 1976)*. 1991;16:429–431

Szepesi K, Rigo J, Poti L, Szucs G. Treatment of leg length discrepancy by subtrochanteric shortening of the femur. *J Pediatr Orthop*. 1990;10:183–185

Part 16: Neuromuscular Disorders, Part 1

TOPICS COVERED

CHAPTER 53

Cerebral Palsy

Introduction/Etiology/Epidemiology

- Cerebral palsy is a collective term to describe a group of disorders resulting in abnormal motor function caused by impairment of fetal or infant brain development.
- The prevalence of cerebral palsy is 1.5 to 2.5 per 1,000 live births.
- The brain pathology in cerebral palsy involves the white matter with periventricular leukomalacia being the most common finding in magnetic resonance imaging (MRI) studies.
- May result from events occurring any time from the prenatal period to 2 years of age.
- *Prenatal risk factors* include infection, drug or alcohol abuse, an incompetent cervix, and third-trimester bleeding.
- *Perinatal risk factors* include multiple births, placental abruption, premature rupture of membranes, infection, birth trauma, and hypoxia.
  - Fewer than 10% of cerebral palsy cases are felt to result from perinatal events during delivery.
- *Postnatal risk factors* include central nervous system infection and any event that results in hypoxia to the immature brain.

Signs and Symptoms

- Increased or decreased muscle tone
- Lack of achievement of early motor developmental milestones (eg, head up, pushes up on forearms at 3 months)
- Gait patterns associated with cerebral palsy include equinus gait (toe walking), scissoring gait, crouch gait, and stiff-knee gait.
- Most patients have neurologic manifestations such as impaired sensation, cognition, communication, perception, and behavior.
- Seizure disorders are common.
- Gastrointestinal problems are also common, including impaired swallowing, gastroesophageal reflux, and disordered motility, which may result in malnutrition.

Differential Diagnosis

- Progressive neurologic disorders must be excluded (ie, genetic syndromes, metabolic disorders, and other neurodegenerative diseases). Unlike in these disorders, in patients with cerebral palsy, the brain lesion is static.

Making the Diagnosis

- The diagnosis is made based on history and physical examination findings.
- Magnetic resonance imaging is usually performed to rule out other neurologic disorders.
  - In cerebral palsy, periventricular leukomalacia is the most common MRI finding.
- Classification can help guide treatment and prognosis.
- *Physiologic classification*
  - *Spastic:* velocity-dependent increase in muscle tone in response to stretch and hyper-excitable stretch reflexes because of upper motor neuron dysfunction
    - Most common form of cerebral palsy
    - Spasticity often results in poor motor control, decreased balance, and weakness.
    - Joint contractures are common.
  - *Athetoid:* uncontrollable writhing movements of the hands and mouth associated with an extrapyramidal brain lesion
    - Joint contractures are uncommon.
  - *Ataxic:* a rare form of cerebral palsy caused by a cerebellar lesion, which results in balance and coordination difficulties
  - *Hypotonic:* infant demonstrates a generalized lack of tone.
  - *Mixed:* a combination of these types in varying degrees
- *Geographic classification*
  - *Hemiplegia:* involvement of one side of the body, usually affecting the upper extremities more than the lower. Associated with equinus and stiff knee gait.
  - *Diplegia:* involvement of both lower extremities
  - *Quadriplegia:* the upper and lower extremities are affected.

Treatment

- *Early intervention*
  - Children up to 3 years of age are eligible to receive therapy services as provided by law in each of the 50 states.
  - Developmental assessment of abnormality determines need for therapy intervention.
- *Treatment of spasticity*
  - *Pharmacologic*
    - Botulinum toxin (Botox) is given as an intramuscular injection and can be used in nearly any muscle with a dynamic (not fixed) contracture.
      - The effects of botulinum injection may last up to 6 months.
      - Used in conjunction with physical therapy to maximize the patient's range of motion.
    - Baclofen may be used orally or intrathecally.
      - Oral baclofen may cause dose-dependent sedation.
      - Confusion, attention deficits, orthostatic hypotension, weakness, and ataxia have also been associated with baclofen use.
      - Intrathecal baclofen has become increasingly popular recently in the treatment of severe spasticity associated with cerebral palsy.

- ◆ Outcome studies of intrathecal baclofen use have shown significantly decreased upper and lower extremity spasticity at 6 months, decreased use of oral medications for spasticity, improvements in patient comfort, and high caregiver satisfaction.
  - ◆ Withdrawal symptoms may occur with abrupt discontinuation of oral or intrathecal baclofen, including increased spasticity, confusion, and fever.
- *Surgical*
  - — Dorsal rhizotomy is a neurosurgical procedure in which afferent sensory rootlets from L1-S2 are transected to decrease lower extremity spasticity and improve motor function.
    - ▪ Selective dorsal rhizotomy has shown greater improvements in strength, gait speed, and gross motor function when compared with physical therapy alone.
    - ▪ Long-term complications of selective dorsal rhizotomy include progressive hip subluxation, scoliosis, heterotopic ossification following hip procedures, spondylolysis, and spondylolisthesis.
    - ▪ The ideal patient for selective dorsal rhizotomy is between 3 and 8 years old, has pure spasticity, is diplegic with the ability to walk, has no fixed contractures, and is mentally and emotionally able to cope with the surgery and rehabilitation.
    - ▪ Rarely indicated today
- *Treatment of common musculoskeletal problems*
  - — *Ambulatory patient*
    - ▪ Primary goal of treatment is to reduce spasticity.
    - ▪ Physical therapy is the mainstay of treatment in children younger than 2 years but should augment other forms of treatment in older children.
    - ▪ For an equinus gait, an ankle-foot orthosis is used if the foot and ankle are in a position that can be braced. More likely, however, an Achilles tendon lengthening or gastrocnemius-soleus recession is needed.
    - ▪ Medications such as baclofen and non-musculoskeletal surgeries such as selective dorsal rhizotomy and placement of intrathecal baclofen pumps may aid in reducing spasticity.
    - ▪ Treatment with a combination of physical therapy, orthopaedic surgery, and rhizotomy results in significantly greater improvements in gait, energy efficiency, and global functioning than any of these treatment modalities individually.
    - ▪ Referral for gait analysis may be suggested by the patient's orthopaedic surgeon prior to treatment. During a gait analysis, the patient is videotaped while walking. Data collected can be used to develop kinetic and kinematic information about the child's gait pattern. This information can help the surgeon plan the appropriate soft tissue or bony procedures necessary to improve a patient's walking ability.
  - — *Non-ambulatory patient*
    - ▪ *Neuromuscular scoliosis* commonly affects non-ambulatory patients with cerebral palsy.
      - ◆ Curve progression depends on severity of neurologic involvement. Severe curves (greater than 60 degrees) occur in 67% of quadriplegic patients, 100% of bedridden patients, and no patients who are ambulatory.

- ◆ Severe untreated curves are associated with increased incidence of pneumonia and require a significant amount of nursing care for dressing, positioning, and personal hygiene.
- ◆ Scoliosis in cerebral palsy patients is likely to progress after growth is completed.
- ◆ Surgery may be recommended for curves greater than 45 to 50 degrees in children older than 10 years.
- ◆ Operative treatment usually involves posterior spinal fusion with instrumentation (fixation) to the sacrum or pelvis.
- ◆ Prior to surgery, the nutritional status must be optimized and in some cases, a gastrostomy tube is required.
- ◆ Complications of spinal fusion in cerebral palsy patients with severe neuro-muscular scoliosis are common.
- ▪ *Hip subluxation and dislocation*
  - ◆ Hip displacement is directly related to gross motor function.
  - ◆ The hips are followed with physical examination and pelvis radiographs every 6 months.
    - ≈ Abduction of less than 30 to 45 degrees puts the patient at risk for subluxation.
    - ≈ *Migration index* is the percentage of the femoral head uncovered lateral to the acetabulum on an anteroposterior radiograph of the pelvis. Migration index of more than 30 degrees is considered a subluxed hip, and a migration index of greater than 90% is considered a dislocated hip.
- ▪ Physical therapy, abduction bracing, botulinum toxin injections, baclofen therapy, and surgery are therapeutic.

Expected Outcomes/Prognosis

- Although the neurologic injury in cerebral palsy is not progressive, the musculoskeletal manifestations of the disorder continue to worsen with time.
- As a result of the constant muscle shortening in spastic cerebral palsy, normal longitudinal muscle growth is impaired, which in turn affects bone growth and development. Bony rotational deformities may develop leading to joint incongruence and early joint degeneration if not addressed.
- The natural progression of cerebral palsy is a decline in the ability to walk, usually beginning in adolescence.
- A combination of operative and nonoperative management can delay or prevent this decline in function.

Prevention

- Prenatal care plays an important role in prevention by educating women about the risks to the baby from certain lifestyle choices such as using drugs and alcohol. Intensive perinatal measures for neuroprotection are under evaluation.

When to Refer

- The medical home for patients with cerebral palsy is with the pediatrician.
- Specialty care is requested as indicated.
- Patients with spasticity should be referred to a physician specializing in physical medicine and rehabilitation (physiatry), a physical therapist, or an orthopaedic surgeon.
- Non-ambulatory patients with scoliosis or hip dislocation should be referred to an orthopaedic surgeon for management of these conditions.

Resource for Physicians and Families

- American Academy of Pediatrics (www.aap.org)

Relevant *International Classification of Diseases, Ninth Revision, Clinical Modification* Codes

- **343.0**   Congenital diplegia or paraplegia
- **343.1**   Congenital hemiplegia
- **343.2**   Quadriplegic
- **343.3**   Monoplegic
- **343.4**   Infantile hemiplegia
- **343.8**   Other specified infantile cerebral palsy
- **333.71** Athetoid cerebral palsy

CHAPTER 54

Myelomeningocele (Spina Bifida)

Introduction/Etiology/Epidemiology

- Myelomeningocele (also called spina bifida) is a spectrum of major birth malformations of the spinal cord caused by failure of closure of the neural tube.
- Affected patients have varying degrees of paralysis of the lower extremities and bladder as well as central nervous system involvement (hydrocephalus and Arnold-Chiari malformation).
- *Meningocele* is a protrusion of the meninges through a defect in the posterior spinal elements, but the spinal cord and nerve roots remain in the spinal canal.
- *Myelomeningocele* is the most severe form of spina bifida, in which the spinal cord is exposed through the opening in the spine. It is associated with partial or complete paralysis of the parts of the body below the spinal opening.
- *Myelocele* (rachischisis or myeloschisis) is a severe form of spina bifida in which the neural plate is exposed with no overlying tissue cover.
- *Lumbosacral lipoma* includes lipomeningocele, intra-spinal lipoma, and lipoma of the filum terminale, and consists of skin-covered subcutaneous lipomas associated with neurologic symptoms and spinal deformity.
- *Spina bifida occulta* is a developmental variant in which one or more vertebrae have defects in the posterior arch without any skin or spine malformation. This incidental form of spina bifida does not cause disability or symptoms and referral for evaluation is not required.
- Risk factors associated with spina bifida
  — Inadequate maternal intake of folic acid prior to conception
  — History of previously affected pregnancy with the same partner
  — Maternal diabetes (not gestational diabetes)
  — In utero exposure to valproic acid or carbamazepine

Table 54-1. Classification of Motor Function Disability

Level	Effects on Mobility	% w/ Scoliosis	% Hip Dislocation/ Subluxation	% Community Ambulator Second Decade of Life
T12	Complete loss of motor and sensory function of both lower extremities. Parapodium and reciprocating braces in early years, wheelchair-dependent later.	90	65	0
L1	Iliopsoas and sartorius muscles present. Ambulatory with knee-ankle orthosis early but wheelchair-dependent in most cases as adolescent.	90	65	0
L2	Strong hip flexion, moderate hip adduction. Prone to develop hip flexion and adduction contracture and hip dislocation. Knee-ankle-foot orthosis early, wheelchair-dependent in most cases as adolescent.	80	75	10
L3	Strong quadriceps. Ability to extend knee. Ambulatory with knee-ankle-foot orthosis. By adolescence, household or community ambulator.	70	55	10
L4	Ankle dorsiflexion and inversion. Prone to develop calcaneal deformities of the foot. Functional ambulator with ankle-foot orthosis or knee-ankle-foot orthosis or crutches. May develop hip dislocation because of muscle imbalance around hip.	60	35	30
L5	Lacks plantar flexion. Also prone to development of calcaneal or valgus foot deformity and late hip dislocation. Ambulatory with ankle-foot orthosis.	25	20	30

Table 54-1. Classification of Motor Function Disability, continued

Level	Effects on Mobility	% w/ Scoliosis	% Hip Dislocation/ Subluxation	% Community Ambulator Second Decade of Life
S1-2	Preservation of some foot and ankle movement; ambulation with minimal support. Scoliosis uncommon. Rule out tethered cord syndrome if present.	5	Rare	>50
S3	Mild loss of intrinsic foot muscular function possible; ambulation without support.			

Adapted with permission from Pillitteri A. *Child Health Nursing: Care of the Child and Family.* Philadelphia, PA: Lippincott Williams & Wilkins; 1999, and Maher AB, Salmond SW, Pellino TA. *Orthopaedic Nursing.* Philadelphia, PA: WB Saunders; 1994:627–634.

Signs and Symptoms

- The level of *neurologic deficit* is the main determinant of disability and is also the method of classifying patients (Table 54-1).
- *Hydrocephalus* occurs in 80% to 90% of children with spina bifida. The incidence of hydrocephalus is related to the neurologic level.
- *Arnold-Chiari malformation* involves caudal displacement of the posterior lobe of the cerebellum into the foramen magnum. Manifestations include dysfunction of the lower cranial nerves presenting as weakness or paralysis of the vocal cords and difficulty with feeding and breathing.
- *Syringomyelia* (cyst within the spinal cord) can cause progressive scoliosis.
- *Tethered spinal cord*
  — Seen on nearly all magnetic resonance imaging (MRI) of persons with spina bifida; however, clinical signs only occur in 15% to 30% of patients.
  — Clinical signs include changes in neurologic function, spasticity in the lower extremities, leg weakness, foot deformity, scoliosis, back pain, increased lumbar lordosis, and sensory changes.
- *Urinary incontinence and infections*

- *Musculoskeletal complications of spina bifida*
  — *Scoliosis and kyphosis*
    - May be neurogenic (because of shunt malformation, Arnold-Chiari malformation, or tethered cord syndrome) or secondary to the paralysis or congenital bony defects.
    - Kyphosis occurs in approximately 8% to 15% of children with spina bifida.
    - Incidence of scoliosis is approximately 60% and is related to the neurologic level, affecting approximately 90% of thoracic-level patients, 44% of L1-L3–level patients and 12% of L4-L5–level patients.
    - Curves greater than 50 degrees affect sitting balance, which can lead to skin breakdown; more severe curves lead to restrictive pulmonary disease.
    - *Hip contractures* are common because of muscle imbalance or spasticity. In wheelchair-dependent children, they may be caused by prolonged sitting.
    - *Hip dislocations* occur in nearly 50% of children with spina bifida.
  — *Knee flexion contractures*
    - More common in thoracic or upper-lumbar–level patients because of prolonged sitting positions.
    - Less common in mid-lumbar–level (L3, L4, L5) patients, and can be a significant hindrance to ambulation.
    - Uncommon in sacral-level patients; may be a sign of spasticity and tethered cord.
  — *Knee extension contractures*
    - May occur in L3- and L4-level patients because of unopposed quadriceps action.
    - Prevent proper sitting and inhibit walking.
  — *Foot deformities*
    - Clubfeet are most common; deformity is typically severe and rigid.
    - Other foot deformities include equinus deformity (heel-cord contracture), calcaneus deformity, and calcaneovalgus deformity.
    - New onset foot deformity in the older child may be a sign of tethered cord.
  — *In-toeing or out-toeing*
  — *Fractures* are unusual in children with spina bifida.
    - Non-ambulatory patients are prone to *metaphyseal fractures* of the *distal femur* and *proximal tibia* secondary to joint contractures and relatively soft and osteoporotic bone.
      - Mechanisms include vigorous physical therapy or inadvertent position changes by a caregiver, such as when the child is lifted out of a wheelchair and the leg gets caught.
      - Present as painless swelling with significant redness of the skin overlying the distal femur or proximal tibia.
    - Ambulatory patients may develop *physeal fractures* or *epiphyseolysis*, which is a non-displaced fracture that can be slow to heal.
      - The physis can appear irregular and widened with exuberant new bone formation around the area, manifesting as painless swelling that makes lower extremity braces tight and ill fitting.

Differential Diagnosis

- *Sacrococcygeal teratomas* may mimic sacral-level spina bifida. Teratomas are usually more heterogeneous and often surround the anal canal.
- *Lipomas* of the midline back may mimic lipomeningoceles; radiographs and MRI can distinguish between the two.

Making the Diagnosis

- Myelomeningocele can be diagnosed prenatally by alpha-fetoprotein determination or ultrasound.
- In the neonate, diagnosis is based on physical examination. Neurologic level is determined by neurologic examination and muscle testing.
- If tethered cord syndrome is suspected, the workup includes MRI and urodynamics. Urodynamics can show signs of tethered cord syndrome before there are orthopaedic manifestations.
- Ultrasound of the head may be performed to evaluate for hydrocephalus.
- *Predicting ambulatory function*
  — Good quadriceps strength, innervated by L2, L3, and L4 nerve roots, is a commonly used positive predictor of ambulation.
    ▪ Patients with weak quadriceps and no patellar reflex are better classified as L2 or L3 and thus are less likely to ambulate as adolescents than those with strong quadriceps and intact patellar reflex.
  — While neuro-segmental level is the best predictor of ambulatory function (Table 54-1), it is not absolute.
    ▪ Some sacral-level patients (who have a 90% chance of walking as adults) can't ambulate secondary to spasticity or shunt problems.
    ▪ Some L3-level patients (who typically use a wheelchair by adolescence) may continue to walk with braces as adults.
  — Patients with grade 2 or better hip abductor strength tend to remain ambulatory as adults.
  — Hip dislocation is not necessarily a detriment to walking. Rather, it is a reflection of the neuro-segmental level, which is the main predictor of ambulation.
  — Balance disturbances, spasticity in the knee and hip joints, and increased number of shunt revisions can adversely affect a child's ability to ambulate.

Treatment

- Intrauterine repair of myelomeningocele is under prospective evaluation. Currently, there is a multicenter randomized trial to determine the benefits of intrauterine repair.
- Shortly after birth, closure of the myelomeningocele is performed. If there are signs of hydrocephalus, a shunt is placed.

- *Tethered cord*
  — Neurosurgical de-tethering has been shown to be beneficial because it stabilizes the neurologic status and prevents further deterioration. Some patients recover lost motor function, whereas a small percentage of patients may lose some function.
  — Tethered cord syndrome can cause scoliosis, and curves less than 40 degrees may benefit from de-tethering.
  — Curves greater than 40 degrees do not seem to have any improvement from de-tethering.
- *Scoliosis*
  — Curves less than 20 degrees are treated with observation; many do not progress.
  — Curves between 20 and 40 degrees typically do not respond to bracing, so spinal fusion is recommended.
  — If spinal fusion is required for non-ambulatory patients, fusion from approximately T2 to the pelvis is preferred.
- *Kyphosis* (myelokyphosis)
  — Kyphosis is usually resistant to bracing.
  — Treatment of kyphosis can be performed in newborns at the time of sac closure, especially if the bone elements are causing tension on the spinal closure. Resection of the kyphotic segment with a short fusion with posterior instrumentation can stabilize the kyphosis, although some recurrence can be expected with long-term follow-up.
  — In older children and adolescents, treatment may involve resection of the kyphotic segment or a subtraction procedure with instrumentation. The instrumentation and fusion must extend from the upper thoracic spine down to the pelvis. Benefits of this procedure include substantial improvement in sitting balance and posture, and elimination of the need to use the hands for support.
  — Complications can be frequent and severe. However, overall parent and patient satisfaction is extremely high, especially with the use of modern surgical techniques such as pedicle screw instrumentation.
- *Hip flexion contractures*
  — Treatment depends on child's functional level; some may benefit from surgical release.
  — Hip flexion contracture is not necessarily a problem in non-ambulatory patients.
  — Contractures of more than 30 to 40 degrees will interfere with efficient ambulation. This can be tolerated in a child walking with a reciprocating gait orthosis, whereas a flexion contracture of 20 degrees or more cannot be tolerated in a lower-lumbar–level patient.
- *Hip dislocation*
  — Treatment of this problem is controversial; however, most orthopaedic surgeons feel that extensive surgical reconstruction is rarely indicated because the failure rate is high.
  — Failed hip surgery worsens function because of resultant hip stiffness.
  — Thoracic and high-lumbar–level patients rarely benefit from extensive hip surgery.
  — Mid-lumbar–level patients may benefit, but the re-dislocation rate is high.
  — Sacral-level patients with a unilateral hip dislocation are the best candidates for relocation surgery.

- *Knee flexion contractures*
  — Surgery is performed to release the contractures if the patient is ambulatory and the contractures are interfering with bracing.
  — In general, knee flexion contractures more than 20 degrees prevent walking, in knee-ankle-foot orthoses or ankle-foot orthoses. These can be surgically treated with hamstring lengthening, hamstring release, or posterior knee capsule release.
  — Most patients in the thoracic and upper-lumbar–level group stop ambulating during adolescence, and extensive surgery rarely changes this pattern.
- *Knee extension contracture*
  — Casting or surgical quadriceps lengthening to obtain better motion
- *Clubfeet*
  — Serial casting may be attempted; however, it is often not completely successful.
  — Tendon releases are usually performed at about 1 year of age, with bracing afterwards.
  — Recurrences can be frequent and bracing is absolutely required to prevent further deformity.
- *Other foot deformities*
  — Can usually be corrected with simple tendon releases.
  — Osteotomies may be required to achieve a plantigrade, flexible foot.
  — Joint arthrodesis (fusion) is not advised because it can result in skin pressure sores and ulcerations.
- *In-toeing or out-toeing*
  — If it impairs walking or there is excessive force across the foot, a tibial and fibular derotational osteotomy may be indicated to bring the foot into a more functional position.
- *Metaphyseal fractures*
  — Simple splinting is recommended rather than casting because the skin has no sensation and is prone to breaking down.
  — The splint must be changed several times a day to ensure that there are no areas of excessive pressure or potential skin breakdown.
- *Physeal fractures*
  — Treatment consists of decreasing activity and splinting to reduce the forces across the physis.

Expected Outcomes/Prognosis

- Ambulatory status varies and is based on neuro-segmental level (Table 54-1).
- Seventy-eight percent of all individuals with spina bifida survive to 17 years of age; 50% survive to 30 years of age. Among survivors, 70% have an IQ of 80 or higher.
- Leading causes of mortality are renal failure, sepsis, and shunt complications.
- Shunt infection, obstruction, or malfunction are serious complications that affect the child's motor and intellectual development.

Prevention

* Folic acid dietary supplementation prior to conception has been shown to reduce the incidence of neural tube defects.
* Pregnant women without a family history of spina bifida are advised to take 0.4 to 0.8 mg of folic acid daily at least 1 month before conception.
* Pregnant women with a positive family history should take 4 mg of folic acid per day at least 1 month before conception.
* Latex allergy occurs in 27% of patients with spina bifida, caused by early and frequent exposure to latex medical products. Latex precautions are advised for all patients with spina bifida to reduce the prevalence of latex allergy.

When to Refer

* On diagnosis, refer to a multidisciplinary team of specialists, including pediatric orthopaedic surgeon, neurosurgeon, urologist, and neurodevelopmental specialist.

Resources for Physicians and Families

* www.ninds.nih.gov/disorders/spina_bifida
* www.sbaa.org

Relevant *International Classification of Diseases, Ninth Revision, Clinical Modification* Codes

* **741.9**   Spina bifida
* **741.0**   Spina bifida with hydrocephalus
* **756.17**   Spina bifida occulta

Bibliography

Adzick NS, Walsh DS. Myelomeningocele: prenatal diagnosis, pathophysiology and management. *Semin Pediatr Surg.* 2003;12:168–174

Albright AL, Turner M, Pattisapu JV. Best-practice surgical techniques for intrathecal baclofen therapy. *J Neurosurg.* 2006;104(4 Suppl):233–239

Banta JV. Combined anterior and posterior fusion for spinal deformity in myelomeningocele. *Spine (Phila Pa 1976).* 1990;15:946–952

Bare A, Vankoski JJ. Independent ambulators with high sacral elomeningocele: the relation between walking kinematics and energy consumption. *Dev Med Child Neurol.* 2001;43:16–21

Bartonek A, Saraste H. Factors influencing ambulation in myelomeningocele: a cross-sectional study. *Dev Med Child Neurol.* 2001;43:253–260

Bax M, Goldstein M, Rosenbaum P, et al. Proposed definition and class of cerebral palsy, April 2005. *Dev Med Child Neurol.* 2005;47:571–576

Bax M, Tydeman C, Flodmark O. Clinical and MRI correlates of cerebral palsy: the European Cerebral Palsy Study. *JAMA.* 2006;296:1602–1608

Berven S, Bradford DS. Neuromuscular scoliosis: causes of deformity and principles for evaluation and management. *Semin Neurol.* 2002;22:167–178

Blickstein I. Cerebral palsy: a look at etiology and new task force conclusions. *OBG Management.* 2003;16:40–50

Campbell WM, Ferrel A, McLaughlin JF, et al. Long-term safety and efficacy of continuous intrathecal baclofen. *Dev Med Child Neurol.* 2002;44:660–665

Crawford AH, Strub WM, Lewis R, et al. Neonatal kyphectomy in the patient with myelomeningocele. *Spine (Phila Pa 1976).* 2003;28:260–266

Delgado MR. Botulinum neurotoxin type A. *J Am Acad Orthop Surg.* 2003;11:291–294

DeSouza LS, Carroll N. Ambulation of the braced myelomeningocele patient. *J Bone Joint Surg Am.* 1976; 58:1112–1118

Dias LS. Surgical management of knee contractures in myelomeningocele. *J Pediatr Orthop.* 1982;2:127–131

Engsberg JR, Ross SA, Collins DR, Park TS. Effect of selective dorsal rhizotomy in the treatment of children with cerebral palsy. *J Neurosurg.* 2006;105(1 Suppl):8–15

Fraser RK, Hoffman EB, Sparks LT, Buccimazza SS. The unstable hip and mid-lumbar myelomeningocele. *J Bone Joint Surg Br.* 1992;74:143–146

Graham HK, Selber P. Musculoskeletal aspects of cerebral palsy. *J Bone Joint Surg Br.* 2003;85-B:157–166

Karol LA. Surgical management of the lower extremity in ambulatory children with cerebral palsy. *J Am Acad Orthop Surg.* 2004;12:196–203

Kirk VG, Morielli A, Brouillette RT. Sleep-disordered breathing in patients with myelomeningocele: the missed diagnosis. *Dev Med Child Neurol.* 1999;41:40–43

Mazur JM, Shurtleff D, Menelaus M, Colliver J. Orthopaedic management of high-level spina bifida. Early walking compared with early use of wheelchair. *J Bone Joint Surg Am.* 1989;71:56–61

McCarthy JJ, D'Andrea LP, Betz RR, Clements DH. Scoliosis in the child with cerebral palsy. *J Am Acad Orthop Surg.* 2006;14:367–375

Morton RE, Scott B, McClelland V, Henry A. Dislocation of the hips in children with bilateral spastic cerebral palsy, 1985-2000. *Dev Med Child Neurol.* 2006;48:555–558

Nieto A, Mazon A, Pamies R, et al. Efficacy of latex avoidance for primary prevention of latex sensitization in children with spina bifida. *J Pediatr.* 2002;140:370–372

Nolden MT, Sarwark JF, Vora A, Grayhack JJ. A kyphectomy technique with reduced perioperative morbidity for myelomeningocele kyphosis. *Spine (Phila Pa 1976).* 2002;27:1807–1813

Ozlem E, Peker O, Kosay C, Iyilikci L, Bozan O, Berk H. Botulinum toxin A injection for spasticity in diplegic-type cerebral palsy. *J Child Neurol.* 2006;21:1009–1012

Paneth N, Hong T, Korzeniewski S. The descriptive epidemiology of cerebral palsy. *Clin Perinatol.* 2006; 33:251–267

Pierz K, Banta J, Thomson J, Gahm N, Hartford J. The effect of tethered cord release on scoliosis in myelomeningocele. *J Pediatr Orthop.* 2000;20:362–365

Renshaw TS, Deluca PA. Cerebral palsy. In: Morrissy RT, Weinstein SL, eds. *Lovell and Winter's Pediatric Orthopaedics.* Philadelphia, PA: Lippincott Williams & Wilkins; 2006

Saito N, Ebara S, Ohotsuka K, Kumeta H, Takaoka K. Natural history of scoliosis in spastic cerebral palsy. *Lancet.* 1998;351:1687–1692

Schoenmakers MA, Gooskens RH, Gulmans VA, et al. Long-term outcome of neurosurgical untethering in neurosegmental motor and ambulation levels. *Dev Med Child Neurol.* 2003;45:551–555

Schwartz MH, Viehweger E, Stout J, Novacheck TF, Gage JR. Comprehensive treatment of ambulatory children with cerebral palsy: an outcome assessment. *J Pediatr Orthop.* 2004;24:45–53

Selber P, Dias L. Sacral-level myelomeningocele: long-term outcome in adults. *J Pediatr Orthop.* 1998;18:423–427

Soo B, Howard JJ, Boyd RN, et al. Hip displacement in cerebral palsy. *J Bone Joint Surg Am.* 2006;88:121–129

Spiegel DA, Flynn JM. Evaluation and treatment of hip dysplasia in cerebral palsy. *Orthop Clin North Am.* 2006;37:185–196

Sponseller PD, Young AT, Sarwark JF, Lim R. Anterior only fusion for scoliosis in patients with myelomeningocele. *Clin Orthop Relat Res.* 1999;364:117–124

Trivedi J, Thomson JD, Slakey JB, Banta JV, Jones PW. Clinical and radiographic predictions of scoliosis in patients with myelomeningocele. *J Bone Joint Surg Am.* 2002;84-A:1389–1394

Tsirikos AI, Chang WN, Dabney KW, Miller F. Comparison of parents' and caregivers' satisfaction after spinal fusion in children with cerebral palsy. *J Pediatr Orthop.* 2004;24:54–58

Verrotti A, Greco R, Spalice A, Chiarelli F, Iannetti P. Pharmacotherapy of spasticity in children with cerebral palsy. *Pediatr Neurol.* 2006;34:1–6

Wren TA, Rethlefsen S, Kay RM. Prevalence of specific gait abnormalities in children with cerebral palsy: influence of cerebral palsy subtype, age, and previous surgery. *J Pediatr Orthop.* 2005;25:79–83

Part 17: Neuromuscular Disorders, Part 2

CHAPTER 55

Neurodegenerative Disorders

Duchenne Muscular Dystrophy

INTRODUCTION/ETIOLOGY/EPIDEMIOLOGY

- X-linked recessive condition characterized by progressive muscle atrophy and weakness, caused by absence of dystrophin
  — Without dystrophin, the sarcolemma (crucial for the stability of the cell membrane) is not protected from injury during forceful contractions; as a result, muscle fibers become necrotic and inflamed and are replaced by fat and fibrous tissue.
- Incidence is 1 per 3,500 boys.
- Rarely, occurs in girls with Turner syndrome.
- Family history is positive in approximately 65% of cases.

SIGNS AND SYMPTOMS

- Becomes clinically evident between 3 and 6 years of age.
- Muscle weakness develops symmetrically and is first noticed in the proximal muscles, often the hip extensors.
- *Early symptoms* include toe walking, delayed ambulation, frequent tripping and falling, and difficulty with running and climbing stairs.
- *Later in the disease*
  — Contractures develop, especially of the hip abductors, then hip and knee flexors and ankle dorsiflexors.
  — Progressive inability to walk and ultimate dependence on a wheelchair by 7 to 16 years of age
  — Scoliosis develops in about 95% of patients with Duchenne muscular dystrophy (DMD) (Figure 55-1).
    - It progresses rapidly, especially after a child loses walking ability.
    - Curves are long, sweeping, and associated with pelvic obliquity (wheelchair sitting is an issue).
    - Spine radiographs are indicated in non-ambulatory patients and those with spinal asymmetry.

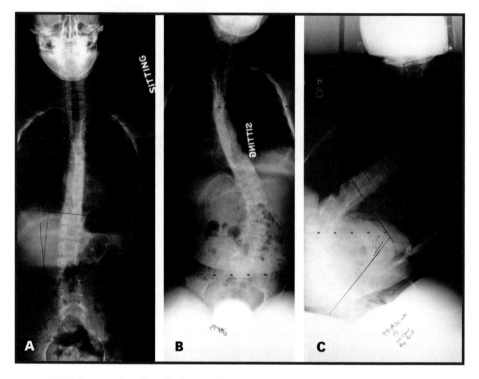

Figure 55-1. Progression of scoliosis in Duchenne muscular dystrophy over a 5-year period after cessation of walking ability. A, 12 degrees. B, 38 degrees. C, 105 degrees.

— Muscle pain accompanies the progressive physical disability, leading to diminished participation and enjoyment of daily activities. Pain may also result from overly zealous passive range of motion therapy and prolonged sitting with inability to shift weight for comfort.
• *Physical examination findings*
— Ankle equinus is an early overt sign of DMD, leading to toe walking.
— Waddling, wide-based gait because of weakness and an attempt to attain stability
— Pseudohypertrophy of the calves, which results from replacement of muscle tissue by fat and fibrous tissue (Figure 55-2)
— *Gowers sign is pathognomonic of DMD*—difficulty rising from a seated position on the floor without using arms to push hips and knees into extension because of weakness of the pelvic girdle and proximal thigh muscles (see Figure 4-3). Some describe this as the child "walking" hands up legs to raise trunk to an upright position from the floor.
— Positive Trendelenburg sign (see Figure 4-24) is also common—when the child stands on one leg, there is a drop in the non–weight-bearing hemipelvis, indicating a weakness of the standing leg's gluteal muscles and hip abductors.
— *Meryon sign* also is a common physical finding, wherein the child slips through when the examiner attempts to lift from under the arms.

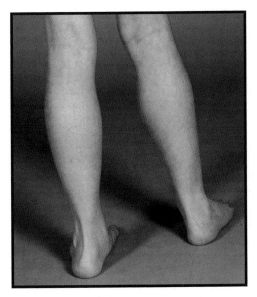

Figure 55-2. Pseudohypertrophy of the calf muscles in a child with Duchenne muscular dystrophy.

- *Associated non-musculoskeletal findings*
  — More than 90% have abnormal electrocardiogram findings such as sinus tachycardia, cardiac hypertrophy, and diminished QRS complex.
  — Mitral valve prolapse is also a characteristic finding because of papillary muscle involvement.
  — Reduced pulmonary function, including diminished expiratory muscle strength
  — Mild mental retardation is common, with the average IQ approximately 80.

DIFFERENTIAL DIAGNOSIS

- Becker muscular dystrophy (BMD)
  — Presents at a later age with less severe symptoms.
  — Dystrophin levels are diminished, not absent as in DMD.
- Fascioscapulohumeral dystrophy
  — Occurs in either sex.
  — Mild involvement
  — Usually presents in the second decade of life.
  — Facial muscles are often affected.
  — Pseudohypertrophy of the calves is very rare.
- Polymyositis
  — Occurs in either sex.
  — Like muscular dystrophies, presents with an elevated creatine kinase (CK).
  — Deep tendon reflexes are preserved longer.
  — Muscular atrophy and pseudohypertrophy are uncommon.

MAKING THE DIAGNOSIS

- Diagnosis is suggested by classic signs and symptoms and *elevated serum CK*, and confirmed by muscle biopsy.
- In DMD, CK levels are elevated more than hundredfold, or even up to 200- to 300-fold.
- Creatine kinase levels are usually highest in the early stages, then approach near normal in the end stages of the disease as muscle is gradually replaced by fat and fibrous tissue.
- Creatine kinase is not specific for muscular dystrophies because levels are elevated in any muscle disease.
- Duchenne muscular dystrophy and BMD cannot be differentiated solely based on CK level.
- Aldolase is elevated in muscular dystrophy, but it is not unique to striated muscle.
- Serum glutamic oxaloacetic transaminase and lactate dehydrogenase may also be elevated but are not specific to muscle disease.
- *Muscle biopsy confirms the diagnosis.*
  — Usually performed on the vastus lateralis or another muscle that is weak but not overly atrophied.
  — A complete absence of dystrophin confirms DMD.
- The role of muscle biopsy is diminishing as the ability to diagnose muscular dystrophies based on *genetic testing* improves.

TREATMENT

- Treatment is focused on maintaining functional capacity involving a multidisciplinary approach, including physical therapy, orthoses, surgery, wheelchair, cardiac and pulmonary management, and genetic and psychological counseling.
- *Corticosteroids*
  — Oral prednisone has been shown to slow the progression of muscle weakness.
  — Because of significant morbidity—weight gain and osteopenia—use of prednisone in muscular dystrophy remains controversial.
- *Physical therapy*
  — May prolong muscle strength and ambulatory potential, and delay or prevent contractures; does not correct established contractures.
  — A program of maximum resistance exercises should be initiated as soon as a diagnosis of DMD is established because progressive weakness leads to adaptive posturing and contractures.
- *Bracing*
  — Night splints for heel-cord and knee-flexor stretching are an adjunct to physical therapy.
- *Surgery*
  — The role of surgery in DMD is for treatment of contractures and scoliosis.
  — Surgical correction of contractures should be considered when ambulation or daily activities are affected.
  — Many studies have shown that correction of contractures and use of orthoses can prolong ambulation for 1 to 3 years.
  — Shapiro and Specht classified approaches to surgical intervention (Box 55-1).

Box 55-1. Approaches to Surgical Intervention in Duchenne Muscular Dystrophy

1. Early, extensive ambulatory approach (Releases at the hip, hamstrings, heel cords, and posterior tibialis transfer before onset of contractures.)
2. Moderate ambulatory approach (no hip releases, and surgery performed when child has difficulty ambulating)
3. Minimum ambulatory approach (correction only of equinus contractures)
4. Rehabilitative approach (surgery after child has stopped walking with the goal of resuming ambulation)
5. Palliative approach (correction of equinovarus for pain relief and improved ability to wear shoes)

- Children with DMD may lose ability to walk between 7 and 16 years of age. As such, it is difficult to determine whether prolonged ambulation was truly caused by surgical intervention, or if those children with prolonged walking simply had milder forms of the disease.
- Once a child has stopped walking, surgery must be performed within 3 to 6 months to make ambulation possible again.
- Ambulatory patients use their equinus deformity to compensate for proximal weakness, and surgical Achilles tendon lengthening may lead to further weakness and loss of ambulation postoperatively.
- Spine fusion in children with DMD is indicated for curves greater than 30 degrees—curve progression is inevitable and pulmonary function will deteriorate over time as the curve progresses; the rationale for surgery is comfortable sitting, improved head control, and independent hand function (Figure 55-3).
- Scoliosis surgery is best tolerated in children whose forced vital capacity (FVC) is above 35% of normal. Some have even recommended surgery for curves greater than 20 degrees in children whose FVC is greater than 40% of normal. The risks of prolonged postoperative mechanical ventilation and pneumonia increase with more advanced pulmonary disease, so preoperative cardiac and pulmonary evaluation are mandatory.
- Surgery is contraindicated when expected life span is less than 2 years.
- *Medical concerns in the perioperative period*
  — Malignant hyperthermia can be associated with muscular dystrophies, so use of inhalational anesthetic agents should be avoided.
  — Anaphylaxis caused by latex allergy, airway obstruction, and intra-operative cardiac arrest have all been described.

EXPECTED OUTCOMES/PROGNOSIS

- Most boys with DMD stop walking around age 12 years and die around age 20 without pulmonary support.

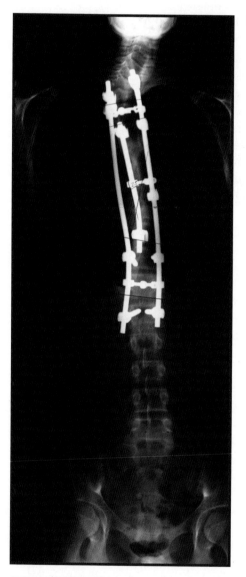

Figure 55-3. Spine fusion.

WHEN TO REFER

— Refer all suspected cases of muscular dystrophy to a pediatric orthopaedic surgeon or neuromuscular specialist for muscle biopsy.
— Refer to an orthopaedic surgeon as soon as diagnosis is made.
— Refer to a geneticist for genetic testing and counseling.

RELEVANT INTERNATIONAL CLASSIFICATION OF DISEASES, NINTH REVISION, CLINICAL MODIFICATION (ICD-9-CM) CODE

• **359.1**   DMD

Clinical Pearls (Duchenne Muscular Dystrophy)

1. Look for pseudohypertrophy of calf muscles and Gowers sign on examination.
2. Creatine kinase is very high early in the disease and decreases with progression of the disease.
3. Refer to geneticist for genetic testing and counseling.
4. Refer to orthopaedic surgeon as soon as diagnosis is made.
5. Spine fusion is indicated for scoliosis greater than 20 degrees and forced vital capacity greater than 40%.
6. Risk of malignant hyperthermia during anesthesia

Becker Muscular Dystrophy

INTRODUCTION/ETIOLOGY/EPIDEMIOLOGY

- X-linked recessive disorder resulting in weakness of proximal musculature
- Unlike DMD, BMD mutation results in a lower molecular weight dystrophin or a normal molecular weight dystrophin in reduced quantities.
- A consistent relationship exists between the amount and quality of dystrophin present and the disease severity.
- Much more rare than DMD; incidence is 1 in 42,000 boys.

SIGNS AND SYMPTOMS

- Similar to DMD except
  — Presents at a later age.
  — Disease progression is slower.
  — Proximal lower extremity weakness is the most prominent early symptom, with some children showing early weakness of the neck flexors.
  — Severe contractures are uncommon before the child becomes wheelchair-dependent.
  — Scoliosis is also relatively rare.
  — Ability to ambulate may be retained beyond 16 years of age, with some ambulating into the early adult years, sometimes as late as 40 years of age.
  — Up to 70% have electrocardiographic abnormalities and may develop cardiomyopathy.

DIFFERENTIAL DIAGNOSIS

- See DMD.

MAKING THE DIAGNOSIS

- Muscle biopsy confirms the diagnosis of BMD.
  — Reveals *diminished, rather than absent,* dystrophin levels.
- Laboratory findings are similar to DMD.

TREATMENT

- Similar to that for DMD.
- Achilles tendon lengthening surgery with or without tibialis posterior tendon transfer is used to treat the equinus foot deformity.
- Because the loss of muscle strength occurs at a much slower rate, lower extremity bracing is an important adjunct to therapy.

EXPECTED OUTCOMES/PROGNOSIS

- Because children with BMD will often live longer than those with DMD, more stress is placed on the already weakened myocardium, resulting in mitral regurgitation and heart failure.
- Restrictive lung disease may occur late, but cardiomyopathy is disproportionately severe and is the major risk of early demise.

WHEN TO REFER

- Refer all suspected cases of muscular dystrophy to a pediatric orthopaedic surgeon or neuromuscular specialist for muscle biopsy.
- Refer to an orthopaedic surgeon as soon as diagnosis is made.
- Refer to a geneticist for genetic testing and counseling.

RELEVANT *ICD-9-CM* CODE

- **359.1** BMD

Clinical Pearls (Becker Muscular Dystrophy)

1. **Similar to Duchenne muscular dystrophy but with milder clinical course**
2. **Longer life span makes follow-up of cardiac and pulmonary disease more important.**
3. **Bracing is an important adjunct to therapy because of preservation of muscle strength.**

CHAPTER 56

Hereditary Neuropathies

Charcot-Marie-Tooth Disease

INTRODUCTION/ETIOLOGY/EPIDEMIOLOGY

- Common form of polyneuropathy considered under hereditary sensory and motor neuropathies
- Manifested by symmetric weakness of distal muscles, especially of the lower extremities
- Hallmark of Charcot-Marie-Tooth (CMT) disease is selective functional loss of the anterior compartment muscles of the lower extremities.
- Incidence is 1 in 2,500 individuals.
- Most common form of inheritance is autosomal dominant, but can also be autosomal recessive or X-linked.
- Charcot-Marie-Tooth 1 and CMT 2 are the 2 main subtypes.
  - Charcot-Marie-Tooth 1 (hypertrophic or demyelinating type) is most common, accounting for 60% to 80% of cases.
  - Charcot-Marie-Tooth 2 (axonal or neuronal type) accounts for 20% to 40% of cases. The disease progresses very slowly, with a highly variable severity.
- Clinical findings in CMT are caused by disrupted axonal transport and impaired intracellular protein trafficking.
- In the past 15 years, more that 30 genes have been identified in cases of CMT, and many more may ultimately be described.

SIGNS AND SYMPTOMS

- Onset of CMT 1 typically occurs in adolescence or early adulthood.
- Charcot-Marie-Tooth 2 presents at an older age, often in the third decade of life.
- Early symptoms include frequent tripping, toe walking, foot pain caused by cavovarus foot deformity, and unstable ankles.
- *Cavovarus foot is the most common orthopaedic manifestation of CMT.*
  - Atrophy and contracture of the intrinsic muscles of the foot, contracture of the plantar fascia, and weakness of the peroneus brevis and anterior tibialis leads to plantarflexion of the first ray, forefoot equinus, and hindfoot varus (Figure 56-1).
  - Probability of a patient with bilateral cavovarus feet being diagnosed with CMT, regardless of family history, is as high as 78%.

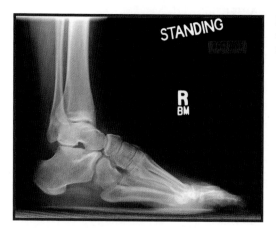

Figure 56-1. Radiograph of cavovarus foot deformity on Charcot-Marie-Tooth disease.

- Weakness of the upper limbs presents later in the disease and slowly progresses proximally, ultimately affecting hands, forearms, and upper arms.
- *Physical examination findings*
  — Cavovarus foot deformity
  — Tight heel cords
  — Inability to walk on heels
  — Calf muscle atrophy causes a stork leg.
  — Claw toes or hammertoes
  — Plantarflexed first metatarsal
  — Intrinsic muscle atrophy of the hand and feet occurs as early as the first decade or as late as the third decade (Figure 56-2).
    ▪ Difficulty with thumb opposition and side-to-side pinch
    ▪ Clawing of the fingers, with ring and small digits affected first
    ▪ In general, *muscles innervated by ulnar and peroneal nerves are commonly affected, while those innervated by the radial and tibial nerves are spared.*
  — Diminished or absent deep tendon reflexes (DTRs), especially at the ankles
    ▪ Knee reflexes are affected after ankle reflexes.
    ▪ Deep tendon reflexes are usually normal in CMT 2.
  — Sensory deficits are less pronounced than motor deficits.

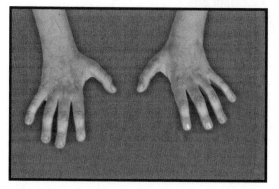

Figure 56-2. Intrinsic muscle wasting of the hand in child with Charcot-Marie-Tooth disease.

- Distal impairment of sensory functions in a stocking distribution, including vibratory sense, light touch, and position sense
- Pain and temperature sensation are also affected, manifesting before or after changes in vibratory sense.
- Because of loss of protective sensation in distal extremities, patients with CMT are susceptible to skin breakdown, burns, and foot ulcers.
— Cranial nerves are usually normal, but hearing deficits may be present.
— Steppage gait (drop foot in the swing phase) is apparent early in the disease. As the dorsiflexors become progressively weaker, the gait becomes more high-stepping, with compensatory increase in flexion of the knee and hip.
— Hip or acetabular dysplasia occurs in 6% to 8%.
- Weakness of the proximal muscles may be the deforming force that, over time, results in a shallow acetabulum and a valgus, anteverted femoral neck.
- Often presents as hip pain between 5 and 15 years of age.
- Radiographic findings are acetabular dysplasia and mild subluxation (Figure 56-3).
- Annual hip radiographs allow for earlier detection.
— Scoliosis occurs in 10% to 50%.
- Tends to occur in adolescents with CMT, rather than in children.
- If scoliosis is observed at a young age, magnetic resonance imaging (MRI) is recommended to evaluate for structural neural abnormalities.
- Left-thoracic curves are more common and there is more kyphosis and a higher rate of progression, despite bracing, compared with idiopathic scoliosis.

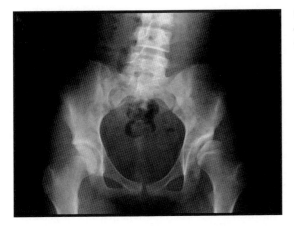

Figure 56-3. Pelvis radiograph of acetabular dysplasia in Charcot-Marie-Tooth disease.

DIFFERENTIAL DIAGNOSIS

- *Chronic inflammatory demyelinating polyradiculoneuropathy*
  — Differentiated from CMT by a negative family history, variable age of onset, and course that may be progressive or relapsing, and rarely associated with skeletal deformities.

— Diagnostic testing reveals nonhomogenous conduction slowing with conduction blocks, high cerebrospinal fluid (CSF) protein levels, and inflammatory infiltrates on nerve biopsy. Similar to CMT 1, onion-bulb formations are also seen on nerve biopsy.

- *Dejerine-Sottas disease*
  — Hereditary sensory motor neuropathy that may be a variant of CMT 1
  — Onset of symptoms by age 2 years with delayed acquisition of motor milestones
  — Severe motor and sensory involvement, with proximal muscles commonly affected
  — Ataxia and scoliosis are common manifestations.
  — Motor conduction velocity is drastically reduced (less than 12 m/second) and nerve biopsy shows severe demyelination and hypomyelination.
- *Hereditary neuropathy pressure palsy (HNPP)* (also known as tomaculous neuropathy)
  — Autosomal-dominant disorder with acute and transient episodes of focal neuropathies
  — Episodes are usually painless, may be recurrent, and often follow trivial trauma or pressure.
  — Patients often complain of paresthesias with compression, eg, on leg crossing, leaning on elbows, carrying plastic bags, or wearing rings.
  — Nerve conduction velocities (NCVs) reveal conduction abnormalities primarily at common entrapment sites.
  — Nerve biopsy shows focal myelin thickenings (tomacula) in several fibers.
- *Refsum disease*
  — Rare recessive disorder with relapsing-remitting generalized sensorimotor polyneuropathy of peripheral nerves
  — Pes cavus is often present.
  — Nerve biopsy reveals demyelination as well as onion-bulb formation.
  — Increased protein concentration in the CSF
  — Unique features include salt-and-pepper retinitis pigmentosa and cerebellar ataxia.
- *Spinal cord lesions*
  — Although CMT is the most common neurologic cause of a cavus foot, other intraspinal causes should be considered, including *tethered cord* and *lipomeningocele*.
  — All patients with suspected CMT should have a comprehensive spine and neurologic examination. If there is hyperreflexia or asymmetry in reflexes, MRI and neurologic consultation is obtained to rule out spinal cord lesion.

MAKING THE DIAGNOSIS

- *Electrical testing:* nerve conduction velocities are the most important first-line diagnostic tool for the classification of CMT disease.
  — Motor conduction velocities may be decreased in CMT even before clinical symptoms manifest.
  — In CMT 1, NCVs are consistently diminished, usually less than 38 m per second, while normal is greater than 42 m per second.
  — In CMT 2, NCVs are normal or only minimally diminished, but the compound muscle action potential is decreased.

- If NCV is inconclusive, *nerve biopsy* is performed to confirm the diagnosis.
  — The sural nerve is commonly used.
  — Charcot-Marie-Tooth 1—onion-bulb hypertrophy of the myelin sheath caused by cycles of demyelination and remyelination
  — Charcot-Marie-Tooth 2—axonal loss and no evidence of demyelination, with few or absent onion bulbs

TREATMENT

- *Medications*
  — Acetaminophen and nonsteroidal anti-inflammatory drugs are used to treat musculoskeletal pain.
  — Neuropathic pain may respond to tricyclic antidepressants, carbamazepine, or gabapentin.
  — Medications known to cause nerve damage (eg, vincristine, isoniazid, nitrofurantoin) should be avoided.
- *Physical therapy*
  — Daily heel-cord stretching can help prevent Achilles tendon contracture.
  — Physical therapists can also assist patients with walking.
- *Orthoses*
  — Shoes with good ankle support or ankle braces may be needed.
  — Forearm crutches or a cane may be necessary to improve gait stability.
  — Ankle-foot orthoses can correct foot drop and help with ambulation.
  — Wrist and hand orthoses can also maintain functional positions.
- *Surgery*
  — *Cavovarus foot deformity*
    ▪ In young patients with flexible deformity, soft tissue surgery (ie, radical plantar fascia release, transfer of the posterior tibialis tendon to the dorsum of the foot, or peroneus longus to brevis transfer) may be sufficient to delay or avoid bone or joint surgery.
    ▪ Forefoot plantarflexion can be corrected with metatarsal osteotomies as long as the hindfoot varus remains flexible.
    ▪ Over time, the foot deformities become fixed so calcaneal, midfoot, or forefoot osteotomies are necessary to correct the deformity. Triple arthrodesis is reserved as a salvage procedure.
    ▪ *Patients and families should be cautioned that recurrence rate of deformity is high after all types of surgery.*
  — *Toe walking*
    ▪ The equinus deformity in CMT is in the forefoot, not the calcaneus; lengthening the Achilles tendon is not part of the corrective operation.

— *Hip dysplasia (silent)*
  ■ Requires surgical correction, even if asymptomatic.
  ■ Redirectional osteotomy of the acetabulum
  ■ Children with weak hip abductors do not function well after femoral (varus) osteotomy: gait abnormality tends to get worse.
  ■ If dysplasia and subluxation are still present after acetabular osteotomy, a proximal femur varus rotation osteotomy may be indicated.
— *Scoliosis*
  ■ Because of failure of orthotic management and high rate of progression, spinal fusion is often recommended (Figure 56-4).
  ■ Monitoring of motor and somatosensory-evoked potentials during surgery is rarely possible because of the underlying demyelinating polyneuropathy.
  ■ Intra-operative wake-up test may not be possible as a result of the lower extremity weakness.
• *Genetic counseling*
— Should be offered so patients understand the potential risk of passing CMT onto their children and can make informed decisions.

EXPECTED OUTCOMES/PROGNOSIS

• Depends on the type of CMT.
• Progression of symptoms is very gradual, but eventually causes disability because of distal muscle weakness and deformities.
• Wheelchair confinement is rare (less than 5%).
• Charcot-Marie-Tooth does not affect normal life expectancy.

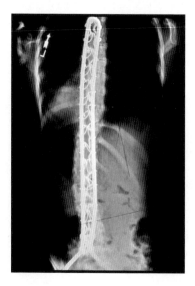

Figure 56-4. After spine fusion.

WHEN TO REFER

* Refer all suspected cases of CMT to a neurologist for further evaluation with electromyography and NCVs.
* Referral to a geneticist is also recommended.

RELEVANT *INTERNATIONAL CLASSIFICATION OF DISEASES, NINTH REVISION, CLINICAL MODIFICATION* CODE

* **356.1**   CMT disease

Clinical Pearls (CMT Disease)

1. Present with cavovarus foot deformity or toe walking.
2. Hip and spine radiographs should be included in the evaluation of cavovarus feet.
3. Refer to geneticist for genetic testing and counseling.
4. Refer to neurologist for nerve conduction testing and electromyography.
5. Hip dysplasia requires treatment even if asymptomatic.
6. Scoliosis is often progressive and requires spine fusion.

CHAPTER 57

Spinal Muscular Atrophy

Introduction/Etiology/Epidemiology

- Though rare spinal muscular atrophy (SMA) is one of the most common inherited neuromuscular disorders of childhood.
- Characterized by degeneration of the anterior horn cells in the spinal cord and lower bulbar nuclei
- Generally transmitted in an autosomal-recessive manner, although de novo mutation can occur with an incidence of 1 in 10,000 live births.

Signs and Symptoms

- Varying degrees of diffuse, symmetric, proximal trunk and limb weakness, greater in lower versus upper extremities
- Tendon reflexes are markedly decreased or absent.
- Sensation and intelligence are unaffected.
- Varying degrees of restrictive respiratory insufficiency
- Cardiac muscle is not involved.
- Classified into 4 subtypes based on maximum attainable physical function (Box 57-1)
- *Musculoskeletal complications of SMA*
  - *Scoliosis* is common (more than 80% of type 2 and 53% of type 3) and can be severe.
  - *Pelvic tilt* as a result of scoliosis tends to occur with significant neuromuscular scoliosis, especially long C-shaped curves (Figure 57-1a, b).
  - *Hip dislocation or subluxation*
    - May be unilateral or bilateral.
    - Occurs in 31% of type 2 and 38% of type 3.
  - *Joint contractures* are especially severe in lower extremities of nonambulatory patients.
  - *Foot deformity* is typically equinus with varus or valgus component.

Differential Diagnosis

- Neuromuscular disorders presenting in infancy are summarized in Table 57-1.

Box 57-1. Classification of Spinal Muscle Atrophy

- *Type 1 (Werdnig-Hoffman/infantile onset disease)*
  - —Most common variety
  - —May be first detected in utero by a decrease or loss of fetal movement in late pregnancy.
  - —Typically severe weakness is present at birth, but some are normal at birth and develop relentless paralysis and absent deep tendon reflexes by 3 to 5 months of age.
  - —Examination reveals an alert expression, furrowed brow, and normal eye movements because the upper cranial nerves are spared.
  - —Weakness of the bulbar muscles results in a poor suck and swallowing reflex, weak cry, and tongue fasciculation.
  - —Weak intercostal muscles lead to respiratory insufficiency and greater susceptibility to aspiration.
- *Type 2 (intermediate or juvenile spinal muscular atrophy)*
  - —Normal developmental milestones until 6 to 15 months of age, when weakness begins
  - —Can sit without support and often present because of failure to walk.
  - —Prone to progressive paralytic scoliosis, which can prevent comfortable sitting and further compromise lung function
  - —Pulmonary care is critical to improve function and prolong survival.
- *Types 3 and 4* are often grouped together *(Kugelberg-Welander disease)*
  - —Mildest forms
  - —Weakness develops after 12 months of age.
  - —While patients with both types can stand independently, ease of ambulation is greater in type 4.
  - —A waddling gait with lumbar lordosis, genu recurvatum, and a protuberant abdomen may be noted in toddlers or later in childhood.

Making the Diagnosis

- To differentiate SMA from other neuromuscular conditions, electromyography (EMG) and nerve conduction velocity (NCV) studies are required (and possibly muscle biopsy).
  - — *Electromyography* demonstrates abnormal spontaneous activity with fibrillations and positive sharp waves.
  - — *Nerve conduction velocity*
    - ▪ The motor unit action potentials have a higher duration and amplitude; many are polyphasic, and the maximum number that can be recruited in a given sampling area is markedly reduced because of massive motor nerve losses.
    - ▪ Sensory nerve tests are normal.
  - — *Muscle biopsy:* large groups of circular atrophic type 1 and 2 muscle fibers interspersed among fascicles of hypertrophied type 1 fibers is typical of SMA.
    - ▪ This pattern may take time to develop, and often the initial muscle biopsy in a neonate shows only widespread muscle fiber atrophy.
- *Genetic testing*
  - — Reveals homozygous deletions in the SMN gene.
  - — May be most useful in neonates or prenatal period in high-risk pregnancies.

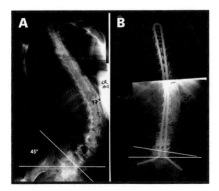

Figure 57-1. A, Pelvic tilt as a result of scoliosis in children with spinal muscular atrophy can have a direct negative effect on physical function and tends to occur in those with significant neuromuscular scoliosis (especially long C-shaped curves) where the pelvis rests lower on the convex side of that spinal deformity. B, Postsurgical radiograph showing correction of scoliosis and pelvic tilt.

Treatment

- Care is best provided by a multidisciplinary team including pediatric orthopaedists, rehabilitation specialists, orthotists, nurses, and other allied health professionals.
- Primary care physicians play a significant role in the early detection and management of the medical complications—pressure sores, intercurrent infections, feeding problems, aspiration, and respiratory insufficiency.
- *Scoliosis and pelvic tilt*
  — Bracing does not seem to prevent scoliosis but slows rate of progression in some cases for a limited period.
  — Surgical intervention may reduce the curvature by as much as 50% to 60% (Figure 57-1b).
     - Generally reserved for non-ambulatory children with SMA type 2 or 3 who have progressive curves of at least 40 degrees.
        - Complications include infection, excessive blood loss, rod breakage, neurologic injury, and rarely, death.
        - Benefits may outweigh the risks of surgery—slower decline in pulmonary function, improved sitting comfort and balance, more spine stability, superior sitting height, less back pain, greater ease of nursing and transport care, and better quality of life.
  — Early surgical repair of the scoliosis with fusion to sacrum provides best correction for pelvic tilt and sustained improvements in seating comfort.
- *Hip dislocation or subluxation*
  — Surgery does not seem to improve function or deformity, so prophylactic repair is no longer recommended.
  — Surgery is indicated for painful hip dislocation.
  — Surgical repairs include soft tissue releases, open reduction, and femoral varus-rotational osteotomy.
- *Joint contractures*
  — Physical therapy for range of motion exercises
  — Adaptive equipment and splinting should be instituted early and continued through-out the life span to maintain adequate physical function.
  — Lightweight long leg braces and crutches may prolong walking.
  — Some may require soft tissue operations to release tight structures.

Table 57-1. Neuromuscular Disorders Presenting in Neonatal Period

Anterior Horn Cell	Spinal muscular atrophy 1 Traumatic myelopathy Hypoxic ischemic myelopathy Neurogenic arthrogryposis

Congenital Hypomyelinating and Axonal Neuropathies	Hereditary motor sensory neuropathy (HMSN)
	  HMSN/CMT 2[a]
	  HMSN/CMT 3
	  Charcot-Marie-Tooth disease
	  Dejerine-Sottas disease
	  HMSN/CMT 4D
	Giant axonal neuropathy
	Hereditary sensory and autonomic neuropathy (HSAN-3; Riley-Day)

Neuromuscular Junction	Neonatal myasthenia gravis Congenital myasthenia Magnesium toxicity Infantile botulism
Congenital Myopathies	Nemaline myopathy Central core disease Myotubular myopathy Congenital fiber type disproportion Multicore myopathy

Muscular Dystrophies	Congenital muscular dystrophy
	  With merosin deficiency
	  Without merosin deficiency
	Congenital muscular dystrophy with structural central nervous system abnormality
	  Ullrich and Bethlem myopathy
	  Walker-Warburg disease
	  Muscle-eye-brain disease
	  Fukuyama disease
	Infantile facioscapulohumeral dystrophy
	Congenital myotonic dystrophy

Metabolic Disorders	Disorders of glycogen metabolism
	  Infantile acid maltase deficiency
	    Severe neonatal phosphofructokinase deficiency
	  Severe neonatal phosphorylase deficiency
	  Debrancher deficiency
	Disorders of lipid metabolism
	  Primary carnitine deficiency
	Peroxisomal disorders
	  Neonatal adrenoleukodystrophy
	    Cerebrohepatorenal syndrome (Zellweger)
	Mitochondrial myopathies
	  Cytochrome-c oxidase deficiency

[a]Hereditary motor and sensory neuropathy/Charcot-Marie-Tooth X-linked.

- *Foot deformities*
  — Ankle-foot-orthoses may slow progression, but surgical repair may be required.
- *Exercise* may be an important adjunct to the treatment of intermediate to mild forms.
  — Children with significant limb weakness are more likely to avoid strenuous activities, leading to lower levels of cardiorespiratory fitness.
  — Swimming encourages joint range of motion and may strengthen extremity muscles in a non–weight-bearing setting.
- *Potential future treatment modalities*
  — Thyrotropin-releasing hormone (TRH) may increase muscle strength in types 2 and 3. Further study is needed before TRH can be recommended.
  — Valproic acid increases fl-SMN protein in vitro and seemed to improve strength in a small number of adult SMA patients in one open label trial.

Expected Outcomes/Prognosis

- Type 1: Never sit independently and generally die of respiratory failure before 1 to 2 years of age.
- Type 2: Some with milder forms may eventually walk with bracing and live well into adolescence and beyond.
- Types 3 and 4: When the onset of weakness appears after 2 years of age, independent walking is possible into the fifth decade and survival is usually normal.

When to Refer

- Refer suspected cases of SMA to a neurologist for EMG and NCV.
- Confirmed cases are best managed by a multidisciplinary team.

Relevant *International Classification of Diseases, Ninth Revision, Clinical Modification* Codes

- **335.10**   SMA types 1 (Werdnig-Hoffman) and 2
- **335.11**   SMA types 3 and 4 (Kugelberg-Welander disease)

CHAPTER 58

Friedreich Ataxia

Introduction/Etiology/Epidemiology

- Neurodegenerative disease characterized by a progressive, mixed cerebellar and sensory ataxia
- Inheritance is autosomal recessive.
- Genetic defect in the frataxin gene on chromosome 9
- Frataxin is a mitochondrial protein expressed at high levels in the brain, heart, and pancreas.
- Pathologically, there is a progressive dying back of the peripheral and central axonal arms of the largest primary sensory neurons. This results in an axonal sensory neuropathy, atrophy of the posterior columns, and neuronal loss in the brainstem nuclei, specifically the cerebellar dentate nucleus and sensory ganglia of the acoustic and vestibular nerves.

Signs and Symptoms

- Truncal ataxia causes imbalance and frequent falls early in the disease.
- Loss of fine motor skills, followed by an inability to control extremity movement and an intention tremor
- Cerebellar dysarthria (slow, jerky speech) appears within 5 years of disease onset.
- Dysphagia, especially for liquids, as a result of brain stem involvement
- Sensorineural hearing loss affects about 20% of patients.
- Visual impairment may be present.
- Loss of vibration and position sense
- Light touch, pain, and temperature sensation deteriorate with advancing disease.
- Deep tendon reflexes are eventually lost in almost all patients but may remain intact in younger children and in those with late-onset disease. A small proportion retain or have exaggerated deep-tendon reflexes.
- Positive Babinski sign is present in most patients.
- Muscle tone is usually normal at onset, but spasms can occur later in disease.
- Nystagmus may be present.
- Pes cavus, pes equinovarus, and hammertoes make ambulation even more difficult.
- Kyphoscoliosis may cause back pain as well as cardiorespiratory compromise.
- Autonomic nervous system dysfunction occurs later in disease, causing cold and cyanotic distal lower extremities and more rarely, decreased heart rate variability and bladder dysfunction.

- Hypertrophic cardiomyopathy occurs in most patients. Affected individuals may be asymptomatic or have shortness of breath and palpitations.
- Pancreatic disease occurs in about 30%. Affected individuals develop impaired glucose tolerance or full-blown diabetes mellitus.

Differential Diagnosis

- *Congenital disorders:* ataxic cerebral palsy; agenesis or hypoplasia of the cerebellum; Dandy-Walker syndrome; hydrocephalus; Arnold-Chiari malformation; cerebellar dysplasia with micro, macro, or agyria; platybasia; and craniovertebral abnormalities
- *Degenerative diseases and hereditary ataxias:* Pelizaeus-Merzbacher disease, neuronal ceroid lipofuscinosis, sialidosis, GM2 gangliosidosis, Ramsay-Hunt myoclonus, metachromatic leukodystrophy, Niemann-Pick disease, argininosuccinic aciduria, juvenile Gaucher disease, pyruvate decarboxylase deficiency, Hartnup and maple syrup urine disease, and spinocerebellar and cerebellar ataxias (Table 58-1).

Making the Diagnosis

- *Essential diagnostic criteria* (defined by Harding in 1981)
  — Onset before 25 years of age
  — Progressive ataxia of gait and limbs
  — Absent ankle and knee reflexes
  — Extensor plantar responses (positive Babinski sign)
  — Dysarthria
  — Motor nerve conduction velocities of greater than 40 m/s^{-1} in the upper extremities with small or absent sensory action potentials
- *Visual-evoked potentials* are reduced in up to 90% of patients.
- *Auditory-evoked potentials* are abnormal in 20% of patients.
- *Neuroimaging* shows thinning of the cervical spinal cord and abnormal signal intensity in the posterior and lateral columns. Cerebellar atrophy is noted in severe and advanced cases.
- *Nerve biopsy* reveals loss of large, myelinated sensory nerve fibers, and secondary axonal degeneration in the later stages of the disease.
- *Electrocardiogram* frequently shows ST-T wave changes and ventricular hypertrophy, with conduction disturbances seen less often.
- *Echocardiogram* is abnormal (ie, concentric left ventricular hypertrophy, asymmetric septal hypertrophy, and decreased left ventricular function) in up to 63% of patients.

Treatment

- Management requires a team of specialists including neurologists, orthopaedists, rehabilitation specialists, orthotists, cardiologists, and endocrinologists.
- Primary care physicians play a significant role in the medical management.
- Orthotics and assistive devices may improve quality of life.

Table 58-1. Autosomal-Recessive Cerebellar Ataxias

Condition	Gene/Protein	Inheritance	Ethnicity	Clinical Features
Abetalipoproteinemia or Bassen-Kornzweig syndrome	MTP	Autosomal recessive	None specified	Malabsorption, pigmentary degeneration of retina, progressive ataxic neuropathy; absent LDL and VLDL
Ataxia telangiectasia	ATM	Autosomal recessive	None specified	Progressive cerebellar ataxia, oculomotor apraxia, oculocutaneous telangiectasia, choreoathetosis, variable immune deficiency, increased malignancy, sensitive to ionizing radiation
Ataxia telangiectasia-like disorder	MREI 1A	Rare	None specified	Similar to ataxia telangiectasia, especially sensitive to ionizing radiation; chromosomes unstable
Ataxia with isolated vitamin E deficiency	α-TTP	Autosomal recessive	North Africa; Mediterranean basin; Japan	Progressive sensory and cerebellar ataxia before 20 y; Friedreich ataxia features but less cardiac and pancreatic disease
Ataxia with oculomotor apraxia 1 and 2 (AOA1 and AOA2)	Aprataxin/ senataxin	Autosomal recessive	Portugal; Japan	AOA1 onset 2–6 y dysarthria, limb dysmetria, oculomotor apraxia, weakness, vibration, and position sense; AOA2 onset 11–22 y spinocerebellar ataxia, choreoathetosis; dystonic posture
Cayman ataxia	Cayataxin	Most autosomal recessive	Grand Cayman Island	Newborn hypotonia, developmental delay, nonprogressive cerebellar dysfunction
Cerebrotendinous xanthomatosis	CYP27	Autosomal recessive	Sephardic Jews of Moroccan origin	Xanthomas of tendons, juvenile cataracts, early arthrosclerosis, progressive cerebellar ataxia after puberty, and spinal cord damage and dementia
Charlevoix-Saguenay-spastic ataxia	Sacsin	Autosomal recessive	French Canadian	Onset 1–2 y progressive spastic ataxia, paraplegia, increased tendon reflexes, nystagmus, positive Babinski, vibration, and position sense
Coenzyme Q$_{10}$ deficiency with cerebellar ataxia	None specified	Autosomal recessive	None specified	Child onset ataxia, cerebellar atrophy, low coenzyme Q$_{10}$ in muscle biopsy, seizures, developmental delay, mental retardation

Table 58-1. Autosomal-Recessive Cerebellar Ataxias, continued

Condition	Gene/ Protein	Inheritance	Ethnicity	Clinical Features
Early-onset cerebellar ataxia with retained tendon reflexes	13q11-12	Autosomal recessive	Northwest Italy	Early onset (first or second decade) cerebellar ataxia with preservation tendon reflexes
Friedreich ataxia	Frataxin	Autosomal recessive	None specified	Ataxia, loss vibration and position sense, nystagmus, areflexia, positive Babinski; deafness, cardiomyopathy, diabetes or glucose intolerance
Infantile onset spinocerebellar ataxia	Twinkle	Autosomal recessive	Finland	Ataxia by 2 y; athetosis, reduced deep-tendon reflexes
Joubert syndrome (JBTS) 1–5	JBTS1; JBTS2; AHII; NPHP1; nephrocystin-6	Autosomal recessive	None specified	Cerebellar agenesis in newborn Nystagmus, vertical gaze paresis, ptosis, retinopathy, mental retardation; apnea of newborn
Marinesco-Sjogren syndrome	SIL1	Autosomal recessive	None specified	Infantile-onset cerebellar ataxia, cataracts, mental retardation, areflexia, sometimes rhabdomyolysis
Mitochondrial recessive ataxic syndrome	Polymerase γ	Autosomal recessive	Finland, Norway, United Kingdom, Belgium	Unsteady gait, nystagmus, seizures, dysarthria, poor deep tendon reflexes, poor vibration and position sense
Posterior column ataxia and retinitis pigmentosa	AXPC1	Autosomal recessive	None specified	Childhood sensory ataxia, pain and temperature preserved, absent tendon reflexes, ring scotoma, eventual blindness
Refsum disease	PAHX; PEX7	Autosomal recessive	None specified	Retinitis pigmentosa, chronic polyneuropathy, cerebellar ataxia; deafness, arrhythmias; onset usually before 20 y
Spinocerebellar ataxia with axonal neuropathy	TDP1	recessive	Saudi Arabia	Seizures, mild brain atrophy, mild increase in cholesterol; albumin
Xeroderma pigmentosum A-G and XP variant	XP A-G and POLH	Autosomal recessive	United States; Japan; Mediterranean	Ataxia, choreoathetosis, deafness, mental retardation, early skin cancer, telangiectasia, keratitis, photophobia, skin photosensitive

LDL, low-density lipoprotein; VLDL, very low-density lipoprotein.

- Exercise can improve function, aerobic fitness, self-esteem, independence, and socialization. Cardiomyopathy is a relative contraindication to exercise.
- Pes cavus, pes equinovarus, and hammertoes
  — Ankle-foot orthoses may increase ambulatory ability, but more severe deformities require surgical correction.
- Kyphoscoliosis
  — Scoliotic curves of less than 40 degrees are closely observed.
  — Curves greater than 60 degrees are surgically repaired.

Expected Outcomes/Prognosis

- Gait progressively deteriorates, becoming wide-based and requiring assistive devices by an average of 10 to 15 years after disease onset.
- Life expectancy varies.
  — Severely compromised patients generally die by 30 to 40 years of age.
  — Longer survival may occur in those with a later onset of disease and adequate treatment of neuromuscular complications, diabetes, and cardiac symptoms.
  — Primary causes of death include cardiomyopathy, arrhythmias, and airway compromise from significant bulbar dysfunction.

When to Refer

- Refer suspected cases to a neurologist for nerve conduction velocity studies.
- Confirmed cases are best managed by a multidisciplinary team.

Relevant *International Classification of Diseases, Ninth Revision, Clinical Modification* Code

- **334.0** Friedreich ataxia

CHAPTER 59

Arthrogryposis

Introduction/Etiology/Epidemiology

- The term *arthrogryposis* is derived from the Greek meaning "curved joint."
- Refers to a group of more than 150 syndromes in which there are multiple joint contractures present at birth.
  - The most recognizable of these syndromes is amyoplasia.
  - All are associated with decreased fetal movement, which results in *multiple joint contractures.*
  - Numerous *primary* etiologies
- The incidence of arthrogryposis is 1 in 3,000
- The incidence of amyoplasia (most common form) is 1 in 10,000.
- About half of the conditions associated with arthrogryposis have a syndromic or genetic abnormality.
- Amyoplasia is thought to be nongenetic.
- Arthrogryposis syndromes may be categorized into 3 major groups.
  - Group I disorders involve all 4 extremities.
    - Arthrogryposis multiplex congenital
    - Larsen syndrome
  - Group II disorders predominantly or exclusively involve the hands and feet.
    - Distal arthrogryposis
    - Freeman-Sheldon syndrome, which also has some facial involvement
  - Group III disorders involve webbing across the joints.
    - Pterygia syndromes

Signs and Symptoms

- Pregnancy history typically reveals decreased fetal movements.
- Loss of skin creases across joints
- Dimples may be present over the extensor surfaces of involved joints.
- Severe muscle atrophy and a decrease in subcutaneous fat
- Joint motion is restricted, and there is a firm inelastic block with passive motion.
- The shoulders are internally rotated and adducted.
- The elbows are extended with the forearms pronated.
- The wrist and fingers are flexed.

- The fingers are thin and tapered.
- Foot deformities are present in 90% of patients.
  — Clubfoot is the most common, especially in amyoplasia.
  — Vertical talus is also seen.
- Seventy percent have knee contractures, both flexion and extension.
- Forty percent have hip deformities including subluxation, frank dislocation, and contracture.
- The incidence of scoliosis in patients with amyoplasia ranges from 2.5% to 70%.

Differential Diagnosis

- Bilateral brachial plexus palsy
- Bony fusion
  — Symphalangism (ie, fusion of phalanges)
  — Coalition (ie, fusion of the carpals and tarsal bones)
  — Synostosis (ie, fusion of long bones)
- Absence of dermal ridges
- Absence of distal interphalangeal joint creases
- Amniotic bands
- Antecubital webbing
- Camptodactyly
- Coalition
- Humeroradial synostosis
- Familial impaired pronation and supination of forearm
- Liebenberg syndrome
- Nail-patella syndrome
- Nievergelt-Pearlman syndrome
- Poland anomaly
- Tel-Hashomer camptodactyly
- Trismus pseudocamptodactyly

Making the Diagnosis

- Diagnosis is based on history and physical examination.
- Electromyograms and muscle biopsies are of little value, although some feel theses tests may help to differentiate between myopathic and neuropathic forms.
- Prenatal ultrasound may suggest the diagnosis when it shows decreased or absent fetal movement in association with oligohydramnios.

Treatment

- Management requires a multidisciplinary team including an orthopaedic surgeon, a rehabilitation specialist, a geneticist, and occupational and physical therapists.
- The goal of treatment is to ensure function and independence.

- In the lower extremities, the goal is alignment and stability for ambulation.
- In the newborn, a program of stretching and bracing can be successful in improving passive range of motion.
  — Careful attention to the birth process is important to make sure there are no long bone fractures before beginning a stretching program.
  — Serial stretching casts applied on a weekly basis are initiated soon after birth.
  — A percutaneous Achilles tenotomy can also be done, as in the Ponseti technique.
- Foot deformities are very difficult to correct, and most will require an extensive postero-medial release.
  — The surgical correction is done at about 1 year of age.
  — High recurrence rate, and long-term bracing postoperatively is required.
  — Talectomy is reserved for severe recurrent deformities.
- Knee contractures
  — Mild knee flexion contractures of less than 20 degrees are compatible with good function.
  — Severe contractures can limit the ability to stand and walk.
  — Early treatment consists of stretching and holding splints.
  — In the newborn period, stretching the quadriceps and serial casting may be beneficial.
  — For more severe contractures, quadricepsplasty can be performed (lengthening of the quadriceps tendon, with a capsular release).
- Hip deformities
  — Closed reduction is rarely successful.
  — Open reduction, if required, is performed at about 1 year of age.
- Upper extremity contractures
  — Limbs are positioned with orthotic devices at tabletop level so that children can feed themselves.
  — Early splinting may prevent deformities.
  — Shoulder contractures can be treated with proximal humeral osteotomy.
- Scoliosis
  — Treatment depends on the curve type and magnitude and may include observation, bracing, or surgical correction.

Expected Outcomes/Prognosis

- Long-standing contractures may lead to undergrowth of limbs.
- Prognosis depends on the underlying condition and the patient's response to treatment.
- Children with amyoplasia have normal intelligence and good prognosis for function and independence.
- Neonates who are ventilator dependent typically have a poor prognosis.

When to Refer

- Patients with arthrogryposis should be referred to a geneticist for diagnosis and a pediatric orthopaedist soon after being diagnosed.

Relevant *International Classification of Diseases, Ninth Revision, Clinical Modification* Code

- **728.3**   Arthrogryposis

Bibliography

Aronsson DD, Stokes IA, Ronchetti PJ, Labelle HB. Comparison of curve shape between children with cerebral palsy, Friedreich's ataxia, and adolescent idiopathic scoliosis. *Dev Med Child Neurol.* 1994;36:412–418

Azmaipairashvili Z, Riddle EC, Scavina M, Kumar SJ. Correction of cavovarus foot deformity in Charcot-Marie-Tooth disease. *J Pediatr Orthop.* 2005;25:360–365

Ballock RT, Skinner SR, Abel MF. Muscular dystrophies and other neurodegenerative disorders. In: Sponseller PD, ed. *Orthopaedic Knowledge Update: Pediatrics 2.* Rosemont, IL: American Academy of Orthopaedic Surgeons; 2002

Ben Hamida C, Doerflinger N, Belal S, et al. Localization of Friedreich ataxia phenotype with selective vitamin E deficiency to chromosome 8q by homozygosity mapping. *Nat Genet.* 1993;5:195–200

Bertorini T, Narayanaswami P, Rashed H. Charcot-Marie-Tooth disease (hereditary motor sensory neuropathies) and hereditary sensory and autonomic neuropathies. *Neurologist.* 2004;10:327–337

Cagnoli C, Mariotti C, Taroni F, et al. SCA28, a novel form of autosomal dominant cerebellar ataxia on chromosome 18p11.2-q11.2. *Brain.* 2006;129:235–242

Cavalier L, Ouahchi K, Kayden HJ, et al. Ataxia with isolated vitamin E deficiency: heterogeneity of mutations and phenotypic variability in a large number of families. *Am J Hum Genet.* 1998;62:301–310

Chan G, Bowen JR, Kumar SJ. Evaluation and treatment of hip dysplasia in Charcot-Marie-Tooth disease. *Orthop Clin North Am.* 2006;37:203–209

Chance PF, Ashizawa T, Hoffman EP, Crawford TO. Molecular basis of neuromuscular diseases. *Phys Med Rehabil Clin N Am.* 1998;9:49–81

Chang JG, Hsieh-Li HM, Jong YJ, Wang NM, Tsai CH, Li H. Treatment of spinal muscular atrophy by sodium butyrate. *Proc Natl Acad Sci USA.* 2001;98:9808–9813

Child JS, Perloff JK, Bach PM, Wolfe AD, Perlman S, Kark RA. Cardiac involvement in Friedreich's ataxia: a clinical study of 75 patients. *J Am Coll Cardiol.* 1986;7:1370–1378

Chng SY, Wong YQ, Hui JH, Wong HK, Ong HT, Goh DY. Pulmonary function and scoliosis in children with spinal muscular atrophy types II and III. *J Paediatr Child Health.* 2003;39:673–676

Cobb JR. Outline for the study of scoliosis. *AAOS Instr Course Lect 5.* 1948:261–275

Cossee M, Durr A, Schmitt M, et al. Friedreich's ataxia: point mutations and clinical presentation of compound heterozygotes. *Ann Neurol.* 1999;45:200–206

Darras BT. Neuromuscular disorders in the newborn. *Clin Perinatol.* 1997;24:827–844

Darras BT, Jones HR Jr. Neuromuscular problems of the critically ill neonate and child. *Semin Pediatr Neurol.* 2004;11:147–168

Deconinck N, Dan B. Pathophysiology of Duchenne muscular dystrophy: current hypotheses. *Pediatr Neurol.* 2007;36:1–7

Durr A, Cossee M, Campuxano V, et al. Clinical and genetic abnormalities in patients with Friedreich's ataxia. *N Engl J Med.* 1996;335:1169–1175

Engel JM, Kartin D, Jaffe KM. Exploring chronic pain in youths with Duchenne muscular dystrophy: a model for pediatric neuromuscular disease. *Phys Med Rehabil Clin N Am.* 2005;16:1113–1124

Evans GA, Drennan JC, Russman BS. Functional classification and orthopaedic management of spinal muscular atrophy. *J Bone Joint Surg Br.* 1981;63B:516–522

Fillyaw MJ, Ades PA. Endurance exercise training in Friedreich ataxia. *Arch Phys Med Rehabil.* 1989;70:786–788

Frischhut B, Krismer M, Stoeckl B, Landauer F, Auckenthaler T. Pelvic tilt in neuromuscular disorders. *J Pediatr Orthop B.* 2000;9:221–228

Gosselin LE, McCormick KM. Targeting the immune system to improve ventilatory function in muscular dystrophy. *Med Sci Sports Exerc.* 2004;36:44–51

Granata C, Magni E, Merlini L, Cervellati S. Hip dislocation in spinal muscular atrophy. *Chir Organi Mov.* 1990;75:177–184

Grondard C, Biondi O, Armand AS, et al. Regular exercise prolongs survival in a type 2 spinal muscular atrophy model mouse. *J Neurosci.* 2005;25:7615–7622

Guyton GP. Current concepts review: orthopaedic aspects of Charcot-Marie-Tooth disease. *Foot Ankle Int.* 2006;27:1003–1010

Harding AE. Friedreich's ataxia: a clinical and genetic study of 90 families with an analysis of early diagnosis criteria and intrafamilial clustering of clinical features. *Brain.* 1981;104:589–620

Harris-Love MO, Siegel KL, Paul SM, Benson K. Rehabilitation management of Friedreich ataxia: lower extremity force-control variability and gait performance. *Neurorehabil Neural Repair.* 2004;18:117–124

Hausmanowa-Petrusewicz I, Vrbova G. Spinal muscular atrophy: a delayed development hypothesis. *Neuroreport.* 2005;16:657–661

Herring JA, ed. *Tachdjian's Pediatric Orthopaedics.* 3rd ed. Philadelphia, PA: W.B. Saunders Co; 2002

Hirtz D, Iannaccone S, Heemskerk J, Gwinn-Hardy K, Moxley R 3rd, Rowland LP. Challenges and opportunities in clinical trials for spinal muscular atrophy. *Neurology.* 2005;65:1352–1357

Johnston HM. The floppy weak infant revisited. *Brain Dev.* 2003;25:155–158

Karol LA, Elerson E. Scoliosis in patients with Charcot-Marie-Tooth disease. *J Bone Joint Surg Am.* 2007;89:1504–1510

Kouwenhoven JW, Van Ommeren PM, Pruijs HEJ, Castelein RM. Spinal decompensation in neuromuscular disease. *Spine (Phila Pa 1976).* 2006;31:E188–E191

Labelle H, Tohme S, Duhaime M, Allard P. Natural history of scoliosis in Friedreich's ataxia. *J Bone Joint Surg Am.* 1986;68:564–572

Lodi R, Tonon C, Calabrese V, Schapira AH. Friedreich's ataxia: from disease mechanisms to therapeutic interventions. *Antioxid Redox Signal.* 2006;8:438–443

McCartney N, Moroz D, Garner SH, McComas AJ. The effects of strength training in patients with selected neuromuscular disorders. *Med Sci Sports Exerc.* 1988;20:362–368

McDonald CM, Abresch RT, Carter GT, Fowler WM Jr, Johnson ER, Kilmer DD. Profiles of neuromuscular diseases. Becker's muscular dystrophy. *Am J Phys Med Rehabil.* 1995;74:S93–S103

Meyer zu Horste G, Prukop T, Nave KA, Sereda MW. Myelin disorders: causes and perspectives of Charcot-Marie-Tooth neuropathy. *J Mol Neurosci.* 2006;28:77–88

Nagai MK, Chan G, Guille JT, Kumar SJ, Scavina M, Mackenzie WG. Prevalence of Charcot-Marie-Tooth disease in patients who have bilateral cavovarus feet. *J Pediatr Orthop.* 2006;26:438–443

Noble-Jamieson CM, Heckmatt JZ, Dubowitz V, Silverman M. Effects of posture and spinal bracing on respiratory function in neuromuscular disease. *Arch Dis Child.* 1986;61:178–181

Palau F, Espinos C. Autosomal recessive cerebellar ataxias. *Orphanet J Rare Dis.* 2006;1:47

Pandolfo M. Friedreich ataxia. *Semin Pediatr Neurol.* 2003;10:163–172

Pareyson D. Differential diagnosis of Charcot-Marie-Tooth disease and related neuropathies. *Neurol Sci.* 2004;25:72–82

Puccio H, Koenig M. Recent advances in the molecular pathogenesis of Friedreich ataxia. *Hum Mol Genet.* 2000;9:887–892

Rice SG, American Academy of Pediatrics Council on Sports Medicine and Fitness. Medical conditions affecting sports participation. *Pediatrics.* 2008;121:841–848

Rodillo E, Marini ML, Heckmatt JZ, Dubowitz V. Scoliosis in spinal muscular atrophy: review of 63 cases. *J Child Neurol.* 1989;4:118–123

Saifi GM, Szigeti K, Snipes GJ, Garcia CA, Lupski JR. Molecular mechanisms, diagnosis, and rational approaches to management of and therapy for Charcot-Marie-Tooth disease and related peripheral neuropathies. *J Investig Med.* 2003;51:261–283

Sarwark JF, MacEwan GD, Scott CI Jr. Amyoplasiaca common form of arthrogryposis. *J Bone Joint Surg Am.* 1990;72:465–469

Schols L, Meyer CH, Schmid G, Wilhelms I, Przuntek H. Therapeutic strategies in Friedreich's ataxia. *J Neural Transm Suppl.* 2004;68:135–145

Shy ME. Charcot-Marie-Tooth disease: an update. *Curr Opin Neurol.* 2004;17:579–585

Silva AC, Russo AK, Picarro IC, et al. Cardiorespiratory responses to exercise in patients with spinal muscular atrophy and limb-girdle dystrophy. *Braz J Med Biol Res.* 1987;20:565–568

Sporer SM, Smith BG. Hip dislocation in patients with spinal muscular atrophy. *J Pediatr Orthop.* 2003;23:10–14

Strober JB. Therapeutics in Duchenne muscular dystrophy. *NeuroRx.* 2006;3:225–234

Sumner CJ, Huynh TN, Markowitz JA, et al. Valproic acid increases SMN levels in spinal muscular atrophy patient cells. *Ann Neurol.* 2003;54:647–654

Thompson GH. Neuromuscular disorders. In: Morrissy RT, Weinstein SL, eds. *Lovell and Winter's Pediatric Orthopaedics.* 4th ed. Philadelphia, PA: Lippincott Williams & Wilkins; 1996

Tzeng AC, Cheng J, Fryczynski H, et al. A study of thyrotropin-releasing hormone for the treatment of spinal muscular atrophy: a preliminary report. *Am J Phys Med Rehabil.* 2000;79:435–440

Wang HY, Ju YH, Chen SM, Lo SK, Jong YJ. Joint range of motion limitations in children and young adults with spinal muscular atrophy. *Arch Phys Med Rehabil.* 2004;85:1689–1693

Weihl CC, Conolly AM, Pestronk A. Valproate may improve strength and function in patients with type III/IV spinal muscular atrophy. *Neurology.* 2006;67:500–501

Zenios M, Sampath J, Cole C, Khan T, Galasko CS. Operative treatment for hip subluxation in spinal muscular atrophy. *J Bone Joint Surge Br.* 2005;87:1541–1544

Zuchner S, Vance JM. Mechanisms of disease: a molecular genetic update on hereditary axonal neuropathies. *Nat Clin Pract Neurol.* 2006;2:45–53

Zumrova A. Problems and possibilities in the differential diagnosis of syndrome spinocerebellar ataxia. *Neuro Endocrinol Lett.* 2005;26:98–108

Part 18: Genetic Diseases and Syndromes

TOPICS COVERED

CHAPTER 60

Skeletal Dysplasias

Introduction/Etiology/Epidemiology

- Skeletal dysplasias (osteochondrodysplasias) are characterized by abnormal cartilage and bone growth, resulting in abnormal shape and disproportionate size of limbs, trunk, or skull.
- There are more than 200 different skeletal dysplasias.
  - The 4 most common are achondroplasia (dwarfism) (see Chapter 64), achondrogenesis, osteogenesis imperfecta (OI), and thanatophoric dysplasia.
- Incidence is approximately 1 in 4,000 live births.
- Etiology generally falls into 1 of 3 categories.
  - Defects in developmental genes
  - Abnormalities of matrix structural proteins
  - Defects in enzymes that process protein
- Modes of inheritance include autosomal dominant, autosomal recessive, X-linked dominant, and X-linked recessive.
- Males and females are equally affected except for X-linked conditions.
- Many skeletal dysplasias involve multiple, seemingly unrelated defects all arising from one abnormal gene.
  - For example, chondroectodermal dysplasia, which is recessively inherited, is characterized by a sixth finger, fine hair, cardiac abnormalities, immune deficiencies, and angular deformity of the lower limbs, with an extreme genu valgum developing over time.
- Some skeletal dysplasias are also associated with abnormalities in other systems (eg, cardiac, neurologic, metabolic, hematologic).

Signs and Symptoms

- Signs of a skeletal dysplasia are usually identified at birth or when the child begins to walk.
- Signs and symptoms will vary depending on the specific syndrome; however, there are many common features of skeletal dysplasias (Box 60-1).

Box 60-1. Features Common to Most Skeletal Dysplasias

Short stature (below third percentile)

Disproportionate limb and body size (relatively short trunk or limbs)

Angular deformity of the limbs

Deformities of the head, neck, hands, and feet (eg, polydactyly, craniosynostosis, disproportionately large head, clubfoot, radial ray defects)

Hip dysplasia

Spinal abnormalities such as kyphosis and atlantoaxial instability

Delayed ossification

Gait disturbances

Developmental delay

Family members with atypical appearance or similar features to affected child

Differential Diagnosis

- Cardiopulmonary disorders such as dysgammaglobulinemia
- Chromosomal disorders such as trisomy 18
- Endocrine disorders such as growth hormone deficiency, Shwachman syndrome, hyperparathyroidism, and hypophosphatasia
- Lysosomal storage disorders
- Inborn errors of metabolism such as cystinosis
- Intrauterine growth retardation
- Severe malnutrition
- Child abuse and neglect
- Constitutional growth delay
- Failure to thrive
- Growth failure
- Down syndrome
- Apert syndrome
- Cornelia de Lange syndrome
- Crouzon syndrome
- Cystic fibrosis
- Cytomegalovirus infection
- DiGeorge syndrome
- Fanconi syndrome
- McCune-Albright syndrome

Making the Diagnosis

- Most skeletal dysplasias are diagnosed based on the history, physical examination (Figure 60-1), and radiographic findings (Box 60-2).
  — When a skeletal dysplasia is suspected, a *skeletal survey* should be performed, including the following radiographic views:
    - Lateral skull
    - Lateral thoracolumbar spine
    - Anteroposterior pelvis
    - Anteroposterior of one arm to mid-humerus
    - Anteroposterior of one leg to mid-femur
  — Family history is a key component in establishing the diagnosis and mode of inheritance.
- An increasing number of skeletal dysplasias now have confirmatory *genetic testing* through select laboratories. This number is expected to grow rapidly over the next decade.
- *Prenatal ultrasound* can diagnose many types of skeletal dysplasias.

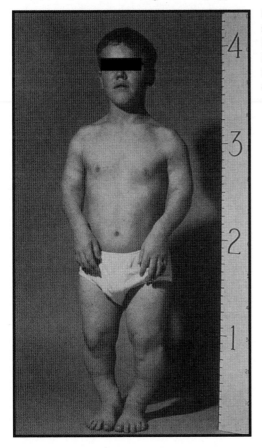

Figure 60-1. Skeletal dysplasia. Note short stature, disproportionate limb and body size, and angular limb deformities. Reproduced from Beals RK, Horton W. Skeletal dysplasias: an approach to diagnosis. *J Am Acad Orthop Surg.* 1995;3:174–181.

Box 60-2. Examples of Radiographic Findings in Skeletal Dysplasias

Oval-shaped lucencies in proximal femur or humerus (achondroplasia)

Dumbbell-shaped long bones (Kniest dysplasia and metatrophic dysplasia)

Bowing of limbs (camptomelic dysplasia, osteogenesis imperfecta [OI] syndromes, thanatophoric dysplasia)

Calcified spikes along lateral femoral metaphyses (thanatophoric dysplasia and achondrogenesis types I and II)

Metaphyseal flaring and cupping at the ends of the rib and long bones (achondroplasia, metaphyseal dysplasias, asphyxiating thoracic dysplasia, chondroectodermal dysplasia)

Long bone fractures (OI syndromes, hypophosphatasia, osteopetrosis, achondrogenesis type I)

Absent epiphyseal ossification centers (spondyloepiphyseal dysplasia [SED] congenita, multiple epiphyseal dysplasia, other SED)

Cone-shaped epiphyses (acrodysostosis, cleidocranial dysplasia, trichorhinophalangeal dysplasia)

Stippling of the epiphyses (chondrodysplasia punctata, cerebrohepatorenal syndromes, warfarin-related embryopathy, trisomy 21, trisomy 18, lysosomal storage diseases, phenytoin-induced embryopathy, Smith-Lemli-Opitz syndrome, anencephaly, cretinism, multiple epiphyseal dysplasia, SED, normal variant hypoparathyroidism)

Rib shortening (short-rib polydactyly syndromes, asphyxiating thoracic dysplasia, chondroectodermal dysplasia, metaphyseal dysplasia [associated with immune defect], metatrophic dysplasia)

Uncalcified vertebral bodies (achondrogenesis types I and II)

Small sacrosciatic notch (achondroplasia, Ellis-van Creveld syndrome, metatrophic dysplasia, thanatophoric dysplasia, Jeune syndrome)

Kyphosis/scoliosis (achondroplasia)

Scapular hypoplasia (camptomelic dysplasia, Antley-Bixler syndrome)

Treatment

- Treatment is supportive. The goal is to prevent neurologic and orthopaedic complications from long bone deformities, spinal cord compression, and joint instability.
- Because overweight and obesity can worsen some deformities or further reduce function, patients and families should be counseled about weight management strategies.
- Mild to moderate scoliosis and kyphosis can be treated with bracing, while more severe forms will often require surgical fusion.
- Bone-lengthening surgery (Ilizarov procedure) may be considered in some cases.

Expected Outcomes/Prognosis

* Lethal dysplasias
  — For infants with skeletal dysplasias identified at birth, approximately 13% are stillborn and 44% die in the perinatal period.
  — *Lethal dysplasias*: achondrogenesis, homozygous achondroplasia, chondrodysplasia punctata (recessive form), camptomelic dysplasia, congenital lethal hypophosphatasia, perinatal lethal type of OI, thanatophoric dysplasia, and short-rib polydactyly syndromes
* Nonlethal dysplasias
  — Have normal or near-normal life expectancy.
  — The natural history and complications depend on the degree of skeletal abnormality and associated non-musculoskeletal conditions (Box 60-3).

Box 60-3. Examples of Specific Complications Seen in Skeletal Dysplasias

* Respiratory
  —Respiratory compromise caused by small chest and lungs or severe kyphoscoliosis, or upper airway obstruction (chondrodystrophy)
* Central nervous system
  —Hydrocephalus (achondroplasia, metatropic dysplasia)
* Musculoskeletal
  —Atlantoaxial instability may lead to spinal cord compression or nerve damage (chondrodystrophies such as achondroplasia, spondyloepiphyseal dysplasia [SED] congenita, and Morquio syndrome).
  —Adult hip and knee arthritis (multiple epiphyseal dysplasia)
  —Frequent fractures (osteogenesis imperfecta)
* Otolaryngologic
  —Recurrent otitis media that may lead to progressive conductive or neurosensory deafness (diastrophic dysplasia and achondroplasia)
* Ophthalmologic
  —Myopia increases risk for retinal detachment (Kniest dysplasia and SED congenital)
* Dental
  —Malocclusion, crowding, and structural abnormalities (chondrodystrophies)
* Nutritional
  —Obesity (achondroplasia)
* Other
  —Anesthesia complications caused by unstable cervical vertebrae or malignant hyperthermia (chondrodysplasias)
  —Obstetric and gynecologic complications caused by pelvic abnormalities

Prevention

- Genetic counseling may be offered to couples with a confirmed family history of a skeletal dysplasia.
- Prenatal diagnosis
  — Ultrasound can identify skeletal abnormalities, which in most cases is sufficient to make the diagnosis.
  — Amniocentesis or chorionic villus sampling can provide DNA diagnosis for some disorders, such as achondroplasia.
- When the diagnosis is known prenatally, cesarean delivery is recommended to reduce the risk for complications due to cephalopelvic disproportion caused by a large fetal head or C1-C2 instability.

When to Refer

- All patients with a suspected skeletal dysplasia should be referred to an orthopaedic surgeon and a geneticist with expertise in this area.
- Many will also require consultation with one or more of the following specialists:
  — Pediatric surgeon
  — Ophthalmologist
  — Otolaryngologist
  — Neurologist
  — Physical and occupational therapists

Relevant *International Classification of Diseases, Ninth Revision, Clinical Modification (ICD-9-CM)* Codes

- **756.0**   Craniosynostosis
- **756.4**   Skeletal dysplasia (includes achondroplasia)
- **756.56**   Multiple epiphyseal dysplasia

Osteogenesis Imperfecta (OI)

INTRODUCTION/ETIOLOGY/EPIDEMIOLOGY

- Osteogenesis imperfecta is a skeletal dysplasia characterized by abnormal collagen synthesis.
- Mode of inheritance can be autosomal dominant or autosomal recessive.
- Prevalence is 1 in 5,000 to 10,000 individuals of all racial and ethnic origins.
- Osteogenesis imperfecta has remarkable clinical variability, ranging from mild forms with no musculoskeletal deformity, to severe forms with frequent fractures of the upper and lower extremities (Table 60-1).
  — Mild forms are caused by a reduced amount of normal collagen, while severe forms result from abnormal collagen.

Table 60-1. Classification of Osteogenesis Imperfecta

Type	Form	Features	Mode of Inheritance
I	Mild	Blue sclerae, mild prepubertal fractures, minimal or no deformities, mild short stature, DI, hearing loss	Autosomal dominant
II	Perinatal Lethal	Extreme bone fragility, beaded ribs, deformed limbs	New dominant mutation
III	Severe Progressive	Severe bone fragility, progressively deforming bones, very short, normal sclerae, frequent fractures, triangular face, hearing loss	New dominant mutation
IV	Moderate	Heterogenous phenotype. Mild to severe bone fragility, moderately deforming, variable short stature, normal sclerae; DI is common.	Autosomal dominant or new dominant mutation
V	Moderate to severe	Variable bone fragility, develop hypertrophic callous after fractures in long bones	Autosomal dominant
VI	Moderate to severe	Moderate to severe skeletal defects similar to type IV with white sclera. Distinguished by unmineralized bone tissue ("fish scale") on biopsies.	Probably autosomal recessive
VII	Moderate or severe	Severe bone fragility, shortening of the humerus and femur	Autosomal recessive
VIII	Severe	Resembles type II or III except with white sclera and severe growth deficiency	Autosomal recessive

DI, dentinogenesis imperfecta.

- Types I through IV are caused by mutations in the type I collagen gene.
- Types V–VIII are rare and do not involve mutations in type I collagen.
- The mildest and most common form of OI is type I.

SIGNS AND SYMPTOMS

- The hallmark of OI is *recurrent fractures after little to no trauma* (Figure 60-2).
- Infants with severe forms of OI are often born with fractures.
- Signs and symptoms can cause significant limitations in physical function (Box 60-4).
- *Bowing of the limbs* can result from recurrent fractures or occur when the muscles and tendons are stronger than the bone during growth (Figure 60-3).
- *Spine deformities* such as scoliosis and kyphosis occur in approximately 70%.
  — Caused by vertebral collapse and joint laxity
  — Appear during growing years but can progress after maturity.
  — Associated with poor sitting and standing balance, chest wall deformities, diminished lung space, and pain

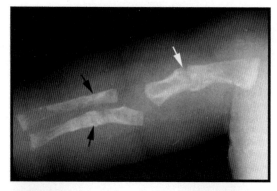

Figure 60-2. Osteopenia and healing fractures in osteogenesis imperfecta. Reproduced with permission from Johnson TR, Steinbach LS (eds): *Essentials of Musculoskeletal Imaging.* Rosemont, IL: American Academy of Orthopaedic Surgeons; 2004.

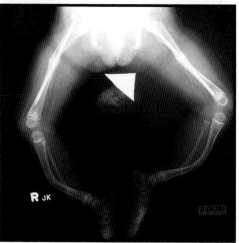

Figure 60-3. Severe limb bowing in child with osteogenesis imperfecta.

Box 60-4. Signs and Symptoms of Osteogenesis Imperfecta

Recurrent fractures
Decreased bone mineral density
Pain
Joint laxity
Easy bruising
Short stature
Brittle teeth
Hearing loss
Blue sclera
Muscle weakness
Spinal curvature
Triangular facies
Bowing of the long bones

DIFFERENTIAL DIAGNOSIS

- Battered child syndrome
- Rickets
- Menkes syndrome
- Camptomelic dysplasia
- Achondrogenesis type I
- Congenital hypophosphatasia
- Idiopathic hyperphosphatasia
- Steroid-induced osteoporosis
- Idiopathic juvenile osteoporosis

MAKING THE DIAGNOSIS

- Diagnosis is based on *history, physical examination, family history,* and *radiographs.*
- Mild cases can be difficult to diagnose.
- Routine laboratory studies are normal, which serves to rule out metabolic bone disease.
- *Prenatal diagnosis*
  - Ultrasound can detect bowing, fractures, shortening, or other bone abnormalities.
  - Diagnosis can be confirmed with chorionic villus sampling, fibroblast analysis, and DNA study.
- *Genetic testing*
  - Detects approximately 90% of all type I collagen mutations.
  - While a positive test for type I collagen defect confirms OI, a negative result does not necessarily rule out the diagnosis.
- *Skin or bone biopsy* may be warranted for those with recessive forms or those without type I collagen mutation.
- *Dual-energy x-ray absorptiometry*
  - Bone density is low in all forms of OI.
  - Useful for evaluating response to treatment such as bisphosphonate.
- *Bone biopsies*
  - Useful for assessing the safety and efficacy of medical therapy.

TREATMENT

- Treatment includes a combination of surgical, medical, and rehabilitative therapies.
  - The goal is to maximize function while controlling and correcting fractures.
  - While ambulation is desirable, it is not essential.
- Acute fractures
  - Minimal immobilization followed by early motion is important to avoid joint stiffness, atrophy of the muscles, and further reduction in bone density.
  - Minimally displaced fractures are best treated by soft dressings or splints.
  - Bulky casts, which create leverage points, should be avoided.
  - Physical therapy facilitates recovery and improves function.
  - Ankle-foot-orthoses may be used to reduce bowing.

- *Bisphosphonates*
  — For example, pamidronate, alendronate
  — Shown to improve vertebral bone density, prevent fractures, improve ambulation, and improve quality of life for those with moderate to severe OI.
  — No observed detrimental effects on growth in short-term studies, but long-term effects are not yet known.
- *Pain management*
  — Often requires a multidisciplinary group of specialists in medicine, psychology, and rehabilitation.
  — Pharmacologic options: nonsteroidal anti-inflammatory drugs, topical pain relievers, narcotic medications (oral or skin patch), antidepressants, and nerve blocks
  — Non-pharmacologic options: ice, heat, transcutaneous nerve stimulation, physical therapy, massage, acupuncture, acupressure, biofeedback, and hypnosis
- *Surgical treatment*
  — Surgical fixation with an intramedullary, expandable, telescopic rod is recommended if nonsurgical treatment fails to slow the progression of bowing.
  — Osteotomies may also be performed to correct some deformities.
  — Posterior spine fusion may be recommended for scoliotic deformities causing constriction of the thorax that do not respond to brace treatment and body jackets. Halo traction before and after surgery may help straighten the spine.
  — Limb-length deformity can be safely corrected toward the end of the growth period with a limb-lengthening procedure.
  — Unfortunately, many patients with severe OI may not be surgical candidates because the expected benefits may not justify the risk of the procedure. Decisions can only be made on an individual basis.

EXPECTED OUTCOMES/PROGNOSIS

- Prognosis varies greatly.
- For mild or moderate types (I, IV, VI), life expectancy is not affected.
- For severe types (II, III, V, VII, VIII), life expectancy may be shortened.
  — The most severe types result in stillbirth or death during infancy.
  — The most frequent cause of death is respiratory failure, followed by accidental trauma.

PREVENTION

- It is imperative for children to stay physically active to prevent bones and muscles from becoming weaker from disuse or during immobilization.
- Swimming and upper or lower extremity strengthening through low-impact physical activities is encouraged to maximize functional abilities and quality of life.
- Current research is investigating intramedullary rods composed of a shape-memory alloy to correct bone deformities, and bone marrow transplantation to increase osteoblast density.

WHEN TO REFER

- Suspected cases of OI should be referred to an orthopaedist and a geneticist.
- Acute fractures should be referred to an orthopaedist for casting, splinting, or surgery.

RELEVANT *ICD-9-CM* CODE

- **756.51**   Osteogenesis imperfecta

CHAPTER 61

Metabolic Bone Diseases

Introduction

- Abnormal bone mineralization and growth
- In the growing child, failure of bone mineralization leads to
  — Growth plate widening and disorganization of the chondrocytes, with loss of the normal straight-columned orientation (eg, rickets)
  — Accumulation of unmineralized osteoid in the trabecular bone of the metaphyses (osteomalacia)
- In skeletally mature adolescents, failure of bone mineralization leads to osteomalacia without rickets.
- Demineralized bone is less resistant to stress and may lead to long bone bowing and increased risk of fracture.

Rickets

INTRODUCTION/ETIOLOGY/EPIDEMIOLOGY

- The most common metabolic bone disease
- A failure of bone mineralization at the growth plate because of a deficiency of calcium (hypocalcemic rickets) or phosphorous (hypophosphatemic rickets)
- Occurs during periods of rapid growth at a time when skeletal tissues require high levels of calcium and phosphate.
- Clinically apparent toward the end of the first year of life, commonly identified because of visible deformities at the wrist, knee, and chest wall
- May be classified according to etiology (Table 61-1).
  — Inadequate dietary intake of vitamin D, calcium, or phosphorous
    ▪ Rare in developed countries (Calcium and phosphorous are found in milk and green vegetables.)
    ▪ Occurs in breastfed infants (human milk is low in vitamin D).
    ▪ Occurs with atypical diets with no milk products (eg, vegetarian, lactose intolerant).
  — Inadequate sunlight exposure (for skin conversion of vitamin D to active form)
    ▪ Dark-skinned infants
    ▪ Infants in northern climates with little sunlight or who stay indoors
  — Because of medical conditions that interfere with the absorption, conversion, or activation of vitamin D, or with calcium or phosphorous homeostasis

Table 61-1. Etiologies of Rickets

Etiology of Rickets	Distinguishing Features
Dietary	
Inadequate calcium intake	
Inadequate phosphate intake	
Inadequate vitamin D intake	Deficient milk products or exclusively breastfed
Poor absorption from GI tract	
Lack of sunlight exposure	
Defect in renal enzyme that converts calcidiol to calcitriol, the active metabolite	Family history of similar bony deformities. Low or normal serum phosphorous, low serum calcium, high PTH, very high alkaline phosphatase, normal calcidiol, very low calcitriol, low urine calcium
End-organ resistance to effect of calcitriol	Family history of similar bony deformities. Low or normal serum phosphorous, low serum calcium, high PTH, very high alkaline phosphatase, normal calcidiol, very high calcitriol, low urine calcium
High phytin formula (eg, soy)	
Antacids (Aluminum binds dietary phosphates, preventing absorption.)	
Anticonvulsants accelerate calcidiol metabolism (eg, phenytoin, phenobarbital).	
Gastrectomy (total or partial)	
Hepatic insufficiency or disease	Elevated liver enzymes
Fat malabsorption (eg, cystic fibrosis, celiac or inflammatory bowel disease)	Steatorrhea
Chronic pancreatic insufficiency	Steatorrhea
Increased renal excretion	
X-linked hypophosphatemic rickets	Do not have tetany, myopathy, rachitic rosary, or Harrison groove, and rarely have enamel defects. Waddling gait and smooth (rather than angular) bowing of the lower extremities. Hypertension and left ventricular hypertrophy possible. Family history of similar bony deformities. Laboratory findings: very low serum phosphorous, normal serum calcium, normal PTH, high alkaline phosphatase, normal calcidiol, normal or low calcitriol, low urine calcium
HHRH	Hypophosphatemia is mild in some cases, without signs of bone disease. Nephrocalcinosis, nephrolithiasis. Family history of similar signs/symptoms. Laboratory findings: very low serum phosphorous, normal serum calcium, normal or low PTH, high alkaline phosphatase, normal calcidiol, high calcitriol, high urine calcium

Table 61-1. Etiologies of Rickets, continued

Etiology of Rickets	Distinguishing Features
Renal insufficiency	Elevated creatinine
McCune-Albright syndrome	Café au lait spots; liver disease; hyperthyroidism; Cushing syndrome; fibrous dysplasia in long bones, ribs, and skull; precocious puberty; advanced skeletal maturity
Fanconi syndrome	Polyuria, polydipsia, dehydration, glucosuria, phosphaturia, proteinuria, hypokalemia, hyperchloremic metabolic acidosis
Diuretic medications (eg, furosemide)	
Renal tubular acidosis with hypercalciuria	
Renal tubular dysfunction (eg, cystinosis, tyrinosisgalactosemia, fructose intolerance, Wilson disease, lead poisoning, other heavy metal poisoning)	
Tumors (usually small, benign mesenchymal tumor)	Very low serum phosphorous, low calcitriol, positive MRI or indium scan
Local effects on bone matrix	
Hypophosphatasia (alkaline phosphatase deficiency)	Low alkaline phosphatase and PTH

GI, gastrointestinal; PTH, parathyroid hormone; HHRH, hereditary hypophosphatemic rickets with hypercalciuria, MRI, magnetic resonance imaging.

Adapted from: Bergstrom WH. Twenty ways to get rickets in the 1990s. *Contemp Pediatr.* 1991;8:88–106

SIGNS AND SYMPTOMS

- Bone pain or tenderness
- Unwillingness to bear weight
- Skeletal deformities
  - Genu varum or valgum
  - Rachitic rosary (enlargement of the costochondral junctions)
  - Thickening of the wrists and ankles (rounded knobs)
  - Pigeon breast deformity of sternum
  - Harrison sulcus (a horizontal grooved depression) along lower border of chest
  - Delayed closure of the fontanelles
  - Craniotabes (skull bone softening that produces a ping-pong ball sensation on palpation over the occiput or posterior parietal bones)
  - Caput quadratum (boxlike appearance of head) from frontal and parietal bossing
  - Pelvic or spinal deformities (scoliosis or kyphosis)
  - Greenstick fractures can occur in the long bones.
- Muscle abnormalities
  - Decreased muscle tone
  - Muscle cramps

- Growth delay and short stature
- Delayed achievement of motor milestones
- Seizures
- Dental abnormalities
  — Delayed dentition
  — Enamel defects
  — Extensive caries and dental abscesses
- Tendency to acquire infections (because of impaired phagocytosis and neutrophil motility)

DIFFERENTIAL DIAGNOSIS

- Other metabolic diseases and epiphyseal lesions (Table 61-2)

Table 61-2. Distinguishing Features of Metabolic Bone Diseases and Epiphyseal Lesions

Metabolic Bone Disease or Epiphyseal Lesion	Distinguishing Features
Scurvy	Decreased density and thinned cortices Increased density near growth plate
Chondrodystrophy	Flared and widened metaphyses V- or U-shaped growth plates Short limbs
Multiple epiphyseal dysplasia	Delayed knee and hip epiphyses Genu valgum
Cytomegalovirus or rubella	Linear lucencies in the long bones Increased densities in metaphyses
Syphilis (rare)	Destructive lesions in long bone metaphyses Increased density of secondary ossification centers
Copper deficiency (rare)	Osteopenia Sickle-shaped metaphyseal spurs

MAKING THE DIAGNOSIS

- Radiographs and laboratory tests establish the diagnosis.
- *Radiographs*
  — Radiographic findings do not appear until after several months of vitamin D deficiency.
  — Radiographic evidence of demineralization first appears at the ends of long bones, and eventually the shafts.
  — *Radiographic views to order*
    ▪ Infants: anteroposterior view of the knees; consider distal ulna radiographs.
    ▪ Older children: weight-bearing knee radiographs will show bowing.

— *Typical findings* (figures 61-1 and 61-2)

▪ Metaphyses are widened with exaggerated concavity (cupping) and irregular calcification.
▪ Along the shaft, the uncalcified osteoid causes the periosteum to appear separated from the diaphysis.
▪ Generalized osteomalacia (observed as osteopenia) with visible coarsening of trabeculae (contrast with the ground-glass osteopenia of scurvy).

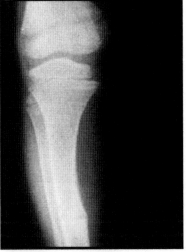

Figure 61-1. Radiograph showing deformed bone and widening of the physis in a patient with osteomalacia. Reproduced from Bostrom MPG, Boskeu A, Kaufman JK, Einhorn TA: Form and function of bone, in Buckwalter JA, Einhorn TA, Simon SR (eds): *Orthopaedic Basic Science,* ed 2. Rosemont, IL: American Academy of Orthopaedic Surgeons; 2000:362.

Figure 61-2. Anteroposterior view displays bowing deformity in the lower extremity as a result of rickets. Additional findings include widening and cupping of the metaphyses, widening of growth plates, and osteopenia.

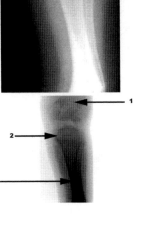

1 = Femoral physis; 2 = Abnormal tibial growth plate; 3 = Bowed tibia.

Reproduced with permission from Bernstein J (ed): *Musculoskeletal Medicine.* Rosemont, IL: American Academy of Orthopaedic Surgeons; 2003.

- *Advanced imaging*
  - Tumor-induced osteomalacia: total body magnetic resonance imaging or scintigraphy using octreotide labeled with indium 111 may be required to locate the occult tumor.
- *Laboratory tests*
  - Serum calcium; phosphate; alkaline phosphatase; parathyroid hormone; 25-hydroxyvitamin D_3 (calcidiol); 1,25-dihydroxyvitamin D_3 (calcitriol); urine calcium
  - Serum creatinine is measured to exclude renal insufficiency.
  - Liver enzymes are measured to exclude liver disease as the etiology of elevated alkaline phosphatase levels.
- *Findings* in rickets caused by inadequate vitamin D intake or sunlight exposure
  - Serum alkaline phosphatase level is elevated.
  - Serum calcium may be normal or low.
  - Serum phosphate level is low or normal.
  - Serum calcidiol is low.
  - Serum calcitriol is low or normal.
  - Urine calcium may be normal or low.
- *If laboratory tests are normal, a diagnosis of rickets is unlikely and another cause for skeletal dysplasia must be explored.*

TREATMENT

- Treatment depends on etiology.
- *General guidelines*
  - For dietary rickets, treatment is replacement of deficient mineral(s).
  - With proper treatment, healing begins within a few days and progresses slowly until normal bone structure is restored.
  - Once the deficiency is corrected, calcium, phosphorus, and parathyroid hormone concentrations should normalize within 1 to 3 weeks.
  - Radiographic evidence of improvement is usually seen within 2 to 4 weeks.
  - If insufficient improvement, evaluate for non-dietary causes of rickets.
- *For rickets caused by inadequate vitamin D intake or sunlight exposure*
  - Preferred treatment is oral vitamin D.
    - Fifty to 150 µg of vitamin D_3 or 0.5 to 2 µg of 1,25-dihydroxycholecalciferol administered daily until healing is evident and the alkaline phosphatase is approaching normal levels
    - Or, a one-time dose of 15,000 µg of vitamin D given as an intramuscular injection or divided into 4 or 6 oral doses (avoids compliance problems)
  - Natural or artificial light can also be effective.

- *For X-linked hypophosphatemic rickets*
  — Forty mg of elemental phosphorus/kg per day in 4 to 5 divided doses
    ▪ If result is inadequate despite good compliance, the daily phosphorus dose is increased in steps of 250 to 500 mg to a maximum of 3,500 mg per day.
  — Calcitriol is administered in 2 doses per day (10–20 ng/kg per dose).
- *For hereditary hypophosphatemic rickets with hypercalciuria*
  — Treatment regimen is phosphorus supplementation alone (as described for the X-linked condition).
  — Calcitriol is avoided because it may increase calcium absorption from gastrointestinal tract, increasing the risk for nephrocalcinosis and nephrolithiasis.
  — Children are monitored every 3 months for progress in height growth.
  — Quarterly laboratories include serum concentrations of calcium, phosphorus, alkaline phosphatase, and creatinine, and urine calcium.
  — Annual renal ultrasound is performed to evaluate for nephrocalcinosis.
  — An annual hand radiograph is performed to exclude reappearance of rickets and determine bone age.

EXPECTED OUTCOMES/PROGNOSIS

- When therapy is issued early and compliance is good, bony deformities can be minimized with little negative effect on activities of daily living and sports participation.
- When detected late
  — Persistent skeletal deformities may prevent development of high-quality gross motor skills and result in short stature.
  — Rarely, pelvic deformities in females may necessitate cesarean deliveries for childbirth.
  — Intercurrent infections may increase morbidity and mortality.

PREVENTION

- Adequate intake of vitamin D, calcium, and phosphorous and exposure to ultraviolet light
- Breastfed infants whose mothers are not exposed to sunlight should receive a supplement of 400 IU of vitamin D daily.
- Monitor dark-skinned, breastfed infants closely at well-child care visits for signs and symptoms of rickets.
- Periodic dental examinations should begin in very early childhood for those diagnosed with rickets.

WHEN TO REFER

- Referral to an endocrinologist is recommended for those with unclear etiologies or poor response to typical treatment.
- Referral to an orthopaedist is recommended for significant bony deformities, especially genu valgum.
  — Bracing is generally not helpful, but surgical correction via osteotomy can be beneficial and may be recommended in moderate to severe cases.
  — Surgical intervention is not recommended until radiographs show healing and the alkaline phosphatase is within normal limits.

RELEVANT *INTERNATIONAL CLASSIFICATION OF DISEASES, NINTH REVISION, CLINICAL MODIFICATION* CODES

- **268.0**   Rickets, active
- **268.1**   Rickets, late effect
- **275.3**   Rickets, vitamin D resistant
- **275.3**   Familial hypophosphatemia
- **588.0**   Renal rickets
- **579.0**   Celiac rickets

CHAPTER 62

Neurofibromatosis-1

Introduction/Etiology/Epidemiology

- Formerly called von Recklinghausen disease
- Autosomal-dominant neurocutaneous disorder seen in all races and ethnic groups
- Incidence is approximately 1 in 3,000 births.
- Penetrance 100%; expressivity variable
- New mutations account for 25% to 50% of cases.
- Caused by mutation in tumor-suppressor gene on long arm of chromosome 17
- Loss of heterozygosity at neurofibromatosis-1 (NF1) tumor locus leads to increased tumorigenesis.

Signs and Symptoms

- *Café au lait spots and intertriginous freckling*
  — Flat, pigmented macules frequently present at birth (Figure 62-1)
  — Increase in number during first 3 to 5 years of life.
  — Not specific for NF1 (Box 62-1)
  — Greater than 95% of children with NF1 will have more than 6 café au lait spots by age 6 years.
- *Neurofibromas*
  — Benign nerve sheath tumors consisting of Schwann cells, fibroblasts, and perineural cells
  — *Cutaneous neurofibromas* protrude just above skin surface or lie just under skin with an overlying violaceous hue.
  — *Subcutaneous neurofibromas* arise from peripheral nerves, lie deeper, and are generally hard and nodular.
  — Generally begin to appear during second decade of life following onset of puberty.
- *Plexiform neurofibromas*
  — Histologically similar to cutaneous neurofibromas that involve single or multiple nerve fascicles arising from branches of major nerves
  — Often have overlying hyperpigmentation or hair.
  — Generally present at birth or become apparent in first several years of life
  — Unpredictable growth rate
  — May lead to disfigurement or organ compromise (eg, blindness, obstructive uropathy).

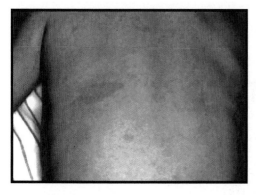

Figure 62-1. Café au lait spots in a black infant with neurofibromatosis-1. From Tekin M, Bodurtha JN, Riccardi VM. Café au lait spots: the pediatrician's perspective. *Pediatr Rev.* 2001;22:82–90.

Box 62-1. Syndromes With Café au lait Spots

McCune-Albright syndrome
Bloom syndrome
Fanconi anemia
Tuberous sclerosis
Russell-Silver syndrome
Ataxia-telangiectasia
Multiple endocrine neoplasia type 2b

- *Lisch nodules*
  - — Slightly raised, well-circumscribed melanocytic hamartomas of iris best seen with a slit lamp
  - — Develop with age; fewer than 30% of children with NF1 younger than 6 years have them, whereas they are present in more than 90% of adults.
- *Optic pathway tumor*
  - — Symptomatic tumors occur in 7% of children with NF1.
  - — Period of greatest risk is during the first 6 years of life; rare to arise after 10 years of age.
  - — May lead to visual loss, proptosis, or development of precious puberty.
- *Orthopaedic manifestations*
  - — Present in 80% of patients with NF1
- *Sphenoid dysplasia*
  - — Pathognomonic of NF1
- *Long bone deformities*
  - — Mesodermal dysplasia
    - ▪ Tibia most commonly affected bone
    - ▪ Bowing is the main deformity (Figure 62-2).
    - ▪ Typically noticed at birth or in the first few months of life.
    - ▪ Dysplastic bones are prone to fracture after minor trauma.
    - ▪ Pseudoarthroses affect approximately 2% of children with NF1, including leg (tibia) and forearm (radius or ulna).

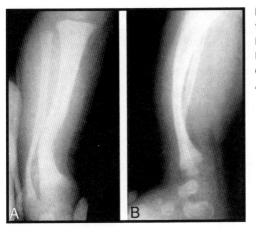

Figure 62-2. Arterolateral bowing of the tibia associated with neurofibromatosis-1. Reproduced with permission from Griffin LY (ed): *Essentials of Musculoskeletal Care,* 3rd edition. Rosemont, IL: American Academy of Orthopaedic Surgeons; 2005.

- Bone hypertrophy or destruction caused by plexiform neurofibromas
- Lytic defects in metaphyses and diaphyses
* *Scoliosis*
  — Affects as many as 10% to 50% of patients.
  — Idiopathic-like juvenile scoliosis
    - Most common form
    - Indistinguishable from that found in non-NF1 patients
  — Dystrophic scoliosis
    - Less common
    - Results from congenital dysplasia of vertebral bodies.
    - Presents with sharply angulated curve at birth associated with rotation and scalloping of the posterior margins of the vertebral bodies.
    - Rapid curvature often develops.
* *Other skeletal manifestations*
  — Short stature
  — Posterior scalloping of vertebral bodies
  — Hemihypertrophy
  — Enlargement of the spinal neural foramina
  — Low bone mineral density

Differential Diagnosis

* Other forms of skeletal dysplasia (see Chapter 60)
* Other syndromes with café au lait spots (Box 62-1)

Making the Diagnosis

* Diagnostic criteria highly sensitive and specific (Box 62-2)
* Genetic testing rarely necessary except in unusual or atypical cases
  — If necessary, RNA/DNA cascade of genetic testing will lead to confirmed mutation in NF1 gene in more than 95% of clinically diagnosed cases.

Box 62-2. Diagnostic Criteria for Neurofibromatosis-1

Two or more required for diagnosis

- Six or more café au lait macules greater than 5 mm in greatest diameter in prepubertal individuals, and greater than 15 mm in postpubertal individuals
- Two or more neurofibromas of any type *or* one plexiform neurofibroma
- Freckling in the axillary or inguinal regions
- Two or more iris Lisch nodules
- Optic pathway tumor
- A distinctive osseous lesion such as sphenoid dysplasia or thinning of long bone cortex with or without pseudarthrosis
- A first-degree relative with neurofibromatosis-1 by these criteria

Treatment

- At present, there are no NF1-specific treatments.
- Children younger than 10 years should have yearly ophthalmologic examinations looking for signs of an optic pathway tumor.
- No other routine testing (eg, neuroimaging, spine radiographs) is warranted.
- *Treatment of orthopaedic manifestations*
  - Early recognition of skeletal dysplasias is important for effective treatment.
  - Long bone bowing can be treated by bracing.
  - Surgery may be necessary for some fractures.
  - Scoliosis is also managed by bracing but commonly requires surgical fusion.

Expected Outcomes/Prognosis

- Mean IQ of the NF1 population is approximately 95. However, as many as 60% of children with NF1 will have some form of learning disability or attention-deficit/hyperactivity disorder.
- Increased incidence of malignancy including malignant peripheral nerve sheath tumor, leukemia, and rhabdomyosarcoma
- Neurofibromatosis-1 vasculopathy may lead to renovascular hypertension or cerebrovascular disease.
- Scoliosis may progress rapidly and may lead to paraplegia.
- Pseudoarthroses usually require surgery; amputation is necessary in severe cases.

When to Refer

- On diagnosis, all children should be referred to an NF1 multidisciplinary clinic for yearly physical examinations and plotting on standardized growth charts.
- Skeletal complications should be referred to an orthopaedic surgeon.

Resources for Physicians and Families

* Children's Tumor Foundation (www.ctf.org)
* Neurofibromatosis, Inc. (www.nfinc.org)

Relevant *International Classification of Diseases, Ninth Revision, Clinical Modification* Codes

* **237.71** NF1
* **733.29** Dysplasia of bone
* **737.30** Scoliosis
* **754.2** Scoliosis, congenital

CHAPTER 63

Hemophilia

Introduction/Etiology/Epidemiology

- Genetically determined coagulation factor deficiencies (Table 63-1)
- Result in prolonged bleeding often after minimal or no trauma.
- Newborns and infants usually present with excessive bleeding after circumcision or hematomas after vaccinations.
- Toddlers present with excessive thick bruises with round, indurated centers along with large intramuscular hematomas from minor falls or trauma.
- Factor levels guide therapy and activity recommendations.
- Factor levels below 2% to 5% of normal can lead to bleeding with relatively minor trauma.
- Factor levels between 5% and 40% of normal produce only a small risk of hemorrhage with daily activities.

Signs and Symptoms

- *Hemarthrosis*
  - Most common in elbow, knee, and ankle joints
  - Acute symptoms are pain, swelling, and stiffness caused by a distended joint capsule.
  - Examination reveals distended joint with limited passive and active range of motion and often tense, shiny overlying skin.

Table 63-1. Etiology and Inheritance Patterns of Common Hemophilia Subtypes

Subtype	Etiology	Inheritance Pattern
Hemophilia A "Classic hemophilia"	Factor VIII deficiency	X-linked 80% positive family history
Hemophilia B "Christmas disease"	Factor IX deficiency	X-recessive
Hemophilia C	Factor XI deficiency	Autosomal recessive
von Willebrand disease	von Willebrand protein deficiency or dysfunction	Autosomal dominant Spontaneous hemarthrosis is rare.

- *Intramuscular hematomas*
  - Present as thick, round, indurated bruises with tense, shiny overlying skin.
  - Can lead to a compartment syndrome characterized by severe pain that is out of proportion to the apparent trauma or other physical findings.

Differential Diagnosis

- *Acute hemarthrosis*
  - Septic arthritis
  - Toxic synovitis
  - Juvenile rheumatoid arthritis
  - Intra-articular injury
- *Intramuscular hemorrhage*
  - Pyomyositis
  - Intramuscular abscess
  - Significant muscle strains
  - Myositis ossificans

Making the Diagnosis

- Radiographs should be obtained in any case of initial joint effusion or in uncertain presentations to rule out intra-articular fracture, loose bodies, or osteochondral lesions.
- Repeated hemorrhage can lead to characteristic radiographic joint changes (Table 63-2).
- Diagnostic ultrasound is a noninvasive and portable modality for evaluation of suspected joint or soft tissue hemorrhage, with greatest value in large joints (hip, shoulder) and deep soft tissues (iliopsoas, retroperitoneum) (Table 63-3).

Table 63-2. Radiographic Staging of Hemophiliac Arthropathy

Stage	Description
I	Soft tissue swelling No radiographic abnormality
II	Overgrowth and osteoporosis of epiphysis
III	Mild to moderate joint narrowing Subchondral cysts Patellar squaring Widening of intercondylar notch of knee and trochlear notch of elbow
IV	Severe narrowing of joint space with cartilage destruction Other osseous changes very pronounced
V	Total loss of joint space with fibrous ankylosis

Table 63-3. Ultrasound Findings in Joint and Soft Tissue Hemorrhage

Soft tissue	Acute (0–3 d)	Increased echogenicity with margins that are well defined (separating muscle planes) or poorly defined (interdigitated with muscle fibers)
	Subacute (4–10 d)	Echo-free appearance may be relative or complete.
Joint		Mixture of echo-free fluid and variable amount of echogenic fluid representing acute hemorrhage. Septic arthritis or toxic synovitis have echo-free joint effusions.

Treatment

- Appropriate management is a multidisciplinary model that involves the primary care pediatrician in concert with orthopaedic surgeons and hematologists.
- First-line treatment for any mild joint effusion or soft tissue hematoma includes ice, elevation, compression, and immobilization for at least 48 hours.
- Aspiration and irrigation of hemarthrosis
  — Controversial
  — The risks of further bleeding and introduction of infection must be balanced with potential benefits of pain relief, ability to send aspirate for diagnostic studies, and possibility of avoiding chronic synovitis by blood removal.
  — Aspiration is generally done by an orthopaedist under strict sterile conditions within 20 to 30 minutes after intravenous (IV) administration of appropriate replacement coagulation factors.
- Home IV therapy—IV administration of appropriate coagulation factors
  — Prime intervention for preventing further pain, disability, or life-threatening hemorrhage
  — On-demand treatment for recurrent hemarthrosis involves elevating appropriate factor levels to a level that secures hemostasis (usually about 50% of normal activity) with treatments daily for 2 to 3 days to control the hemarthrosis.
  — For factor VIII, a typical daily dose of 15 to 25 IU/kg is sufficient.
  — For factor IX, 25 to 50 IU/kg/day is generally recommended.
  — For von Willebrand disease, cryoprecipitate (contains factor VIII) and fresh frozen plasma (contains factor IX) can be used.
  — Desmopressin (0.3 µg/kg body weight) can be used to treat mild bleeding episodes (oral bleeding, dental work, or small hematomas) in patients with factor VIII deficiency.
  — Self-administration of coagulation factor replacement therapy can be used by well-informed parents and older patients to allow earlier intervention and reduce risk of significant complications.
  — Remind all patients and caregivers that severe joint bleeding leading to a marked joint distension is a medical emergency and patients should be receive medical treatment within 4 hours of the onset of bleeding.
- Because pain is a primary indicator of continued hemorrhage, select narcotic mediations with caution so they do not diminish the patient's ability to judge symptom progression.

- Physical therapy including application of cold and hot modalities combined with joint range of motion and strengthening exercises can help prevent and treat the sequelae of recurrent hemorrhages.
- Orthopaedic surgeons can perform open or arthroscopic synovectomy or recommend radionucleotide or chemical synovectomies to decrease recurrent bleeding from target joints.

Expected Outcomes/Prognosis

- Prolonged or repeated hemarthrosis may create an inflammatory synovial reaction leading to cartilage destruction and joint degeneration and contracture, known as secondary hemophiliac arthropathy, which results in a fixed, unusable joint.
- Sequelae of a compartment syndrome include underlying muscle ischemia potentially leading to necrosis, neurapraxia, and myostatic contractures.
- Multiple exposures to blood products increase the risk for HIV, hepatitis B and C (universal hepatitis B immunization reinforced for hemophilia patients and caregivers), chronic active hepatitis, and cirrhosis.
- Other long-term sequelae include osteoporosis and muscle atrophy.
- Patients with hemophilia also suffer higher risks of hypertension and renal disease of uncertain etiology.

Prevention

- *Prophylactic factor replacement*
  — May reduce recurrent hemorrhage and subsequent arthropathy, especially in younger patients without history of repeated hemorrhage.
  — Hematologist calculates the appropriate factor replacement dose based on patient weight and plasma volume, with a treatment goal of 30% to 40% of normal factor activity.
  — Randomized, controlled studies are ongoing to assess concerns about proper initiation and frequency of prophylactic therapy, costs, and efficacy versus placebo and on-demand factor replacement.
  — Once joint damage has occurred, secondary prophylaxis can retard but not prevent ongoing joint damage.
- *Education of patients and caregivers*
  — Pad cribs and play areas.
  — Provide close supervision of toddlers learning to walk.
  — Avoid giving aspirin, antihistamines, and other medications that inhibit platelet function.
  — Avoid giving nonsteroidal anti-inflammatory medications.
  — Learn to recognize early signs of abnormal bleeding into joints and soft tissue.

- *Sport or activity recommendations*
  — Children with hemophilia should be encouraged to be as active as possible within general restrictions on not engaging in any impact or collision sports.
  — An emergency plan to treat bleeding is required, including immediate application of cold compresses or ice to the affected area and rapid replacement of deficient clotting factors.
  — Protective pads in clothing and equipment can help reduce the bleeding risk.

When to Refer

- Significant bleeding into a joint is an orthopaedic emergency warranting immediate orthopaedic evaluation.

Relevant *International Classification of Diseases, Ninth Revision, Clinical Modification* Codes

- **286.0** Hemophilia A
- **286.1** Hemophilia B
- **286.2** Hemophilia C
- **286.4** von Willebrand disease
- **719.15** Hemarthrosis, hip
- **719.16** Hemarthrosis, knee
- **719.17** Hemarthrosis, ankle or foot
- **719.12** Hemarthrosis, elbow
- **719.11** Hemarthrosis, shoulder

CHAPTER 64

Achondroplasia

Introduction/Etiology/Epidemiology

- Achondroplasia is the *most common* skeletal dysplasia.
- Incidence is 1 in 30,000 live births.
- Mutations of fibroblast growth factor receptor 3 (FGFR3) on *chromosome 4* result in the inhibition of chondrocyte growth and proliferation, with underdevelopment and shortening of bones formed by endochondral ossification. Articular cartilage is unaffected.
- Patients with achondroplasia display manifestations in the spine, upper and lower extremities, and midface hypoplasia.
- Inheritance is autosomal dominant.
- *More than 80% of cases are sporadic.*
- High paternal age (older than 35 years) is associated with sporadic mutations.

Signs and Symptoms

- *The primary feature of achondroplasia is short stature,* defined as a height at least 2 standard deviations (SD) below the population mean.
  - Short stature is caused by rhizomelic (proximal extremity) shortening, as trunk length is in the lower range of normal.
  - Patient length on average is -1.5 SD at birth, -4.4 SD at 1 year, and -5.0 SD at 2 years.
  - The final adult height is 6 to 7 SD below the mean of 52" (range, 46–57") in males and 49" (range, 44–54") in females.
- There may be frontal bossing and midface hypoplasia.
- During infancy, patients may develop *foramen magnum stenosis.*
  - Stenosis may present as sleep apnea, excessive snoring, signs of chronic brain stem compression (ie, lower cranial nerve dysfunction, swallowing difficulty, hyperreflexia, hypotonia, weakness, developmental delay, and clonus), or sudden infant death syndrome (SIDS).
  - When developmental delay is present, foramen magnum stenosis must be ruled out by magnetic resonance imaging (MRI) screening.

The views expressed in this article are those of the author(s) and do not necessarily reflect the official policy or position of the Department of the Navy, Department of Defense, or the US Government.

- Most neonates develop thoracolumbar kyphosis as sitting begins.
  - The normal thoracolumbar junction is straight in the sagittal plane; the newborn with achondroplasia typically has 20 degrees of thoracolumbar kyphosis.
  - When sitting begins, these newborns slump forward because of their large heads and poor trunk control.
  - Repeated slumping can increase the kyphosis and result in anterior wedging of the vertebral bodies (Figure 64-1).
  - Examination reveals a gibbus or prominence of the thoracolumbar junction when the neonate is in the sitting position.
  - When walking begins and trunk postural control improves, most kyphoses resolve, resulting in a frequency of 87% in 1- to 2-year-olds, 39% in 2- to 5-year-olds, and 11% in 5- to 10-year-olds.
  - Persistent thoracolumbar kyphosis may result in deformity progression and neurologic symptoms, including paresthesias, incontinence, and inability to walk.
- Genu varum
  - The primary manifestation in the lower extremity
  - May be asymptomatic or associated with knee pain or instability.
  - A fibular thrust may be evident with walking.
- Lumbosacral hyperlordosis
  - May be seen during childhood in up to 80% of patients.
  - Secondary to increased pelvic tilt while standing
  - Presents as a prominent abdomen and buttocks with hip flexion contractures.
- Symptomatic spinal stenosis
  - Occasionally develops during adolescence, but more often in adulthood.
  - Symptoms include leg pain, numbness or weakness, and neurologic incontinence.
  - Occurs as a result of endochondral ossification defects along the entire spinal column, producing short, thickened pedicles and a narrowing of the interpediculate distance from L1 to L5 (Figure 64-1). Mismatch between the smaller spinal canal and the normal-sized neural elements increases risk for spinal stenosis.
- Flexion contractures of the elbow and subluxated radial heads
- Trident hand
  - Extra space between the third and fourth rays
  - Trident hand alone does not cause functional impairment, but because of rhizomelic shortening, the fingertips may reach only to the greater trochanters, creating difficulties with personal hygiene.
- Medical complications
  - Up to 95% of patients with achondroplasia have abnormalities of the midface or otolaryngeal system, including frequent otitis media and adenotonsillar hypertrophy. Surgical intervention may be required.
  - Speech acquisition may be delayed.
  - Hydrocephalus may be present, and shunting is required in approximately 11% of patients.
  - Overweight and obesity are not uncommon.

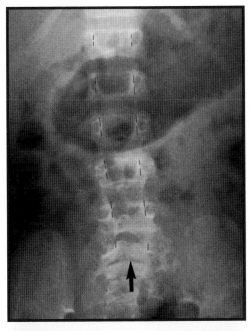

Figure 64-1. Decreasing interpediculate distances consistent with spinal stenosis of lumbar spine in achondroplasia. Reproduced with permission from Johnson TR, Steinbach LS (eds): *Essentials of Musculoskeletal Imaging.* Rosemont, IL: American Academy of Orthopaedic Surgeons; 2004.

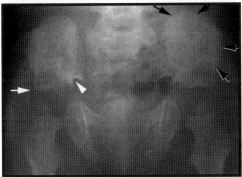

Figure 64-2. Horizontal acetabular roof and squaring of sciatic notch in achondroplasia. Reproduced with permission from Johnson TR, Steinbach LS (eds): *Essentials of Musculoskeletal Imaging.* Rosemont, IL: American Academy of Orthopaedic Surgeons; 2004.

- Achievement of motor milestones may be delayed.
  — Developmental delay may be the result of joint laxity, hypotonia, or foramen magnum stenosis.
  — On average, achondroplasty patients are able to sit at 10 months, stand at 18 months, and walk independently at 20 months.

Differential Diagnosis

- Hypochondroplasia (milder form of achondroplasia)
- Severe achondroplasia with developmental delay and acanthosis nigricans

Making the Diagnosis

- Diagnosis is based on the combination of clinical findings and radiographic findings from a skeletal survey, often in infancy.
- The diagnosis may be made via prenatal testing, which can detect the FGFR3 G380R point mutation.
- Radiographic findings
  — Narrowing of the interpediculate distance from L1 to L5 (Figure 64-1)
  — Squared iliac wings (Figure 64-2)
  — Rhizomelic shortening
  — Flared metaphyses of the long bones
  — Genu varum is demonstrated on standing anteroposterior radiographs by an increased femoral-tibial angle (the angle between the shafts of femur and tibia) or a mechanical axis (line from the center of the femoral head to the center of the ankle) that passes medial to the medial compartment of the knee.
  — Lateral sitting spine radiographs are obtained to determine the degree of the kyphosis and to evaluate for vertebral wedging (Figure 64-1).

Treatment

- *Health supervision*
  — Weight, head circumference, and occipitofrontal circumference are measured monthly during the first year.
  — Careful neurologic and spine examinations are performed at each well-child care visit.
  — Speech evaluation by 2 years of age.
  — All newborns with achondroplasia are screened for foramen magnum stenosis with a sleep study and MRI for visualization of brain stem compression.
  — In an effort to prevent persistent kyphosis, neonates with achondroplasia should be prohibited from sitting without support, or at an angle greater than 60 degrees, even with support, and from being curled into a C position. Sitting at an angle of 45 degrees is sufficient to allow the newborn to interact with others. When holding the newborn, hand counter pressure should be placed on the thoracolumbar junction.
- *Weight control*
  — Difficult for patients with achondroplasia
  — Physical activity is encouraged, with the exception of collision sports, which are hazardous in patients with potential cervical stenosis.
- *Stature augmentation*
  — Because short stature may result in impairments of daily activities, such as conducting business at countertops, using public restrooms, and playing sports, stature augmentation may be considered.
  — May be achieved by medical or surgical means, but the latter method produces greater height increases.
  — Not advocated by the Little People of North America

- *Surgical limb lengthening*
  — Can be challenging due to potential for worsening body size disproportion because upper and lower extremity lengthening is required.
  — Lengthening typically occurs at 2 intervals, at approximately 7 and 12 years of age.
  — The total treatment and rehabilitation duration may be as long as 3 years.
  — Complications of lower extremity lengthening may be as high as 40%.
- *Upper extremity manifestations*
  — Intervention is typically not needed for flexion contractures of the elbows or subluxated radial heads because these rarely cause functional impairments.
- *Genu varum*
  — Surgical treatment is indicated for pain, fibular thrust, or substantial malalignment.
  — An osteotomy of the femur or tibia, or both, corrects malalignment, which ameliorates the pain and fibular thrust.
  — Many patients with genu varum also have in-toeing because of internal tibial torsion, which is corrected at the time of surgery.
- *Foramen magnum stenosis*
  — When the signs or symptoms of stenosis are present in combination with MRI evidence of compression, a referral to neurosurgeon for surgical decompression is necessary.
  — Decompression before 4 years of age is required in approximately 7% of patients.
- *Thoracolumbar kyphosis*
  — If the kyphosis persists or severe anterior wedging is seen, bracing is considered but not always used because it may be disadvantageous in a small child with poor trunk control.
  — If the kyphosis progresses to greater than 50 degrees, spinal arthrodesis is indicated to prevent further progression with potential neurologic compromise.
- *Lumbar hyperlordosis*
  — Although nonoperative treatments for hyperlordosis are unsuccessful, surgical treatment is usually not indicated because the neurologic significance is not clear.
- *Symptomatic spinal stenosis*
  — Magnetic resonance imaging is necessary to localize areas of spinal stenosis.
  — Surgical intervention, which consists of a long, wide decompression, is required to avoid recurrence.
- *Frequent otitis media and adenotonsillar hypertrophy*
  — Surgical intervention may be required.

Expected Outcomes/Prognosis

- Depends on disease severity.
- Infants who receive the abnormal gene from both parents often do not survive beyond a few months.
- Increased rate of SIDS during the first 2 years of life, with a 2% to 5% mortality in the first 12 months of life

- Most people with achondroplasia have a normal life span and normal intelligence.
- Very few people with achondroplasia reach a height of 5 feet.

When to Refer

- Refer to a geneticist and a pediatric orthopaedic surgeon on diagnosis.
  — These specialists will evaluate the child during the first few months of life to establish a baseline examination and educate parents about the manifestations that may develop.
- Refer patients with foramen magnum stenosis to a neurosurgeon.
- Refer patients with frequent otitis media and tonsillar hypertrophy to an otolaryngologist.

Relevant *International Classification of Diseases, Ninth Revision, Clinical Modification* Code

- **756.4**   Achondroplasia

CHAPTER 65

Down Syndrome

Introduction/Etiology/Epidemiology

- Genetic disorder associated with mental retardation and musculoskeletal, cardiovascular, endocrine, gastrointestinal, immune, and visual abnormalities (Box 65-1)
- Affects 1 in every 800 to 1,000 live births.
- Common physical characteristics include microcephaly, epicanthal folds, hypotonia, short neck, flattened nasal bridge, single transverse palmar crease, shortened limbs, and a protruding tongue.

Musculoskeletal Manifestations

- Ligamentous laxity increases risk for shoulder, hip, and patellar dislocations (see Chapter 27), pes planus (see Chapter 43), and atlantoaxial instability (AAI) or laxity at C1-C2 (see Chapter 7).
- Slipped capital femoral epiphysis (SCFE) (see Chapter 20)
- Scoliosis (see Chapter 11)
- Treatment of musculoskeletal manifestations is *similar* to that for those without Down syndrome and is discussed in previous chapters.

Participation in Sports and Physical Activities

- Because of increased risk for obesity, physical activity is encouraged.
- The Special Olympics is an international organization that offers children and adults with intellectual disabilities year-round training and competition in 30 Olympic-type winter and summer sports.
- Special Olympics requires lateral radiographs of the cervical spine for participation. Those with AAI are restricted from certain sports (see Chapter 7).
- If ligamentous laxity is present in other joints (see Figure 4-2), counsel patient and family on increased risk for recurrent traumatic subluxations and dislocations. Some individuals may choose not to participate in sports that increase risk of dislocation, including, but not limited to, basketball, football, wrestling, soccer, and hockey.

Box 65-1. Medical Concerns for Individuals With Down Syndrome

Mental retardation, varies

Obesity

Obstructive sleep apnea

Hearing loss

Epilepsy

Leukemia

Musculoskeletal
• Atlantoaxial instability
• Joint instability/laxity
• Hypotonia
• Pes planus
• Scoliosis

Cardiovascular
• Congenital heart defects (atrial septal defect, ventricular septal defect, atrioventricular septal defect, patent foramen ovale, patent ductus arteriosus, tetralogy of Fallot)
• Lower cardiovascular fitness level

Endocrine
• Thyroid disease

Gastrointestinal
• Tracheoesophageal fistula
• Duodenal atresia
• Annular pancreas
• Hirschsprung
• Anal atresia
• Umbilical hernia

Visual
• Cataracts
• Severe refractive errors

Relevant *International Classification of Diseases, Ninth Revision, Clinical Modification* Codes

• **758.0**   Down syndrome
• **728.4**   Ligamentous laxity
• **718.31**   Recurrent shoulder dislocation
• **718.35**   Recurrent hip dislocation
• **718.36**   Recurrent patellar dislocation
• **737.9**   Scoliosis
• **820.01**   SCFE
• **754.69**   Pes plano valgus

Bibliography

Aldegheri R, Dall'Oca C. Limb lengthening in short stature patients. *J Pediatr Orthop B.* 2001;10:238–247

Alman BA. A classification for genetic disorders of interest to orthopaedists. *Clin Orthop Relat Res.* 2002;401:17–26

American Academy of Pediatrics Committee on Sports Medicine and Fitness. Atlantoaxial instability in down syndrome: subject review. *Pediatrics.* 1995;96:151–154

Antoniazzi F, Mottes M, Fraschini P, Brunelli PC, Tato L. Osteogenesis imperfecta: practical treatment guidelines. *Paediatr Drugs.* 2000;2:465–488

Arnold WE, Hilgartner MW. Hemophiliac arthropathy: current concepts of pathogenesis and management. *J Bone Joint Surg Am.* 1977;59:287

Boyadjiev SA, Jabs EW. Online Mendelian Inheritance in Man (OMIM) as a knowledgebase for human developmental disorders. *Clin Genet.* 2000;57:253–266

Brockmeyer D. Down syndrome and craniovertebral instability. Topic review and treatment recommendations. *Pediatr Neurosurg.* 1999;31:71–77

Burnei G, Vlad C, Georgescu I, Gavriliu TS, Dan D. Osteogenesis imperfecta: diagnosis and treatment. *J Am Acad Orthop Surg.* 2008;16:356–366

Byers PH, Steiner RD. Osteogenesis imperfecta. *Annu Rev Med.* 1992;43:269–282

Chen H. Skeletal dysplasia. Available at: http://emedicine.medscape.com/article/943343-overview. Accessed February 18, 2010

Corrigan JJ. Hemorrhagic and thrombotic diseases. In: Behrman RE, Kliegman RM, Nelson WE, eds. *Nelson's Textbook of Pediatrics.* 15th ed. Philadelphia, PA: WB Saunders; 1996:1424–1428

Dreyer SD, Ahou G, Lee B. The long and short of it: developmental genetics of the skeletal dysplasias. *Clin Genet* 1998;54:464–473

Herring JA. *Tachdjian's Pediatric Orthopedics.* Philadelphia, PA: WB Saunders; 2002:1879–1892

Horton WA, Hall JG, Hecht JT. Achondroplasia. *Lancet.* 2007;370:162–172

Hunter AG, Bankier A, Rogers JG, Sillence D, Scott CI Jr. Medical complications of achondroplasia: a multicentre patient review. *J Med Genet.* 1998;35:705–712

Kopits SE. Orthopedic complications of dwarfism. *Clin Orthop Relat Res.* 1976;114:153–179

Kristiansen LP, Steen H, Terjesen T. Residual challenges after healing of congenital pseudarthrosis in the tibia. *Clin Orthop Relat Res.* 2003;414:228–237

Land C, Rauch F, Montpetit K, Ruck-Gibis J, Glorieux FH. Effect of intravenous pamidronate therapy on functional abilities and level of ambulation in children with osteogenesis imperfecta. *J Pediatr.* 2006;148:456–460

LeBlanc CMA. Chronic conditions. In: Anderson SJ, Harris SS, eds. *Care of the Young Athlete.* 2nd ed. Elk Grove Village, IL: American Academy of Pediatrics; 2010

Listernick R, Charrow J. Neurofibromatosis-1 in childhood. *Adv Dermatol.* 2004;20:75–115

Lofqvist T, Nilsson IM, Berntorp E, Pettersson H. Haemophilia prophylaxis in young patients—a long-term follow-up. *J Intern Med.* 1997;241:395–400

Oberklaid F, Danks DM, Jensen F, Stace L, Rosshandler S. Achondroplasia and hypochondroplasia. Comments on frequency, mutation rate, and radiological features in skull and spine. *J Med Genet.* 1979;16:140–146

Pauli RM, Breed A, Horton VK, Glinski LP, Reiser CA. Prevention of fixed, angular kyphosis in achondroplasia. *J Pediatr Orthop.* 1997;17:726–733

Pueschel SM, Scola FH. Atlantoaxial instability in individuals with Down syndrome: epidemiologic, radiographic, and clinical studies. *Pediatrics.* 1987;80:555–560

Rauch F, Munns C, Land C, Glorieux FH. Pamidronate in children and adolescents with osteogenesis imperfecta: effect of treatment discontinuation. *J Clin Endocrinol Metab.* 2006;91:1268–1274

Sanyer ON. Down syndrome and sport participation. *Curr Sports Med Rep.* 2006;5:315–318

Sillence DO, Senn A, Danks DM. Genetic heterogeneity in osteogenesis imperfecta. *J Med Genet.* 1979;16:101–116

Spranger JW, Brill PW, Poznanski A. *Bone Dysplasias: An Atlas of Genetic Disorders of Skeletal Development.* 2nd ed. New York, NY: Oxford University Press

Stobart K, Iorio A, Wu JK. Clotting factor concentrates given to prevent bleeding and bleeding-related complications in people with hemophilia A or B. *Cochrane Database Syst Rev.* 2006;2:CD003429

Trotter TL, Hall JG, American Academy of Pediatrics Committee on Genetics. Health supervision for children with achondroplasia. *Pediatrics.* 2005;116:771–783

Van den Berg HM, Dunn A, Fischer K, Blanchette VS. Prevention and treatment of musculoskeletal disease in the haemophilia population: role of prophylaxis and synovectomy. *Haemophilia.* 2006;12(Suppl 3):159–168

Vitale MG, Guha A, Skaggs DL. Orthopaedic manifestations of neurofibromatosis in children: an update. *Clin Orthop Relat Res.* 2002;401:107–118

Winell J, Burke SW. Sports participation of children with Down syndrome. *Orthop Clin North Am.* 2003; 34:439–443

Part 19: Rheumatologic Diseases

TOPICS COVERED

CHAPTER 66

Juvenile Idiopathic Arthritis

Introduction/Etiology/Epidemiology

- The term *juvenile idiopathic arthritis* (JIA) replaces the older term, juvenile rheumatoid arthritis.
- A family of diseases characterized by chronic inflammation and overgrowth of the synovial membranes
- Conservative estimates suggest as many as 300,000 children in the United States have a form of JIA.
- The etiology of JIA remains unknown.
- Once thought to be autoimmune, newer data suggest that JIA pathogenesis involves complex interactions between innate and adaptive immunity.
- The 3 major JIA subtypes (pauciarticular, polyarticular, systemic-onset disease) are best considered distinct and separate diseases.

Signs and Symptoms

- Signs and symptoms are specific to the JIA subtype (Table 66-1).
- *Pain is almost never a prominent feature of the presentation of JIA.*

Table 66-1. Signs and Symptoms of Juvenile Idiopathic Arthritis Subtypes and Other Diagnoses Consistent With Joint Pain or Swelling

Disease Entity	Demographics	Distinguishing Features	Clinical Pearls
Pauciarticular JIA	Preschool children (usually girls)	Present with lower extremity swelling or gait disturbance. The gait disturbance is better with activity and more prominent after periods of rest.	This entity is rare in non-European populations. Think of other disease entities (eg, tuberculous arthritis) in such populations.
Polyarticular JIA	Ages 1–15 y Figure 66-1	Present with swelling in multiple joints, including fingers or wrists. Morning stiffness may be prominent.	Thickened synovial membranes may obscure extensor tendons as they cross the wrist.
Systemic-onset JIA	Ages 1–10 y Figure 66-2	Fever and rash are prominent. Synovitis may not be present. Brisk acute phase response common (ESR >50 mm/h, WBC count >20,000/mm³, platelets >500,000 per mm³).	Child usually feels and appears well when the fever is absent, very ill when the fever is present. Fever typically occurs daily at specific times and does not last all day.
Acute lymphocytic leukemia	Preschool and school-aged children	May present with very painful joint swelling. Pain awakens the child at night or keeps the child up all night.	First complete WBC count may be normal. May need to be repeated. Serum LDH may be elevated.
Benign hypermobility syndrome	Late preteens and early teens Girls > boys	Diffuse musculoskeletal pain made worse with activity and better with rest.	Hypermobile joints and mild ligamentous laxity of the ACL and MCL of the knee.
Adolescent sleep and stress disorder (ie, fibromyalgia)	Usually adolescents	Diffuse musculoskeletal pain not prominent at any particular time of day and not made better or worse by activity	History of disturbed sleep usually points toward the diagnosis.
Apophysitis (eg, Osgood-Schlatter disease)	School-aged children and adolescents	Localized musculoskeletal pain made worse with activity and better with rest	Tenderness ± swelling at the affected apophysis
Infectious arthritis	Any age	Usually acute onset and very painful. Fever may or may not be present.	Tuberculous arthritis may be indolent. Have a high index of suspicion in non–European-descended children presenting with a relatively painless monoarthritis.
Acute rheumatic fever	Arthritis as a presenting manifestation is rare before age 10 years.	Very painful, migratory arthritis	A given joint will stay swollen for about 12 h. Another joint will frequently become symptomatic as symptoms in the first joint subside.

JIA, juvenile idiopathic arthritis; ESR, erythrocyte sedimentation rate; WBC, white blood cell; LDH, lactate dehydrogenase; ACL, anterior cruciate ligament; MCL, medial collateral ligament.

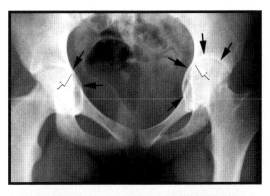

Figure 66-1. Anteroposterior view of the hips and pelvis shows bilateral protrusio acetabulae (black arrows) with axial narrowing of the joint space (white arrows). Reproduced with permission from Johnson TR, Steinbach LS (eds): *Essentials of Musculoskeletal Imaging.* Rosemont, IL: American Academy of Orthopaedic Surgeons; 2004.

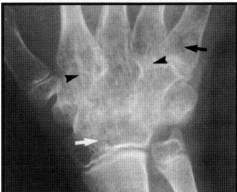

Figure 66-2. Anteroposterior view of wrist of skeletally immature patient shows generalized osteopenia (black arrow). Note spontaneous fusion of the carpal bones to each other and to the distal radial epiphysis (white arrow) and the proximal metacarpals (arrowheads). Reproduced with permission from Johnson TR, Steinbach LS (eds): *Essentials of Musculoskeletal Imaging.* Rosemont, IL: American Academy of Orthopaedic Surgeons; 2004.

Making the Diagnosis

- *The diagnosis is made on the history and physical examination.*
  - The hallmark sign on physical examination is *overgrowth of the synovial membranes.*
    - Easily palpable
    - Often described as warm and doughy
    - The overgrown synovium may obscure other anatomic structures such as the extensor tendons of the hand as they cross the wrist joint.
  - *Muscle atrophy* and *joint contractures* may be present in cases in which the diagnosis has been delayed.
  - Juvenile idiopathic arthritis can be safely excluded in a child with musculoskeletal pain and a normal physical examination.
- *Laboratory studies have little utility in making the diagnosis of JIA,* except to exclude other causes of joint swelling (eg, acute lymphocytic leukemia).
  - *Rheumatoid factor* tests have a very poor positive and negative predictive value and should *never* be ordered as a diagnostic test in children.
  - *Antinuclear antibody* (ANA) tests have limited ability to distinguish children with JIA from healthy children.
    - As many as 35% of normal children have "positive" ANA tests.
    - Antinuclear antibody tests should not be ordered if the suspected diagnosis is JIA.
- Radiographs may show characteristic findings in late-stage JIA (figures 66-1 and 66-2).

Treatment

- Pauciarticular JIA
  — Combinations of nonsteroidal anti-inflammatory drugs (NSAIDs) and local joint injection with triamcinolone
- Polyarticular JIA
  — Becoming increasingly aggressive as sustained remissions are extremely difficult to achieve with NSAIDs and oral glucocorticoids.
  — Methotrexate and therapies directed against the pro-inflammatory cytokine, TNFα (eg, etanercept, infliximab) are becoming the standard of care
- Systemic-onset JIA (Still disease)
  — Combinations of glucocorticoids and anti–interleukin-1 agents (eg, anakinra).

Expected Outcomes/Prognosis

- Early, aggressive therapy improves outcome in children with JIA.
- In all subtypes, sustained remission is rare.
- Recurrences in adulthood are common.

Prevention

- There is no known prevention for JIA.

When to Refer

- All children with JIA should be referred to a pediatric rheumatologist as soon as the diagnosis is made or suspected.

Resource for Physicians and Families

- Arthritis Foundation (www.arthritis.org)

Relevant *International Classification of Diseases, Ninth Revision, Clinical Modification* Codes

- **714.30**   Systemic-onset JIA
- **714.31**   Polyarticular JIA
- **714.32**   Pauciarticular JIA
- **714.33**   Monoarticular JIA
- **728.5**   Benign hypermobility syndrome
- **729.1**   Fibromyalgia

Bibliography

Aggarwal A, Misra R. Juvenile chronic arthritis in India: is it different from that seen in Western countries? *Rheumatol Int.* 1994;14:53–56

Eichenfield AH, Athreya BH, Doughty RA, Cebul RD. Utility of rheumatoid factor in the diagnosis of juvenile rheumatoid arthritis. *Pediatrics.* 1986;78:480–484

Gortmaker SL, Sappenfield W. Chronic childhood disorders: prevalence and impact. *Pediatr Clin North Am.* 1984;31:3–18

Jarvis JN. The unique clinical presentation of children with chronic arthritis: putting the pediatrics in pediatric rheumatology. *Curr Probl Pediatr Adolesc Health Care.* 2006;36:80–82

Jarvis JN, Cleland SY. Rheumatic disease in Native American children: opportunities and challenge. *Curr Rheumatol Rep.* 2003;5:471–476

Jarvis JN, Jiang K, Petty HR, Centola M. Neutrophils: the forgotten cell in JIA disease pathogenesis. *Pediatr Rheumatol Online J.* 2007;5:13

Malleson PN, Sailer M, Mackinnon MJ. Usefulness of antinuclear antibody testing to screen for rheumatic diseases. *Arch Dis Child.* 1997;77:299–304

McGhee JL, Burks F, Sheckels JL, Jarvis JN. Identifying children with chronic arthritis based on chief complaints: absence of predictive value for musculoskeletal pain as an indicator of rheumatic disease in children. *Pediatrics.* 2002;110:354–359

McGhee JL, Kickingbird LM, Jarvis JN. Clinical utility of antinuclear antibody tests in children. *BMC Pediatr.* 2004;4:13

Pascual V, Allantaz F, Arce E, Punaro M, Banchereau J. Role of interleukin-1 (IL-1) in the pathogenesis of systemic onset juvenile idiopathic arthritis and clinical response to IL-1 blockade. *J Exp Med.* 2005;201:1479–1486

Singsen BH. Rheumatic diseases of childhood. *Rheum Dis Clin North Am.* 1990;16:581–599

Wallace CA. Current management of juvenile idiopathic arthritis. *Best Pract Res Clin Rheumatol.* 2006;20:279–300

Wallace CA, Huang B, Bandeira M, Ravelli A, Giannini EH. Patterns of clinical remission in select categories of juvenile idiopathic arthritis. *Arthritis Rheum.* 2005;52:3554–3562

Pediatric Orthopaedic Terms and Definitions

Pediatric Orthopaedic Terms and Definitions

Adductor tenotomy: Soft tissue release is a release of a muscle on the inside of the thigh next to the groin used to alleviate developmental hip dysplasia.

Adductus: Deviation of a body part toward the midline and one or both legs from moving.

Anisomelia: Limb-length inequality.

Ankylosis: Marked stiffness of a joint.

Anomaly: Abnormality.

Apophyses: Cartilaginous structures at the insertion of major muscle groups into bone that may be susceptible to overuse syndromes and acute fractures in pediatric athletes.

Arthrography: A dynamic study typically performed in the operating room that involves injecting contrast dye into the joint to view the outline of the cartilage and soft tissue structures of the joint.

Basilar invagination: Occurs when the top of the second vertebrae moves upward. It can cause the opening in the skull where the spinal cord passes through to the brain (the foramen magnum) to close. It also may press on the lower brainstem.

Blount disease: A pathologic cause of varus deformity at the knee.

Brachydactyly: Abnormal shortness of the fingers.

Brodie abscess: Oval or round lesion walled off in a fibrous capsule with a sclerotic rim.

Bunion: Valgus deformity of the metatarsophalangeal joint.

Cauda equina: Intraspinal nerve roots found at the termination of the spinal cord, usually at the L1-L2 level.

Cavus: Increased height of the medial longitudinal arch.

Chiari malformations: Structural defects in the cerebellum. Chiari malformations may develop when the bony space is smaller than normal, causing the cerebellum and brain stem to be pushed downward into the foramen magnum and into the upper spinal canal. The resulting pressure on the cerebellum and brain stem may affect functions controlled by these areas and block the flow of cerebrospinal fluid to and from the brain.

Clonus: Repetitive, rhythmic contractions of a muscle when attempting to hold it in a stretched state

Compartment syndrome: Increased pressure within a myofascial compartment; may be acute or chronic and can lead to compromised blood flow to muscle and nerves, causing tissue damage.

Congenital muscular torticollis: Most common form of torticollis.

Constitutional growth delay: Weight and height decrease toward the end of infancy, remain stable during middle childhood, and decrease toward the end of adolescence, resulting in normal adult stature.

Coxa vara: A deformity in which an inward curvature of the hip takes place where the angle between the upper femur and ball joint is reduced and the femoral neck shaft angle is less than 120 to 135 degrees, causing pain and stiffness, resulting in one leg being shorter than the other. Causes a limp.

Cubitus varus: A deformity of the elbow resulting in a decreased carrying angle so that, with the arm extended at the side and the palm facing forward, the forearm and hand are held at less than 5 degrees.

Deficiency: General term connoting absent structures or parts of structures, inclusive of all mechanisms of dysmorphogenesis.

Deformity: Alteration in shape or position of a structure that differentiated normally.

Delta phalanx: Classic delta phalanx is characterized by a triangular or trapezoidal shaped bone with a C-shaped epiphyseal plate.

Dermatome: A localized area of skin that has its sensation via a single nerve from a single nerve root of the spinal cord.

Developmental deviation: Development of skills out of the usual sequence.

Developmental dissociation: Achievement of developmental spheres at different rates.

Developmental variations: Resolve with time and seldom require treatment. Examples include flatfeet, in-toeing, out-toeing, bowlegs, and knock-knees.

Diaphysis: Shaft of a long bone.

Diplegia: In cerebral palsy, indicates involvement of both lower extremities.

Diskitis: Inflammation of the disc space, typically caused by infection.

Dislocation: Complete separation of humeral head from glenoid fossa; may spontaneously reduce, but more often requires manual relocation.

Dorsiflexion: Extension of the ankle, foot, or toes superiorly in the sagittal plane.

Dysplasia: Abnormal growth or differentiation.

Effusion: The presence of fluid within a joint.

Electromyogram: Measures the electrical impulses of muscles at rest and during contraction.

Endochondral ossification: Type of bone formation in which cartilage is replaced by bone with accompanying longitudinal bone growth.

Epiphyseal plate (physis): Growth plate at the end of a long bone, where the epiphysis meets the metaphysis. Composed of cartilage cells. Contributes to longitudinal growth. Subject to pressure or axial forces.

Epiphysiodesis: Pediatric surgical procedure in which the epiphyseal (growth) plate of a bone is removed.

Epiphysis: Rounded end of a long bone.

Eversion: Motion in the coronal plane where the heel is turned outward.

Exostosis (osteochondroma): A benign bony growth projecting outward from a bone surface.

Facet joints: Facet joints occur in pairs at the back of each vertebra. The facet joints link the vertebrae directly above and below to form a working unit that permits movement of the spine.

Failure to thrive: Weight is less than the fifth percentile or declines more than 2 major percentile lines (eg, declines from the 80th percentile to the 40th percentile).

Familial short stature: The child and parents are small, and the child's growth remains below but parallels the normal curves.

Fat-free mass (lean body mass): Percentage of body weight composed of water, bone, and muscle.

Foot progression angle (FPA): The angle made by the foot with respect to a straight line plotted in the direction the child is walking. Determines whether the child is in-toeing or out-toeing.

Goniometer: An instrument that quantifies joint range of motion.

Gowers sign: Exhibited by children with proximal lower extremity weakness (eg, muscular dystrophy). Will rise from a seated position by walking hands up thighs.

Grisel syndrome: The occurrence of atlantoaxial subluxation in association with inflammation of adjacent soft tissues.

Hangman fracture: Fracture of the pedicles of C2.

Hemiatrophy: Atrophy of one side of the body.

Hemihypertrophy: Asymmetric overgrowth (hypertrophy) of the skull, face, trunk, limbs, or digits, with or without visceral involvement.

Hemiplegia: In cerebral palsy, indicates involvement of one side of the body, usually affecting the upper extremities more than the lower.

Hemivertebrae: Developmental anomaly in which one side of a vertebra is incompletely developed.

Heterotopic ossification: The formation of bone in any nonosseous tissue; often after trauma.

Hip arthroplasty: Surgical replacement of the hip joint with an artificial prosthesis.

Hypertonia: Increased resistance to passive joint range of motion.

Hypotonia: Decreased resistance to passive joint range of motion.

Iliotibial band: Thickening of the iliotibial tract that inserts directly into the lateral tubercle of the tibia.

Impingement: Shoulder pain caused by tendinosis of the rotator cuff tendon or irritation of the subacromial bursa.

Inversion: Motion in the coronal plane where the heel is turned inward.

Involucrum: In osteomyelitis, a sheath of live bone that forms around a piece of dead bone, the sequestrum. *See also* Sequestrum.

Isometric strengthening: Muscle contraction against resistance without a change in muscle length.

Joint hypermobility: Also called ligamentous laxity; defined as the ability to extend a joint beyond its range of motion.

Klippel-Feil syndrome: Represents 50% of all congenital cervical abnormalities. Patients have an abnormal number of cervical vertebrae or fusion of hemivertebrae into one osseous mass, leading to the clinical triad of short neck, low posterior hairline, and limited range of neck motion.

Kyphosis: Angular curvature of the spine in the sagittal plane with the apex of the curvature being posterior; usually in the thoracic spine. The thoracic spine normally has 20 to 40 degrees of kyphosis.

Ligamentous laxity: Also joint range of motion. Tends to be hereditary and highly variable among individuals.

Lipomeningocele: An intraspinal lipoma associated with a spina bifida.

Listhesis: Forward slippage of one vertebrae over the vertebrae below it.

Lordosis: Spinal curvature in the sagittal plane with convexity on the patient's ventral aspect.

Malformation: Interruption of morphogenesis without return to normal.

Meningocele: Protrusion of the meninges through a defect in the posterior spinal elements, with the spinal cord and nerve roots remaining in the spinal canal.

Meralgia paresthetica: Neurologic disorder characterized by disturbance of sensation in the anterolateral aspect of the proximal thigh.

Metaphysis: Broad portion of the long bone adjacent to a joint. In children, includes the epiphysis, physis, and the metaphysis.

Mid-parental height: Child's predicted adult height. For boys, paternal height + maternal height + 5 (inches)/2. For girls, paternal height + maternal height − 5 (inches)/2.

Milestone regression: A serious developmental problem indicated by a loss of developmental skills, suggesting an ongoing neurologic condition.

Miserable malalignment syndrome: A condition in which medial femoral torsion combines with external tibial torsion to create patellofemoral dysfunction and pain.

Muscle contusion: Injury to muscle tissue caused by blunt trauma that results in leakage of blood from damaged capillaries.

Myelocele: A severe form of spina bifida in which the neural plate is exposed with no overlying tissue cover.

Myelomeningocele: Most severe form of spina bifida, in which the spinal cord is exposed through an opening in the spine. It is associated with partial or complete paralysis of the parts of the body below the spinal opening.

Myositis ossificans: Non-neoplastic, heterotopic proliferation of bone and cartilage occurring within muscle that has suffered major or repetitive trauma.

Nonossifying fibroma (fibrous cortical defect): Osteolytic and sometimes painful proliferative lesions composed of spindle (fibrous) cells.

Ocular torticollis: A compensatory mechanism that children with strabismus, ptosis, or nystagmus adopt to obtain the best vision.

Ossification: Process of the synthesis of bone from cartilage.

Osteomyelitis: Inflammation of bone caused by bacterial or fungal infection.

Osteonecrosis: Disease resulting from the temporary or permanent loss of blood supply to the bones. The bone tissue dies, and ultimately the bone may collapse. If the process involves the bones near a joint, it often leads to collapse of the joint surface. Also known as avascular necrosis, aseptic necrosis, and ischemic necrosis.

Osteopenia: Generalized thinning of bone structure.

Paroxysmal torticollis of infancy: Benign paroxysmal torticollis is a cause of torticollis of early infancy. The attacks usually last for less than 1 week, recur from every few days to every few months, improve by age 2 years, and end by age 3. There very frequently is a family history of migraine.

Peak height velocity (PHV): Maximum rate of growth in height during the adolescent growth spurt.

Peak weight velocity (PWV): Maximum rate of growth in body weight during adolescent growth spurt.

Periosteal reaction: Formation of new bone in response to injury or other stimuli of the periosteum surrounding the bone. It is most often identified on radiographs of the bones.

Physeal obliquity: Risk factor for slipped capital femoral epiphysis associated with obesity.

Physiatrist: Physician who specializes in physical medicine and rehabilitation.

Physiologic: Within normal physiologic limits as defined for age and developmental status.

Plagiocephaly: Malformation of the head marked by an oblique slant to the main axis of the skull.

Plantarflexion: Flexion of the ankle, foot, or toes inferiorly in the sagittal plane.

Planus: Flattening of the medial longitudinal arch.

Polydactyly: Presence of more than 5 digits on a hand or foot.

Pronation: Describes a position, or motion, where the heel is everted and the midfoot is abducted and dorsiflexed. The sum of this motion tends to flatten the longitudinal arch.

Puberty: Transitional period between childhood and adulthood during which growth spurt and maturation of sex organs and reproductive system occurs.

Pyomyositis: Rare, purulent soft tissue bacterial infection of muscle occurring most commonly in the lower extremities.

Quadriplegia: In cerebral palsy, indicates involvement of upper and lower extremities.

Radiculopathy: Pain caused by nerve root impingement that radiates down the extremity in a dermatomal pattern.

Radiodense (radiopaque): Exhibiting relative opacity to, or impenetrability by, x-rays or any other form of radiation.

Radiolucent: Anything that permits the penetration and passage of x-rays or other forms of radiation.

Rhizomelia: Disproportion in the length of the most proximal segment of the limbs (upper arms and thighs).

Sandifer syndrome: Torticollis without spasm of the neck muscles, dystonic body posturing and movements in association with gastroesophageal reflux, with or without a hiatal hernia.

Scapular dyskinesis: Asymmetry or winging with scapular movement, noted while watching arm elevation and lowering from behind.

Scheuermann kyphosis: Scheuermann disease (juvenile kyphosis) is a deformity in the thoracic or thoracolumbar spine in children. Patients have an increased kyphosis in the thoracic or thoracolumbar spine with associated backache and localized changes in the vertebral bodies.

Scoliometer: An instrument used to estimate the amount of curve in a patient's spine. It may be used as a tool during screening or as follow-up for scoliosis.

Scoliosis: Lateral curvature of the spine in the coronal plane—on frontal radiograph—of at least 10 degrees, described according to the location (eg, lumbar, thoracic) and direction (right or left) of the convexity. Curves less than 10 degrees are considered normal anatomic variants that may be described as mild spinal asymmetry.

Septic arthritis: Also called suppurative arthritis (pus); results from bacterial invasion of a joint and subsequent inflammation, usually as a result of transient bacteremia, spread into the joint from a skin lesion, or extension from adjacent tissue.

Sequestrum: In osteomyelitis, the necrotic portion of bone walled off by the involucrum. *See also* Involucrum.

Skeletal age (SA): Bone age. Estimated by comparing the appearance of the physes on a hand radiograph to published norms.

Slap-foot or drop-foot gait: Seen with tibialis anterior weakness resulting from nerve impingement.

Somatosensory evoked potentials (SSEP): A series of waves that reflect sequential activation of neural structures along the somatosensory pathways.

Spica casting: A spica cast is used to keep the lower body and one or both legs from moving.

Spina bifida occulta: A developmental variant in which one or more vertebrae have defects in the posterior arch without any skin or spine malformation; rarely causes disability or symptoms.

Spondylolisthesis: Displacement in the sagittal plane of one vertebral body on the adjacent level.

Spondylolysis: Pars interarticularis defect (Scotty dog sign).

Spondyloptosis: When the posterior aspect of the cranial vertebral level "falls off" the anterior aspect of the inferior vertebral body.

Sprain: An injury to a ligament.

Sprengel deformity: Congenital elevation of the scapula.

Strain: An overstretching or overexertion of some part of the muscle-tendon unit.

Subluxation: An incomplete or partial dislocation that usually reduces quickly and spontaneously.

Supination: Describes a position, or motion, where the heel is inverted and the midfoot is adducted.

Symbrachydactyly: Fused short digits.

Symphalangism: Failure of separation of the digits in which there is fusion of one phalanx to another within the same digit.

Synchondrosis: Type of cartilaginous joint that is temporary and exists during the growing phases. Synchondroses consist of hyaline cartilage that becomes progressively thinner during skeletal maturation and ultimately become obliterated by bone union.

Syndactyly: Webbing or fusion between fingers or toes.

Synostosis: Conjoined bones.

Syringomyelia: A cyst within the spinal cord.

Tandem walking: Walking with one foot in front of the other; part a 6-point gait examination quick check.

Tarsal coalition: Fusion of 2 or more of the major tarsal bones (talus, navicular, calcaneus, and cuboid).

Thigh-foot angle (TFA): The angle between the axis of the foot and the axis of the thigh when the child is prone with knees flexed to 90 degrees.

Torsion: Rotation that exceeds 2 standard deviations from the mean.

Torticollis (wry neck): Condition in which the head is tilted toward one side and the chin is turned toward the other.

Undernutrition: Weight for age typically declines (wasting) before height for age (stunting) and weight for height.

Valgum: Angulation of the junction of 2 body segments or fracture fragments toward the midline.

Varum: Angulation of the junction of 2 body segments or fracture fragments away from the midline.

Version: Rotational variation within normal limits for age.

Vertebra plana: A condition of spondylitis in which the body of the vertebra is reduced to a sclerotic disk.

Winking owl sign: Characteristic obliteration of the pedicle on anteroposterior radiograph that typically resolves over the course of several years, although may benefit from surgery. Requires referral to an orthopaedic specialist.

Index

Index